THINNER WINNERS

The Complete All-in-One Guide to Lifetime Weight Control

Roseanne Welsh Strull, B.A.
Howard Strull, M.A.

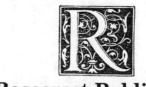

Rosecrest Publishing
Brookings, Oregon

THINNER WINNERS
The Complete All-in-One Guide to Lifetime Weight Control

Published by:
Rosecrest Publishing
22745 Carpenterville Road, Suite 4
Brookings, Oregon 97415
Tel/Fax (503) 247-7255

Library of Congress Catalog Card Number: 95-68218

Library of Congress Cataloging-in-Publication Data
    Strull, Roseanne Welsh
        THINNER WINNERS: The Complete All-in-One Guide to Lifetime Weight Control
            by Roseanne Welsh Strull and Howard Strull
    Includes bibliographical references and index.
    ISBN 0-9634934-3-4 : Soft cover $19.95
    1. Diet 2. Reducing 3. Health 4. Fitness 5. Psychology 6. Self-help
    I. Title: THINNER WINNERS
    II. Strull, Howard III. Title: The Complete All-in-One Guide to Weight Control
    613.2   1995   95-68218

Notice

The information and ideas in this book are in no way intended as a substitute for medical counseling. The information is designed to help you make informed choices about your health, and thus is meant to be supplemental to the advice and care you are receiving from your physician or other health care professionals.

Anyone may have a special health problem, and it is advisable to check with your physician before beginning this or any other weight control program. If you suspect that you have a medical problem, or have any existing medical conditions, seek competent medical care.

Printed in the United States of America.

10 9 8 7 6 5 4 3 2 1

Cover design by:
Lightbourne Images
Ashland, Oregon

Illustrations courtesy of Dover Publications

Dedication

To those of you who feel you are alone
in your quest for health and thinness.
You are not.
We're all in this gravy boat together.

And for Delores.

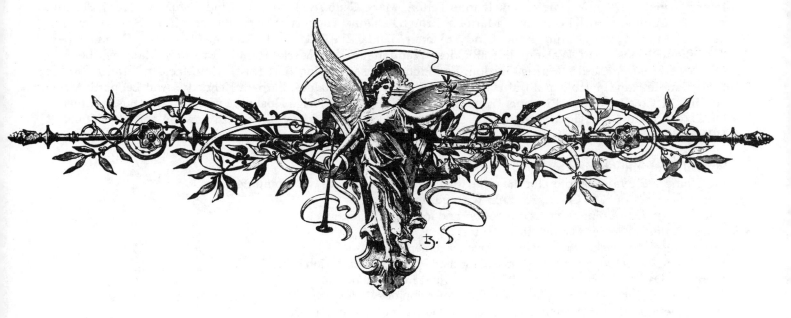

Acknowledgments

We are deeply grateful for the vast amount of wonderful, loving support from family, friends and associates that we have received over the years it has taken to complete this book. Special thanks to every one of you for your encouragement and unconditional love. We're grateful for your belief in our abilities to bring this book to the people who need it. It would not be a reality without you.

The following very special THINNER WINNERS supporters get our whole-hearted thanks: Mary Jo Anderson, Dorice Gustafson, Rosemary Sieve, Delores and Glenn Van Winkle, John and Cindy Golding, Marjorie Stadelman, Tiny Caudell, Rose and Roger Gabrielson, Marsha and Wayne Reum, Peggy Mirabel, June Gustafson, Dee Dee Wood, Diane and Don Gillin, Betty and Paul Rettig, Florence Henry, Lynda McDonald, Marilyn Rempfer, Sue Oliver, Richard Stolz, Pat Oden, Joanna Yax, Tracey McReynolds, Eleanor Cook, Angie Breece, Lynda Timeus, Deanna Harrington, Joanne Felton, Mary Cello, A. J. Mason, Linda Murray, Tracy Placido, Annette Cooley, April Rosenthal, Marjorie Brown, Dianne Halbert, Marge Barrett, Judy Stringham, Pat Silveria, Mary Wallace, Audra and Cindy Skinner, Linda Zia R.D., Darla Moore, Liz James, Donna Bibey, Ethyellene Jones, Gail Watson, Jim Buckles, Wandah Fowler, Merle Haney, Roxanne Ramsey, Beverly McNamara, Suree Gould, Martie Gordon, Leo Lightle, Susan Taylor, Bart Kast, Ann Maclean, Fran Bollinger R.N., Bonnie Hand, Nicole and Bill Hand, Vella Stover, Becky Hodges, Barbara Kennedy, Ann Leonard, Marie and Jim McCoy, Joye Kerr, Risa and Truman Durley, Jill Fairchild, Helga Hoehne, Lynn McCann, Susan Miller, Dr. David Young, Dr. Thomas Martinelli, Sheri Legat, Glenda Brockway, Elyzabeth Lawson and all THINNER WINNERS across the country ...

Special appreciation goes to:

Ed, Elaine and Evan Compton for the more than generous assistance with computers.

William Appel of Edit Cetera for help with editing.

Dan Poynter for helping us chart our course and for flying so high.

Marie Keifer for generous, practical advice.

Eileen and Kathy Jaskol for consistent encouragement.

Phyllis and Sol Alfassa for always knowing that we would get the job done.

Margaret Davis Welsh for unconditional love and inspiration.

Gailyn and Glenn Nemhauser for too much to mention or ever forget.

Vivian Nemhauser for cheerful support and never forgetting those muffins.

Jay and Michele Breuner for helping us through the early days.

Kerry Greene for high energy, unending support and unique ideas galore.

Wendy and Chris Greene for sticking with us through the sticky years.

Lue Morrison for wonderful letters and riding out the tornado with us.

Heather Leigh Welsh for an energetic, unique perspective.

Victoria Welsh (and Scout) for remembering the best times and leading the fan club.

Toastmasters Club #1215, the Chetco Chatterers, for listening to and helping us clarify our views.

Kathy and Steve Cadwalader of Bayside Fitness in Brookings for encouragement and generosity.

Penny Starr, Bill Schlichting and Marge Woodfin of the Curry Coastal Pilot for getting the word out.

Norm Suiter of KURY Radio for believing in our message and for sharing it "on the air".

Betty DeCicco for always remembering us on special occasions.

Our lifelong Missouri friends: Janice Crane, Jane Mann, Dick and Teresa Babcock, Marla and Randy Little.

And the multitude of friends, relatives and powerful forces contributing to our life-affirming work ...

We give unending gratitude to Jamison, HR, Rivienne and Satrienne who help us daily to stay focused on living our lives to the "greatest glory" of the God in each of us and everywhere.

Introduction

"If you have knowledge, let others light their candle from it."
Margaret Fuller

When it comes to successfully controlling your health and weight there are just two kinds of people: those who know how and those who don't. Those who don't know how continue to struggle, strain, huff and puff their way to intermittent temporary success and subsequent disheartening backslides. Classic stressed-out, burned-out, over-dieted, cynical, frustrated desperate yo-yo's. I can only say it takes one to know one. Power to sustain true health is elusive for them because of confusion over both the actual underlying process and the application of the natural laws of health

THINNER WINNERS are the ones who understand that losing their excess unhealthy weight is a result of applying exact laws of thinness. Every person who understands and activates these principles must inevitably become thin permanently. Failure is impossible. These laws, once mastered, flow into all areas of your life because they are universal success principles. Weight loss was merely my vehicle for learning these fundamental truths and it may be yours as well. THINNER WINNERS are not only thinner, they are winners in life and can direct and shape their lives into exactly what they choose because of this knowledge. It's time for you to become one if you can answer "yes" to a simple question: Are you finally ready to learn and apply the true laws of success when it comes to weight control? If you are, read this book and do exactly as it tells you to do. You will become a THINNER WINNER, too.

The debate rages on over the health ramifications of losing weight and whether "dieting" even works or not. It makes for great headlines and a thriving "diet industry". Meanwhile you want to get your weight under control and could care less what the academics choose to argue about or what the tabloids print. In spite of poor success people continue dietary struggling to lose their unwanted extra pounds because of simple misinformation about the real process. In reality, what you eat is only a small portion of the big picture.

Going far beyond any weight related programs you've been exposed to in the past, this book is a complete mind/body strategic system. What you will discover is that it takes your mind to get your body into shape. Many people find it easier to stick with a program when they understand the "why" of a system. That's the whole point of this book. Studying it, you will come to thoroughly understand why it is to your advantage to get your weight under control and you'll learn exactly how to do it.

Of the millions of people who are desperately seeking solutions to their weight problem only a small number succeed at present. This will change drastically in the next few years as people come to understand and apply these principles. I predict that obesity will be a relic of the past as THINNER WINNERS everywhere develop and practice their craft ... sharing it, instructing and nurturing others. People who get thin permanently do so for very specific reasons and by following a certain strategy. You are about to learn those liberating principles.

Here are a few suggestions on how to make the best use of this book:

1) Your best shot ever at getting off the diet roller coaster for good is contained in the information on these pages. Read it. Better yet, study it with a group or support person. This isn't just another book to add to your collection, it's your proven key to a thinner, healthier future. Master the principles to master your life.

2) Once you have reviewed the concepts and strategies in this book, make them your own. Weight control is a highly personal realm and you need to adapt new information to suit your situation. Take what you learn, customize it within the guidelines of the laws of thinness, then use it.

3) Don't overload yourself by trying to do everything at once. There is a step by step plan to follow. You will be most successful by gradually easing into changes, understanding them fully. This is a developmental process, like the growth of a mighty tree. Sink your roots deep.

4) Don't skip anything. If you were learning to fly, would you skip a few days of flight training because you didn't see the need for those particular lessons at the time? Hopefully not. You never know when you might need that missing information! Some of these ideas might surprise you. I was sometimes surprised when they worked! Try to keep an open mind. Come back to something if it doesn't click the first time. Every piece is essential.

THINNER WINNERS is designed to take your focus off weight as the primary issue and put it on improving your health ... physical, emotional and spiritual. One of the wonderful fringe benefits of this healthy lifestyle is having a normal weight. You don't have to struggle, deprive yourself or "live to get thin". When you know how, it will happen naturally.

Getting healthy is a gradual process and can be a lot of fun. Really! Stripping off the old fat shell and the negative thinking that goes along with it feels incredibly liberating. You'll learn how to encourage and allow this ultimate acceptance of yourself and gain respect for the extraordinary person that you are. That we all are. May you enjoy this gift of awakening.

Roseanne's Preface

When I was born, fat babies were "in". Those chubby, pinchable cheeks were considered healthy in the abundant post-war years. Unfortunately it backfired. The taste I developed for rich, sweet foods quickly turned me into a fat, unhappy, "socially unacceptable" little girl.

At age nine I was taken to my first "diet doctor" and began my official dieting career. Over the next 30 years, like many of the women around me, I bought all the diet books, traipsed in and out of countless doctor's offices, followed all the advice and still was fat most of the time. Sometimes I succeeded temporarily at losing weight with strange regimes that undoubtedly compromised my health, and got a maddeningly brief but glorious taste of what thin felt like. Clothes fit, I fit. However, as soon as I started eating "normal" food again ... well, the search for a new diet started all over. And there was always another one to try. It sounds ludicrous now, but that was all anyone had to hope for; that was the way it was done. A vicious, cruel trap.

I remained fat, on and off, until I was nearly forty years old. Of course, during my lifetime I did lose lots of weight and occasionally got close to "normal". It was inevitable since I was constantly striving with all my willpower. It was the one thing in life I wanted ... to be normal. Sometimes I even stayed at a reduced weight for as long as two or three months before the pounds and inches would start creeping back on again. Each time I "failed" my self-esteem sank lower until I almost believed I just didn't have what it took to be "normal". This was a complete mystery to me and many of my friends who were likewise yo-yoing up and down frantically pursuing stability. Nobody was winning.

Finally the endless frustration drove me to a different course of action. I set out to beat the system and educate myself on the way things really work. Forget the "experts". They obviously didn't know the difference between girdles and griddle cakes and they didn't weigh 272 pounds either. So when I was 39 years old I finally found the right combination of factors. And they were not what I had been led to believe. In fact, they were a lot different and a lot more enjoyable. I began to lose weight for the last time. I went from 220 pounds at age 39 to 135 pounds at age 40. I am the "genuine article" ... a fat-my-whole-life, chronically obese person who found a way to beat the odds for good. In my eyes, a miracle. Think of yourself right now at your perfect weight, with perfect health and being there happily, without deprivation, enjoying food and life every day ... no obsession, no striving, no fear of regain, just perfect balance. A miracle? It happened to me ... it can happen for you, too.

To make a long story short, *I lost nearly 140 pounds of fat from my top weight and, most importantly, have maintained at goal for over six years to date.* I no longer have several sizes in my wardrobe to handle weight fluctuations, because my weight doesn't fluctuate much. I wear a perfect size 8 for my 5'7" frame (even in a bathing suit!). And I'm not just a bag of skin either, like you might suspect. I'm athletic and trim, full of health and energy. And lest you think I eat only grass and water to maintain my svelte figure, perish the thought! My yummy recipes should convince you that I still love to eat well! And another miracle, I actually eat more now than I ate at my top weight! Now I know what to eat and how to eat ... and you will learn, too.

But this program isn't about me. It's about you ... and how you can achieve your weight and health goals. This book shares the insights that finally lifted me to the peak of permanent thinness and excellent health. The information is here to help you do the same. If a miracle happened to you, wouldn't you want to tell everyone about it? I want to share it with you! As you're reading, imagine that I'm sitting right there with you, personally talking to you, giving you a helping hand with all that I've learned. That's the way this book was written. I wrote it for you.

My goal was to rebuild my body, metabolism, self-esteem and my life after so many years of tearing down and abuse. Now my greatest desire is that this program will help teach you the principles and the skills for controlling your weight and health forever ... and rebuilding your self-image as well. The thin and healthy life does exist, right now. You just have to uncover the path and it can be your reality, too. You have the power already. I'll help you find it within yourself.

A question I'm often asked is, "How did you do it?" or "What's your secret?". The questioner then waits expectantly for me to tell them, in a sentence or two, the secret formula for weight control and good health that took over 35 years to discover, test and perfect. I usually, with a shrug and a sweet smile, deny the existence of such a formula. But I'm going to confess. Just between you and me, there really is a secret. I looked long and hard and finally found it ... and it's in this book. As a matter of fact, loving a good mystery the way I do, I've left clues for you in nearly every chapter.

Why the intrigue? Because you'll benefit most by discovering it on your own. When the light dawns you'll be out of the overweight darkness forever. Maybe you've even heard the secret before. Nevertheless, it has little effect until you discover it for yourself ... in your own context and on your own terms.

My real purpose in developing this program is this: to give you the hope and the courage to begin again ... and to help you build the skills that it takes to be a THINNER WINNER. To give you back the "bright promise" of thinness and good health, and a life you can love. Your dream can come true, too! You're about to learn the way.

Lots of standard diet information is just plain wrong. In other words, it doesn't work. Maybe you've found this out for yourself. Losing fat and getting healthy is a lot more fun and empowering than you have been led to think. In reality, when you see it for what it is, it's not a chore, a "hard row to hoe" or anything of the sort. It's a "get to", not a "have to" kind of attitude. Just don't let "hard" in. Choose to perceive health as your choice, your preference. You're in for a wonderful awakening to a new world of health and freedom, personal choice, respect, acceptance and joy. Believe it or not, your obesity is a wonderful gift for you, as it was for me. Really, how many people ever get to weigh 272 pounds? I'm in an elite group with this incredible experience. It was, and is, my path to awakening, my light to follow. The Rubik's Cube of weight loss was given to me to solve because I had the ability to solve it! What a privilege. I had to know this and accept it before I could allow it to be.

Positively and without a doubt, knowing what I do now, I can honestly say there is no reason for anyone who can follow the straight-forward directions in this program and sincerely wants to be thin, to have to stay fat. If I could get thin ... then anyone can. Take a look at my "before and after" pictures. Miracles do happen if you know how to bring them about. And I do. Read carefully. Listen and learn ... and you will, too!

Now is the time to recommit to getting your weight and life under control. Everything you need is here now. With this program, you'll learn how to fly solo, so you can take off in your own direction. You will then have empowered yourself for success. You will, like me, have evolved into health and out of fat. And maybe we'll have a little fun along the way.

Most people who start a weight control program hope to lose weight and gain happiness for their efforts. As you learn the principles in this program, and discover the THINNER WINNERS "secret", you'll develop the power and skills to build for yourself, permanently, both a new body and a new life.

Health, Happiness and Love,

Roseanne
"Rosecrest"
Brookings, Oregon, 1995

Howard's Preface

In 1980 I married a fat girl. Like the old song goes, I must have wanted a girl just like the one who married dear old Dad. My mother seemed to be perpetually fighting to lose the 30 pounds she put on after she had her two kids. Mom was always trying to regain the slenderness of her youth. And she had a lot of friends in the same boat. I grew up surrounded by overweight women who were always on diets. So the fact that I chose to marry a girl with a "weight problem" is no big surprise. I was used to it.

Conquering this problem was central to Roseanne's purpose in life. Not surprising from a girl who had topped the scales at 272 pounds. From the time I met her, twenty-one years ago, she told me that someday she would be thin and "normal". And she was determined to meet this objective (several years before our marriage, when we were studying psychology together, I watched her lose 50 pounds in three months by consuming nothing but liquid protein).

From 1977 (when our courtship began) to 1988 her weight fluctuated between 175 and 220 pounds depending on the stresses of our circumstances. Some of the high-stress events included the deaths of my Mother, Father and younger sister. Health awareness gained a new focus for us during those years and Roseanne really began paying a lot more attention to what we were eating, as opposed to merely how much food we were shoveling down.

Shortly after my sister died in 1988, Roseanne came to me with a request. She said, "I don't want to be fat when I'm 40". And she asked for my help. She told me she would stop playing the "diet game" if I would keep her honest and help her design a plan she could follow. Neither of us was in much of a mood for games at that point when it came to health. So we took a good long look at all we had learned about weight loss over the years and devised a basic comprehensive program.

To the expected food and exercise components we added specific behavior changes. Then we looked at the most critical
factor of all ... attitudes. Everyone knows that when you make up your mind to lose weight, you can always do it ... at least for a while. We designed this program so your mind will stay made up. And by following this four-part
"mind/body" strategy Roseanne went from 220 pounds at age 39 to 135 pounds at her 40th birthday. She did it. Other THINNER WINNERS have done it. And so can you!

One of the proudest moments of my life was lifting Roseanne into my arms when her weight dropped below mine for the first time since I had known her. I could truly say "half of my wife is missing!".

When Roseanne reached her goal we were faced with a new issue ... weight maintenance. It became a matter of weight "control", not merely weight loss. Different factors come into play. So we expanded the program to address these issues.

After a year at her goal Roseanne began work on a book because she wanted to share our successful techniques with other people who were risking their health with obesity. She feels that it's a horrible waste of human potential to spend a lifetime unsuccessfully fighting against fat ... all that energy can be put to better uses. I agree.

After researching and working on the project for several years Roseanne again asked for my help. Together we finished fine-tuning and completing the book.

Even though I played an active role, this book is, more than anything, a gift of love from Roseanne to you. It's her story, told in her words, of how she overcame a lifetime of chronic obesity. Today Roseanne has been at her goal weight for over 6 years and the THINNER WINNERS weight control program has helped many people get their weight under control.

So if you're ready, willing and able to stop playing the diet game, and are serious about controlling your weight and improving your health and attitudes, you'll find the answers in this book.

Howard Strull
Brookings, Oregon

Table of Contents
Brief Version

Table of Contents

I. Introductory Section

II. Attitudes and Personal Development

III. Behavior Changes

IV. Activity and Exercise

V. Nutrition and Food

VI. Additional Tools And Resources

Part I

Introductory Section

Welcome to THINNER WINNERS!   1

"Nothing astonishes men so much as common sense and plain dealing."
Ralph Waldo Emerson

Welcome! You are now a member of the THINNER WINNERS Weight Control Program. Congratulations on taking your first step towards a healthy, permanently thin future! In this unique program you will be learning proven weight control techniques which will allow you the ultimate luxury of an improved level of health, and looking and feeling better in the process. You will be an active participant in designing and implementing your own successful, personalized weight control and maintenance program ... one that you can understand, live with and use for the rest of your life. The more actively you get involved in the program's many features the more you will benefit. All will become clear as you read and learn just what to do.

Solutions vs. Miracles

It's only fair to tell you right up front what this program is, and what it isn't. THINNER WINNERS offers an array of solutions to the weight-related problems you may be experiencing. It contains a variety of methods from which you can choose to learn to lose excess fat and control your weight for good. It is designed to be used as a four-part plan. By following the recommended steps, you'll get the maximum benefit. The parts fit together like a puzzle to reveal a well-balanced picture of health and fitness for you. Comprehension is the glue that holds them all together. If you choose to follow only selected portions of the program you will derive fewer benefits overall. This is as honest and straight-forward as I can get. The program worked, and continues to work, for me. It also works for program members who follow the complete plan and allow themselves to evolve through the changes they need to make. This takes courage, belief and faith which all get stronger as you begin to experience your success. It also takes a good dose of stick-to-it-iveness. This is a long-term program ... which means you need to develop a long-term attitude towards weight control.

THINNER WINNERS does not promise miracles, although to me it is a miracle that I wake up skinny everyday. But if you're looking for instant miracles, like so many dieters are, I'm afraid you're doomed for disappointment. All the one-food miracle diets, magic pills and potions, and all the shiny, expensive exercise machines offer promises of miraculous, instant results. If their promises held any truth there wouldn't be fifty million Americans who go on diets every year. If you're looking for an instant solution to what is a long-term problem, I suggest you look elsewhere.

On the other hand, if you're finally fed up with all the bogus claims and are ready to get down to the business of true self-improvement, positive change and being thin for life by knowing how and what to do, you've come to the right place. The THINNER WINNERS program was designed to help you accomplish these important goals. During the course of my "dieting career" I rode the "diet roller coaster" countless times, just like you may have. I fell for those promises of instant, miracle weight loss more times than I care to remember. Then I started waking up. I began to read, study and learn all that I could about losing and controlling weight. This program is a refined version of the best mind and body research available, put together in a unique way. There are some unorthodox concepts that step far beyond the typical weight loss mentality. That's why THINNER WINNERS works. It doesn't do what everybody else does ... and it's a good thing, because nobody has ever come up with a program that really works for long-term weight control. Until now.

But what you really want to know is how long it's going to take you to lose your excess weight, right? The only honest answer I can give is "it depends on you". If you follow the program as recommended, and make a serious effort to learn and apply all the principles, it is probably safe to say that you can average a weight loss of about 1 to 1.5 pounds a week. This is after the first week or two when you may lose more due to dropping "water weight". Also, larger people, "virgin dieters", serious exercisers and men tend to lose more. It is not recommended that you lose at a rate any faster than this because the weight you lose will probably not be fat (which is what you want to lose). Rather it will be muscle (which you want to keep). Also, fat lost at a more moderate rate tends to stay off because your body has a chance to adjust to the changes. A pound a week doesn't sound like much, does it? Well, 50 or more pounds in a year is fairly substantial, and it looks a lot better when you know that you can keep the weight off ... forever. Never to return.

THINNER WINNERS isn't just a weight loss program. It's a weight control program. The focus and philosophy are very different. Any well-intentioned "expert dieter" can lose weight. However, weight control, that is keeping it off forever without suffering, involves understanding how and why your body and mind work. Why? Because until you become aware of and understand the working principles of your own body and mind (the way you gain, lose and react to foods and situations) you will continue to act in counter-productive, fat-producing ways. You will undermine all your best efforts, without even knowing why or how you can change. Thus, THINNER WINNERS is an educational program. If you study it, learn the lessons well and get an "A" you will derive many benefits additional to simple weight loss. First, you'll gain the knowledge and understanding to control your weight for life. That's pretty good right there. Next, you'll become healthier in body and mind. Finally, you will get the greatest benefit of all ... a self-aware, self-accepting, loving attitude towards yourself. The deep effects this will have on your life are no less than profound.

I can't do it for you, but I can help you do it for yourself. You have the power already as you will discover in these pages.

Each chapter is designed to teach you different variations of the essential principles. As the following list shows, the program is organized into four major parts:

1)   **Attitudes and Personal Development**
2)   **Behavior Changes**
3)   **Exercise and Activity**
4)   **Nutrition and Food**

If you want an easy way to remember the program parts, think "BEAN": Behavior, Exercise, Attitude, Nutrition. However, attitude is critical and needs to come first.

Additional Tools and Resources has supplemental information about various topics. The whole set is needed to ensure that you have all the tools necessary for keeping your excess weight off permanently.

Important themes are emphasized in different ways throughout the program to help you learn the essential lessons. But please note carefully, it's up to you to take the responsibility for learning them.. Don't be like the proverbial horse who gets led to the water, but won't drink. Drink your fill of the information in this program. Then be like the truly "good students" of the world ... if you don't understand something, ask questions until you do!

It is the specific objective of the THINNER WINNERS program to help you advance at your own pace. Take your time and apply the principles you learn along the way. A major key to your success is that you acquire an understanding of why certain attitude, behavior, activity, and food choices will bring you successful results ... and why others won't.

Once you have successfully mastered the principles, you will have the necessary skills to control your weight and lead a healthful lifestyle. You will be empowered to choose permanent health, including weight control for life. That's a promise to yourself that's worth making and keeping.

What to do first

Keep reading! Chapter 2 is an entertaining look at "Myths That Keep You Fat".

1)   Then read Chapter 3 "Your Personal Success Plan". This chapter gets you going with a step-by-step plan. What to eat and do, it's all in there.

2)   Sign your "Weight Control Commitment" (at the end of the Success Plan).

3)   Complete your "Self-Assessment" (Chapter 4) to determine your eating habits, diet history, general health, family eating style, etc. to help pinpoint your specific strengths and needs.

4)   Complete a 3-day "Food Journal" (I know, but it really will be useful. Trust me.) and record everything you eat during that time. This will be the basis for your personalized "food analysis".

5)   Then you will begin a series of lessons designed to help you understand and master the skills needed to overcome the obstacles you're having in losing pounds and maintaining your ideal weight. Be teachable and you will learn what it takes!

Again, congratulations on your decision to face your "weight problem" sensibly and permanently! Now you're on your way to becoming a THINNER WINNER!

Myths That Keep You Fat   2

*"We have forty million reasons for failure, but not a single excuse.
So the more we work and the less we talk the better results we shall get."*
Rudyard Kipling

Let's start by taking a closer look at some of the most common excu ... er, myths that some people might use to keep themselves from beginning or sticking with a program of weight management and health enhancement. It's a rare dieter indeed who hasn't come up with at least a few fanciful reasons as to why their last diet just didn't do the trick. Some "valid justification" as to why they're standing there with a cheesy slice of pizza in one hand and a quarter of a chocolate cake in the other.

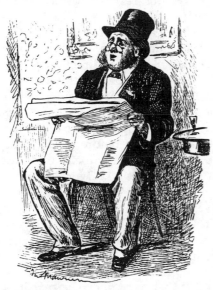

*"But it's not the croissants at all, dear.
It's that new "fat gene" they discovered."*

Perhaps you've used one or more of the following at one time or another (just like I have):

Myth #1:
Diets should be serious, hard work. After all, your health and future depend on it.

Bull-oney. I considered calling this program "Fun With Food". Food needs to be fun at all times, when cutting corners or not. I love to play with my food ... touch it, mold it, arrange it, smell it, hide it, sneak it and enjoy every bite. Food used to be the center of my life, my solace, my faithful companion. It is not reasonable to think that it will become

merely sustenance to me, now that I'm thin. It is like asking me to fall out of love! I love the smell of baking cookies or bread (and licking the spoon!). I love to fix a big holiday meal for my family with all the trimmings. I love to lick a nice cold frozen yogurt cone. I enjoy it and I don't feel guilty any more. I have learned to pick the best foods for me and still have a great time enjoying the wonders of food. Food is entertaining ... so enjoy! Never let it get boring or tedious. If you find yourself slipping into "serious hard work" mode, then do something to break out of it that is silly and fun. Eat lollipops, make a heart-shaped ricotta cheesecake, have popcorn for a snack, have a fun food for your next meal such as tacos or burritos, pizza or an ice cream sundae.

You will learn how to make all of these foods in versions that you can have and enjoy guilt-free. Good food is not your enemy any more. It is the best friend you will ever have in reaching and stabilizing at a weight where you look and feel wonderfully healthy ... and are satisfied at the same time.

Myth #2: Sneaking food is bad.

I enjoy sneaking! And when I can have fun with food, I do it! I still hide goodies or eat them in the car and get some kind of thrill by eating a yummy cookie or chocolate all alone. If I didn't do this, I would be constantly thinking about how much I miss doing it. So instead of delving into your deep, dark past to find out why, why, why you love to eat an apron full of cookies while hiding under the dining room table (it just happens to be that you and your cousin used to hide there during family get-togethers and giggle and eat) just do it, if it keeps you from feeling deprived. It's a lot cheaper than therapy, too.

Myth #3: I don't have the time to cook, prepare special foods, exercise, etc.

You have to cook and eat anyway. Why not do it right? Yes, being in this program and changing some old habits may take a little extra time on your part initially. But not as much as you may think when you get it down pat ... and have applied the principles a few times. You'll soon have some of your favorite recipes memorized and you'll whip them out almost automatically. A lot of the recipes in the THINNER WINNERS program can be doubled and eaten at two or more meals ... or can be frozen for later use. The microwave and the freezer will become your fast-food buddies instead of the drive-through greasy spoons. Besides, by cooking your own meals you'll get to spend more time around your new friend ... healthy food. I like that part.

Myth #4:
My family won't eat diet food.

This isn't diet food. This is great food. I once taught a series of cooking classes called "The Healthy Gourmet". I love good, gourmet foods, so do you think I'm going to show you how to fix junk? Think again. Besides, I'm not going to tell them if you're not.

Myth #5:
My family likes me the way I am.

Of course they like you the way you are. You're a wonderful person! If they like you now, just wait until you're a slim, athletic and healthy mom (dad, sis or bro ...) who serves them fun foods and is in a great mood all the time! And since they love you so much, wouldn't they want you to be the best you're capable of ... healthy and happy? You bet.

Myth #6: I'm too old or too young to worry about weight.

Come on. Too old to want to look and feel your best? Too old to want to be happy and feel free of the extra burden of excess weight? Too old to care about how you look and how others look at you? I just don't believe it. And you're never too young to want to join in the activities and feel like you belong with the rest of the gang ... without worrying about what they think of your weight. You who are young should really strive to make these changes now, because they just get easier with time, whereas the extra weight just gets harder to deal with. The things you do become habits, and you want to spend most of your life thinking about better things than being overweight. The sooner you start, the better. Excess weight affects you from the start. It is the single most important factor in unhealthy cholesterol levels, raising the LDL (bad) cholesterol and lowering the HDL (good) cholesterol. That can mean an increased risk of heart disease. It also raises your insulin levels at any age, and that can lead to diabetes and high

blood pressure. Your body's balance of hormones can be affected increasing risk of breast and endometrial cancer and throwing your cycles off, increasing PMS. All overweights regardless of age have increased risk of developing gallstones, arthritis and joint problems from the extra work that the body must do to carry the weight. Back problems, knee strain and foot problems abound in the obese. And of course, that means you sure don't feel like exercising much. That's a real problem because to bring your body back to normal weight and increase mobility, and positively affect moods exercise is the #1 ticket to health.

As you get older, these problems all begin to pile on top of one another. They don't go away unless the weight is lost. They just get worse. So a "minor" cholesterol elevation at age 25 or 30 could easily develop into high blood pressure at 35 or 40 and full blown heart disease or diabetes or cancer at age 50 or 60. After that, you could live a miserable life keeping track of all your medications and symptoms, feeling rotten most of the time and betrayed by your body.

It's never too early to start heeding the warning signs of impending disease. Read the writing on the wall, take charge of the direction your health is headed and choose to be healthy and fit into your 80's and 90's! If you already have health problems, choose now to halt the progression of disease and reverse the trend of degenerative conditions. I was a mess with a capital M before taking charge of my health. So much so that my doctor told me to get my affairs in order! I was 24. Over 20 years later, my doctor can't find a single thing I could change or do to improve! So hang in there, you can do it, too. My THINNER WINNERS program shows you how.

If you are under 12 years old, be sure to get an adult to help you out.

Myth #7: I've got so much to lose I'll never lose enough to be healthier.

If you are 50-100 pounds or more overweight like I was, the tendency to not even get started is common. It seems like such a big job! Actually, losing even a few pounds can make a huge difference in your health and how you feel. That can then encourage you to try for a little more and pretty soon you'll have the "snowball" effect working for you instead of against you. Studies have shown that for every 2 pounds of excess weight you lose, your cholesterol drops by an average of 3 points. As little as 10 pounds can help lower blood pressure, too. As you begin to feel better, then exercise and healthier foods take on a different meaning to you. They are not just a way to lose weight, but a way to feel better, live longer without disease, and increase self-esteem by giving you a choice over your life. My method of losing a few pounds, then reveling in the joy of accomplishment for awhile, maintaining the loss without pressure to keep losing allowed me to ultimately cut my body weight in half in a healthy way! You can, too.

Myth #8 To stay thin, you can't eat much except rabbit food.

Just the opposite is true with a THINNER WINNERS lifestyle. This time you have all the means at your fingertips to really do it right. No fad diets and starvation that strip you of your fat burning machinery and lowers your metabolism. You will be building up that machinery to its highest level ever, because now you will understand how important a role it plays in letting you eat all the healthy, wholesome food you need to be dynamically thin.

I didn't really believe this until I got thin using these techniques. But now that I am thin I can make a truly unbelievable statement: I eat more food now than I ate when I was 272 pounds! Sometimes I wonder how I can possibly stay thin with all the food I eat. I used to wake up in the morning and expect to be 20 pounds heavier because of all that I had consumed the day before. "How can that possibly be true?", you ask. The secret lies in the types of food I eat (great stuff, believe me), and the fact that I have stripped off the fat from my body and added muscle in its place. In this program you will learn how to do the same thing. It's really incredibly simple once you grasp the concepts. Once you understand, you will do everything possible to live the THINNER WINNERS principles. Get your appetite ready because you will be able to eat more than you can even dream of now. And stay thin forever! Honest!

Myth #9:
You can't eat the food you really love.

On the contrary, I have found that in order to reduce and eliminate my cravings and obsessions about food, I absolutely must identify the food specifically ... and then go ahead and eat it, either the real thing or a reasonable facsimile. If I don't, I continue to be haunted by thoughts of that food until I burst through the gates of reason and devour everything in sight even remotely similar to the food in question! And usually consume far more than I would have if I just went ahead and had a serving. By learning your own cravings and devising healthier versions of those foods you can even enjoy your favorites more often. There are wonderful healthy versions of ice cream, pizza, sweets of all kinds, chips and dip, etc.

An occasional indulgence of the real thing is not a tragedy either. Choose to let yourself have it, really enjoy every bite (after all, it is an indulgence) and nix the guilt. It's not a weakness, but a strength to be able to recognize your particular cravings and consciously choose to reasonably indulge. And it gives you a great feeling of control to know that you made the choice yourself.

I think that the biggest mistake made by most people on "diets" is to deprive themselves. It's no wonder they get bored to tears without their favorite tastes ... and then chuck the whole program. Deprivations only lead to binges and overindulgence later on. So eat what you want.

Myth #10: I have to do "The Plan" perfectly or not at all.

Even though it may seem like changing habits and "working on" a program is rigid and restrictive, the reality is that the truly permanent lifestyle of the THINNER WINNER is anything but rigid. Life throws you all sorts of curves and twists. It zigs and zags like crazy at times! Learning to be flexible and bend while not snapping in two is the real skill that will keep you thin and healthy for a lifetime.

Who says you can't have pancakes or an omelet for dinner? A sandwich for breakfast? Exercise at midnight? Meditate while in the dentist's chair? Go ahead and learn the basics of what it takes, then I encourage you to throw in your own style get creative! The lifestyle you end up with is ultimately going to reflect your individual style anyway if it's to be successful, so know that going in with your eyes open. You and I are two different individuals and our healthiest lifestyles will be different, too. If I say eat breakfast, understand the reasoning behind it, then devise your own plan if you want to eat at 10 P.M. because you aren't hungry for breakfast until then! Shocking? Maybe. But the truth is that it works.

Nothing is set in stone, so don't let that hold you back. You may begin to feel resentment and "fall off" the wagon of "must do's". There are some basic laws of physics that can't be changed, but you have a lot of leeway here, much more than you think. Use it to avoid boredom, express your individuality and have fun with your food and your life. (Yes, this really can be fun!)

Think about other programs you've tried. When did you stop following them? When you stopped following their suggestions to the letter, right? Well, THINNER WINNERS isn't a followers program. It's a solution from someone who has succeeded at doing what most people only dream of doing, found the basic success guidelines and teaches you how to put them to work for yourself in the best way possible. Take the ideas and run with them. Make them your own and you will permanently succeed (with style!), too. Not by following on the dotted line, but by using the basics to change your processing of the "pizza and ice-cream" world that we all live in (including little old size 8 me!)

Myth #11 I don't need to exercise. I'm already dieting.

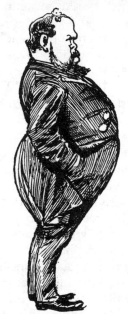

"I am sucking it in!"

First of all, with THINNER WINNERS you are not "dieting". You're learning about the healthiest foods to choose for your body to return naturally to a normal weight. No foods are off limits unless you choose to make them. So no more diets ... just healthier food choices.

Studies have shown that average weight loss is about 7-8 pounds if you simply limit foods alone, even fat. After that initial loss, it gets really tough ... often to the point of discouragement. This may encourage eating disordered behavior such as fasting or skipping meals, using diuretics, laxatives, diet pills, over-exercising or tiny food portions in order to continue losing.

To go beyond that 7-8 pounds, safely and permanently, exercise is the key. It does more than just burn up calories. It re-educates your cell systems by producing enzymes during aerobic exercise that help your body permanently burn excess fat and actually change your way of metabolizing it. Building muscle through anaerobic weight-training can also permanently increase your rate of fat-burning. An exerciser burns more calories, the right kind of calories and stores less fat even while sleeping than a non-exerciser!

All this adds up to the permanent kind of fat and weight loss that leads to a lifetime of slimness and health. Far easier and healthier than constantly struggling to maintain a small, tenuous food-only based loss ... which gets tougher the older you are or the more times you have "dieted".

You need both exercise and healthful dietary changes to lose that weight forever. Follow the THINNER WINNERS program and you'll maximize your fat loss in the right way ... the way that can lead you to permanent weight maintenance at the weight you want. I can honestly tell you, exercise feels good when you're healthy and at your ideal weight. It's a natural urge that just asks to be fulfilled every day, like a fine car that begs to be driven. The reason you resist exercise so much is that it hurts and is hard right now because of your extra weight. As you begin to lose weight it will get easier and a lot more fun. Trust me.

Myth #12: I don't need to diet. I'm already exercising.

This myth is the direct opposite of the preceeding one and is just as misleading. Again, you are not "dieting". You are learning to eat for health and that leads to a healthy weight as well as numerous health profile improvements. Of course regular exercise is a fundamental necessity for positive health and achieving a healthy weight.

If you already know that and are exercising, that's great. But you can't just shovel in the old junk or high-fat non-health-promoting foods and expect the exercise to counteract the effects. Exercise does a lot of good, but it doesn't perform miracles. If you're treating your body to the wonderful effects that exercise can bring, why in the world would you want to undo all that benefit with junk food anyway? When you exercise you'll be able to eat a bit more calories and you will be able to eat a few goodies now and again without it being the undoing of your svelte form (for reasons discussed in the Exercise section), but that does not give you wholesale carte blanche to scarf up the world and then "work it off"! So keep exercising and work on giving the highest quality food to your body as possible. Follow the well-balanced THINNER WINNERS guidelines and you can have it all ... great food and a well-toned, fit body, too.

Myth #13: It's selfish to spend all this time, effort and money just on me.

Many people, especially women, have been brought up to believe that it's selfish to do special activities for themselves because it somehow takes away time and energy that they can be spending on "more important" people such as their children, families and spouses. In this philosophy, to work yourself to the bone until you can barely stand means to be selfless and sacrificing, an admired martyr who puts all others above herself.

Let me ask you this: what are you really giving to them if you are functioning at less than your potential? How much do you have to give to your loved ones and the world if you are overweight and unhealthy and have never bothered to develop your talents, abilities and potential that you were born with?

Who is the most important person in the world? Is it your child? Many women say yes. Your spouse, parents or siblings? Well, the truth is that it's none of those other people. The answer is YOU. You are the most important person in your world and when you realize this then you will stop trying to do everything for the people you love. Instead, you will begin to be everything you can be for yourself and also for them. That is the ultimate love and your first duty in life. Not only to them but to yourself. Then you will begin developing the self-esteem to blossom and grow even more. And by being even more you will become the truly fulfilled person they need you to be to foster their growth.

Concentrate your efforts and strength on achieving the positive self-development skills that are laid out in this book. Truly be all that you can be by concentrating on your own inner enrichment. Then you will have the best to give to yourself, your world and all the people in it. You will be the one who can truly help others by being a strong, aware and caring role model for everyone you encounter and influence. You can help others more by making the most of yourself than in any other way. In the long run, that is the highest, most genuine and richest contribution you can ever make to others.

Myth #14: I don't wanna do all those weird things. I just wanna be thin!

If you are reluctant to do some of the program exercises, if they seem "odd" to you, or "not your style" or even useless (Heaven help me!), then just consider this: You bought this book because you believed that I was successful and I could help you be successful, too. You choose well. When it comes to weight control I am an Olympic champion ... the gold medal genuine article. So congratulations, you've got a good coach. Now let me help you.

If you hired a gold medal Olympic skier to coach your skiing, would you say to them, "That's just not me", or "That's weird. I'll just skip it and only do the things that appeal to me"? That athlete knows what works and what doesn't through years of experience, trial and error and ultimately hard-won success. That's why he or she does the things they do (weird or not) in training, recommends the same for others in training and wins gold medals. And that's why I do it, too. It works. I've crashed and burned a billion times and I've learned from every mistake. I know how to get that gold. Let me help you be a gold medal THINNER WINNER, too.

Myth #15: I'm perfectly happy the way I am, thank you.

So why are you reading this book?? Come on. There are tons of excuses out there for you to not get started on a program that will really get you thin and keep you there for life. Face them one by one and get rid of them. Then let's get going.

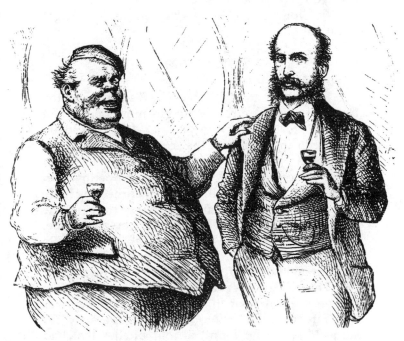

" ... and my father had big bones, too."

Your Personal Success Plan   3

"Never mistake motion for action."
Ernest Hemingway

A Balanced Plan of Action

THINNER WINNERS uses a balanced approach to losing weight and keeping it off. Why? Because chances are good that before you ever heard of THINNER WINNERS you were already something of an expert at losing weight. If you're like most "dieters" you've been riding the weight loss roller coaster for years and you've already lost a lot of weight, and gained it back again ... many times! But your focus was on losing weight, period, and so your plan was unbalanced. You were leaving out essential ingredients for permanent success, so you couldn't succeed! This time it's going to be different. When you finish studying these materials and fitting the information you learn into your lifestyle, you're going to know how to avoid regaining the weight that you lose. You can lose weight in a hundred different ways (the banana diet was fun until I started swinging from the chandelier), but maintaining your goal weight long-term requires a specific, balanced set of indispensable attitudes and skills. You're going to wind up a lot smarter about controlling your weight than you've ever been before.

But you can't get all this by osmosis. You've got to take it ...

Step by Step

Remember the fable of "The Tortoise and the Hare"? Weight control reality has more in common with the tortoise. Before you get discouraged by this, keep in mind that the tortoise won the race. Controlling your weight and improving your health is not a race, however. You're not competing with anyone. The simple truth is that over the long haul, and we're talking about years here, your relationship with your body is a personal issue. There isn't anybody living in your skin but you. So forget about getting thin before someone else ... just get thin and healthy for yourself, in your own time.

There's another ancient fable that applies here as well. A poor thirsty raven was flying over the parched land. After looking desperately for signs of water he found an old pitcher that had some rain water down in the very bottom, beyond his reach. Being an intelligent bird, he started dropping pebbles into the pitcher. With each pebble the water level rose slightly higher. Finally, after dropping in 77 pebbles, the water was within his reach and he took a well-deserved drink. He reached his goal by completing the process step by step. If he had stopped at ten pebbles he would still be a thirsty bird. Twenty, thirty, forty, fifty and even sixty pebbles wouldn't have been enough. He was tired after forty pebbles and it was taking some effort to find more of them, but he knew that in spite of all his work he wasn't going to get any water until he put in enough pebbles to do the job. He had to complete the process in order to get the reward for his efforts.

You can use a similar strategy to succeed. If you think of the lessons in this program as the pebbles you need to find, you'll have a pretty good idea of what you need to do. I discovered and developed the principles while trying to find the solution to my personal obesity problem. Each one is important for success. I lost my weight by progressively following these principles. They will work just as well for you.

These days it's easy for me to maintain my goal weight. That's because I follow the principles set forth in this program. They're simple and straightforward and they will work for you if you take them step by step. Talking about losing weight won't get you thin. Doing something about it will. Doing what it takes ... whatever it takes for you. Doing half of the steps will only get you half of the benefits, if that. So be like the successful raven ... keep picking up those pebbles and watch the water rise.

How to Use this Program

This book consists of a series of lessons, grouped into four main subject areas (remember BEAN: Behavior, Exercise, Attitude, Nutrition). You'll find that these lessons overlap and blend into each other. Nearly all of the chapters will refer you to other chapters for additional information and elaboration on a particular topic. After you complete the exercises in Chapter 4 "Self-Assessment" you can really start anywhere, but we recommend that you read it straight through the first time. A second complete reading will help you get a better grasp of the balance of the four parts. Then you can use the book as a reference source anytime you need to look up something.

This program is meant to be used! Read it with a highlighter in hand. Underline the concepts that are important to you. Read the materials a number of times ... until you understand the concepts completely. Make this program your own! Avoid using unproductive study methods ... the ones that don't work. Some people get their hands on new materials and either say "I already know all this" and stick it on the shelf with all their other "diet" books, or they think it looks like too much to do ... so they don't do anything. Make it one of your objectives to avoid these problems. Use your highlighter and learn!

Reading the lessons from a certain point of view will help you get the most from them, too. What point of view is that? In the last century a man named Russell Conwell made a famous speech called "Acres of Diamonds". The story he told was of a number of people who went on fruitless searches for fortunes only to find out later that the greatest fortunes of all were right under their feet before they ever left. One man went chasing all over Africa looking for diamonds ... which he never found. However, the man who bought the searcher's old farm discovered that it was covered with acres of diamonds in the rough, and he became exceedingly rich.

You may not realize it yet, but the book you're holding in your hands is your "acres of diamonds" in terms of weight control. Just like real diamonds you're going to have to dig them out, cut and polish then to your own taste. Read the materials carefully. Use what you learn. Find your diamonds.

You may be tempted to refer to sections of the program that you think are the most important. That's great! In fact, that's one of the "secrets" of your eventual success ... you need to turn the concepts you learn into "your own plan". But don't make the mistake of leaving out any of the other sections because you don't understand them, they seem hard or because you've already "been there, done that". It's hard to drive a car on only one, two or three wheels. You will need all the concepts ... just like you need all four wheels.

I'd also like to toss in a small reminder for you. If your approach to the THINNER WINNERS weight control program is to race through and get it over with ... then to put it simply, put the book in a box and send it right back. If you bring your old "instant result" mentality to this program you are absolutely guaranteed to fall right on your nose. So why waste your time? If you're not going to take what we have to say seriously we'd much rather refund your money and wish you bon voyage.

This is a long-term program. And you will learn skills that will get you long-term results. You can't learn long-term skills without long-term commitment! This means that you are going to have to put in the time and the work to see the results. Are you still with me? Good! Because ...

You Are One-of-a-Kind!

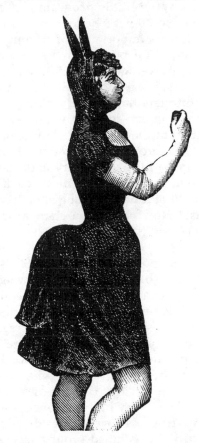

Weight control's most intriguing challenge, and the place where dieters often get trapped, both emotionally and physically, is the area of individual differences. A single, rigid weight control plan does not fit all. It can't. The exact combination of factors that works perfectly for you may not work very well for your neighbor across the street, or even your twin sister. You have different bodies and minds, and different relationships with them. You bring an individual set of needs to this program. The answers are here but it's up to you to fine-tune your individual working plan. Tailor the basics to fit only you and you will succeed big time!

You and I both know that most people don't follow instructions to the letter. That goes for everything from weight loss plans to putting bicycles together at Christmas. Everybody wings it. You look at the instructions for about 2 seconds, and then race along in the direction we think is going to get it done the fastest. Similarly, you may not follow the model Start-Up Plan to the letter although it's sensible, progressive and painless. That's good, because you need to find your own style of relating to the basic principles if it's going to work for you, using the plan as a general outline. You have to personalize it. There are as many ways to do this as there are people on the planet.

Keeping that in mind, let's look at how different people have chosen to approach the THINNER WINNERS program ... and their motivations. You'll get a better sense of perspective and see the real importance of finding your own flexible way. The people in these examples are composites of average dieters. They have some of the basic qualities and attitudes that potential weight controllers have. Look for qualities in these people that you can identify with. See if you can figure out what they're doing right and what they might do to improve their situation. If any of these people sound a bit like you, try and identify what you can do to propel yourself most steadily towards your goal. What kind of dieting style have you had in the past? How could you change or rearrange things to succeed this time?

A) Amy is 60 pounds overweight. She's relatively new to the ways of serious long-term weight control. She has played the diet game for several years but has never had any really good results. She has always lacked a strong sense of drive regarding her weight, preferring to buy into "complete" programs ... all laid out neatly and with the work done for her. She's been willing to pay "whatever it takes" for this "custom service". Her self-esteem is weak on the best of days. Amy has developed the bad habit of anticipating failure ... and she's rarely disappointed. She's joined groups several times in the past and always quits within a few months. She doesn't feel a part of things, and it's easier for her to "hide". She likes the idea of the THINNER WINNERS program because she can do it at home. She has reservations of course, but none-the-less she has committed to following the Start-Up Plan for 8 weeks. She has an "I'll see" attitude. She's optimistic about the part of the program having to do with attitudes and building self-esteem. She's going to concentrate on her attitudes. Nobody has ever talked to her about goals in the past and she is filled with a new sense of hope. (I recommend that Amy focus on the Attitudes and Personal Development section, and point her right away to the Chapter 6 "Great Expectations").

B) Bob has a stronger sense of resolve than Amy. He takes his weight loss seriously. But his self-esteem is chained firmly to his weight at the wrists and ankles. When he's feeling trim he's on top of the world. All confidence and good cheer. On the other hand, when he's up 20 pounds or more (which he often is) a mouse could kick him around. He has lost weight successfully in the past, but usually through sheer strength of will. He's the kind of person who will live on bread and water for a month just to prove he can. Unfortunately it's easy to knock him off balance. If he thinks somebody is being critical of him (especially about the way he looks) he loses his fragile control and reverts to excessive eating. He's also resistant to the idea of changing his habits. He insists on being "right" about what he knows, and this doesn't allow a lot of room for new ideas slipping in. He hates to exercise and likes those fast food burgers. However, now he's up about 75 pounds and even he has to admit that he's not fooling anybody by wearing long jackets or with talk about "carrying his weight well". He also suffers from indigestion a lot. He's made up his mind to try what looks like something different. He's skeptical about Roseanne's 6 year claim but he is impressed with the before and after photos. His philosophy is "If she can do it, so can I". Bob has decided to take another look at the whole concept of exercise and also has committed to filling out a Daily Success Planner for at least 3 months. He also likes the idea about the rewards. (I point Bob to the Nutrition and Food section, particularly Chapter 26 "Real Nutrition". He needs to learn more about what he's actually putting in his body. He should also look at Chapter 25 "Creating An Active Lifestyle" to get started with exercise in his daily routine. Then he should concentrate on his attitude about being "on" a diet, then "off").

C) Carol is a real yo-yo woman. She's yo-yo'd herself up an extra 120 pounds. She's a binge style eater and a binge style dieter as well. She eats, drinks and makes merry until she wakes up one day feeling downright embarrassed and scared about her obesity. She knows that the mirror doesn't lie ... especially when it's too small to see her whole body. When that happens she usually cuts back her eating to the bone for about 6 months and drops as much as 100 pounds. She has done this several times. In terms of dieting, Carol has done it all from liquid protein to toughing it out at well under 1000 calories a day. She always "knows" that she can lose weight when she really chooses to. She's a big, "large-boned" gal and she fancies that her business clients respect her more because of her size ... both her physical "largeness" and her "larger than life" personality. But deep down in her core she knows that she's pushing her luck. Her family tree is full of obese people who have died relatively young. Carol is almost 50 now and she's starting to worry about her health. She is also acutely aware that her teenage daughter is fat and very unhappy. This brings back a lot of unpleasant memories. She wants to do what she can for her, and being fairly self-aware she knows that she has contributed to her daughter's problem by setting an unhealthy example. Carol is interested in learning to change her behavioral patterns in terms of eating. Being in management she already knows the importance of the right attitudes and working towards goals. (Carol needs to slow down the pace. She needs to gradually lose about 30 pounds and then stabilize there for at least a month before she tries to lose any more. She can then repeat this process. She also needs to start an exercise program. Strengthening her heart with mild aerobics will head her in a much healthier direction. Keeping a weight graph over a long period may help her see the long-term yo-yoing of her weight. She might start with Chapter 14 "Taming Your Stress").

D)   Debbie is ready to get to her goal weight , once and for all. She's had a lifelong tendency towards being a bit chubby, and has been as much as 50 pounds overweight. But for the last three years she's been able to stabilize at about 10-15 pounds above her goal weight. She has not been able to make the additional effort to lose those last 10 pounds. She was willing to stay one step removed from the spotlight and let her slender friends attract the most dating interest . Sometimes she had to bite her lip from envy but she always feared that she would somehow risk more by competing head to head with her flamboyant, slender, popular friends. But now she's getting married in about 4 months and she's concerned that if she has children she might really lose control of her weight. She's determined to get down to her goal weight for the wedding. But she also made a pact with herself that she will stay at her goal for at least a year. She has decided to follow the Start-Up Plan to the letter. And then use it as the basis of her own continuing program. She filled out her weight control commitment and it made her feel really good to be doing something important and healthy for herself. She's been at the sidelines for so long that she has a real good feel for the meaning of long-term. (Debbie needs to look at the wonderful trimming benefits of exercise and also at the joys of those oh-so-reinforcing rewards. Since she's getting married soon we also recommend that she start learning how to convert some of her own and her fiancé's favorite recipes into healthier versions.)

Did any of these examples remind you a bit of your own weight history? You know yourself better than anyone. And only you know what your real motivation is to get your weight under control. All the chapters in this book will prove important to you if you have truly made the commitment to long-term weight control. Put all four program elements to work and you've got an unstoppable powerhouse that will get you to your goal safer and healthier than any other program ever. Take some time to think about your style and how you can flex the program to work with it.

An important thing we can't provide is a personal supporter for you. Before too much time goes by, you need to find a friend, spouse or group that can give you the emotional support that you need to carry you through the periodic tough times. See Chapter 18 "Creating A Powerful Support System", then choose and "train" your supporter. With a strong support and this plan you will ...

Build a Solid Foundation in 8 Weeks! The THINNER WINNERS Start-Up Plan

Whether you're a relative beginner to the world of weight control or a seasoned veteran, more or less following the model Start-Up Plan will get you off to a good start. There are enough innovative elements in this program that even the old pros will learn some important new tricks. The emphasis is on learning the essential principles and establishing positive habit patterns according to a graduated format ... in an 8-week program for you to follow step by step. It takes the guesswork out in the beginning and helps you establish a solid foundation of knowledge in order to make better, more informed choices. You'll learn why a certain choice is better than another.

At the end of the 8 weeks you'll have developed enough knowledge and skills to continue the program effectively on your own. Once your positive new habits are in place you'll be able to stay on track with periodic fine-tuning. That's the idea ... for you to be confidently independent .

THINNER WINNERS is a solution oriented program. The goal is to help you find solutions to your weight control challenges and obstacles. If you're a "reader" by nature, go ahead and read the whole text ... then follow the step-by-step plan. The Start-Up Plan will allow you to gradually build up to speed. In eight weeks you'll be well on your way to successful long-term weight control. Remember, long-term means years. The quality of your life, your health and your happiness are on the line. Take your time and do it right. Complete all of the steps, even if you can't see the immediate value. This will assure that you'll be prepared when a difficult situation does come up.

Please note that this weekly format is only to be considered a guideline. This is what we recommend in terms of an ideal plan, but if it takes you longer to get going don't worry about it, you'll still be fine. Take it at your own pace ... it is your program after all. The most important thing is to just keep going, Whatever your pace.

Also feel free to interchange the order that you choose to read the chapters. After you complete your self-assessment in Chapter 4 start with the lessons that you feel are going to do you the most good. But be sure to read them all ... at least twice.

There are a few pieces of basic support equipment that you'll need. First, you'll need a notebook of some type. Plain or fancy is up to you. You can order the THINNER WINNERS Workbook that goes along with this program if you like. All of the exercises are nicely laid out for you. See the coupon at the back of the book to order. Next we recommend that you obtain a book of food counts which includes fat, protein, carbohydrates, cholesterol, fiber, sodium and calories. "T-Factor" has a small, inexpensive one. Also handy is "The Complete Book of Food Counts" by Corrine Netzer. Refer to the Bibliography for additional reading material. Now, let's get on the road!

Week 1

1) Buy a food composition book as described in the paragraph above.
2)   Find a support person who will help you stay focused
      (see Chapter 16 for guidelines on this very important step).
3) Read the following chapters, one from each section:
   a)   #5 "Motivation and the Success Mindset"
   b)   #17 "Rewards - A Feather In Your Cap!"
   c)   #20 "The Basics About Exercise"
   d)   #25 "What To Eat"
4) Complete your self-assessment (Chapter 4).
5) Weigh and measure yourself. Start your charts.
     (See Chapter 19 "Keeping Track of Your Progress").
6) Take your "before" picture. I know this is tough,
     but if you don't have one you'll be glad you did later.
7) Choose a breakfast, lunch, dinner and snack each day
     from the sample menus (Chapter 29).
8) Exercise at least once (for at least 10 minutes) ...
     preferably walking.
9) Start writing down your self-observations in your
     Personal Journal (see Chapter 12).
10) Call the THINNER WINNERS "Pep Talk" Hotline
     New updates every other week.
     (503) 471-3922 (It's FREE!).
11) Give yourself a nice, reinforcing reward.

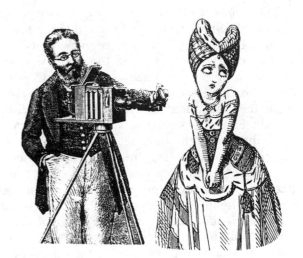

"Come on now... smile!
Before pictures aren't that bad."

Week 1 is fun and exciting. With a new program there's hope. So ride it for all it's worth! Did you complete all the items? If you did, give yourself a gold star!! If you somehow managed to leave out an item or two, maybe you need a good talk with yourself or your support person. There's nothing here that a THINNER WINNER can't do. Complete all the items on week 1 before you go on to week 2 (even if it takes longer than a week).

Week 2

1) Read the chapters in the section on Attitudes and Personal Development.
2) Choose a breakfast, lunch, dinner and snack each day from the sample menus.
3) Exercise at least two times (for at least 10 minutes). Be sure to warm-up, stretch and cool-down.
4) Meditate at least once (for 20 minutes).
5) Begin your Dream Book or Treasure Map.
6) Start monitoring your self-talk (try to keep it positive only).
7) Write to THINNER WINNERS with any questions or comments you have about the program.
8) Give yourself a nice, reinforcing reward.

Yes, week 2 is a bit more intense. There are things to do that you may never have done before. Don't worry ... gradually developing positive habits is good for you and your health. You can do this!

Week 3

1) Read the chapters in the section on Behavior Changes.
2) Pick your favorites from the sample meals and design your own meal plan for the week.
3) Exercise at least three times (for at least 10 minutes a session).
4) Meditate at least two times (20 minute sessions).
5) Identify your primary stressors (see Chapter 14 "Taming Your Stress").
6) Write down your weight control goals (be optimistic but realistic).
7) Keep working on your Dream Book and Treasure Map. Add Affirmations.
8) Keep monitoring your self-talk. Write positive affirmations at the top of your Daily Success Planner.
9) Call the PepTalk Hotline.
10) Write to THINNER WINNERS with any comments or questions.
11) Give yourself a nice, reinforcing reward.

By the end of the third week you are developing the seeds of new habits. Do you have any positive new habits that you're aware of yet? Make some notes in your Personal Journal. What's happening with your weight? Are you losing pounds or inches? How do you look in the mirror? Is your clothing any looser? Try to determine which factors are having the greatest affect on your weight and your attitude.

Week 4

1) Read the chapters in the section on Activity and Exercise.
2) Pick your five favorite choices from the sample meals. Pick out two days worth of recipes from your favorite health-oriented cookbooks or magazines and design your own meal plan for the week.
3) Exercise at least three times (for at least 15 minutes). See if you can find at least two aerobic activities you might enjoy (for cross-training benefits).
4) Calculate your target heart rate range.
5) Meditate at least three times (20 minute sessions).
6) Keep working on your Dream Book, Treasure Map and Affirmations.
7) Begin visualizing yourself at your goal weight if you haven't already.
8) Keep monitoring your self-talk and using your affirmations daily.
9) Write to THINNER WINNERS with your comments or questions.
10) Give yourself a nice, reinforcing reward (isn't this fun?).
11) Spend some time talking to your support person about what you're learning and doing.

Now you're starting to get into the swing of things. You're beginning to gain some independence about what you're going to eat ... so watch it. Avoid falling back into your old food habits. How do you feel about your "mental work"? Are you more aware of the kinds of thoughts you allow into your mind? Remember ... you're in charge of all those thoughts, so if you don't like what you're thinking, double up your efforts to plug in positive thoughts. Are you calling the Hotline for your regular pep talk? We want to know how you're doing ... if you haven't written to us yet, do it now. Allow yourself a "FREE DAY" where you don't keep track of anything if you want (see Chapter 26 "How To Eat"). Relax, have a treat, think about your month and enjoy the work you've done! Great Job!

Week 5

1) Read the chapters in the section on Nutrition and Food.
2) Pick your three favorite choices from the sample meals. Pick out two days worth of recipes from your favorite health-oriented cookbooks or magazines. Convert two days worth of your personal favorite recipes into healthier versions. Design your own meal plan for the week.
3) Weigh and measure yourself.
4) Exercise at least three times (for at least 20 minutes).
5) Meditate at least four times (20 minute sessions).
6) Keep working on your Dream Book, Treasure Map, Affirmations and Visualizations.
7) Keep monitoring your self-talk and using your affirmations.
8) Call the PepTalk Hotline.
9) Write to us with any comments or questions that you have.
10) Give yourself a nice, reinforcing reward.

This is a good time to make some journal notes about what seems to be working for you. Are you doing well and dropping pounds or inches? Remember, on this program the idea is to lose weight slo-o-owly and steadily. That way it will stay off. What are your feelings about meditation? Have you noticed any changes in your stress levels? Your energy level? Have your cravings for food diminished?

Week 6
1) Read the chapters in the section on Additional Tools and Resources.
2) Pick out four days worth of recipes from your favorite health-oriented cookbooks or magazines. Convert three days worth of your personal favorite recipes into healthier versions. Design your own meal plan for the week.
3) Exercise at least three times (for at least 25 minutes).
4) Meditate at least five times (20 minute sessions).
5) Keep working on your Dream Book, Treasure Map, Affirmations and Visualizations.
6) Keep monitoring your self-talk and using your affirmations.
7) Write to us with any comments or questions that you have .
8) Give yourself a nice, reinforcing reward.

Are you falling into the groove of this program? Or are you in danger of falling "off the wagon"? Many people only last about this long before they begin thinking that it's just "too much work". So you were expecting some big payoff without having to work for it? Come on ... this is your life here. If your attitude is slipping, re-read Chapter 5 "Motivation and the Success Mindset". Pay particular note to the quality of persistence. It won't always be this intense ... you're developing new habits!

For those of you (hopefully all) who are getting into the groove, we congratulate you! You're on your way to long-term weight control! As you can see, once you establish new habits it's not so hard to keep them going. Having the right attitude is 99% of it. Think of all the potential at your fingertips now. You're learning how to control your thoughts. Amazing, isn't it?

When you've finished your first reading of the book, start the second pass. This time read it slower. Concentrate especially on the concepts that are pertinent to your own lifestyle. Take your time and make a real effort to understand the information. It is not a complicated program, but there is a lot to learn. Take notes and write down any questions that you have. If you have trouble understanding any of the concepts let us know by writing, calling or faxing (Tel/Fax 503-247-7255).

Week 7
1) Start re-reading the entire text. Highlight the dickens out of it. Remember, this information is for you to use! If you don't learn it and apply what you've learned, it won't do you any good.
2) Pick out three days worth of recipes from your favorite health-oriented cookbooks or magazines. Convert four days worth of your personal favorite recipes into healthier versions. Design your own meal plan for the week ... daily is best.
3) Exercise at least three times (for at least 30 minutes each time).
4) Meditate at least six times (20 minute sessions ... daily is best).
5) Keep working on your Dream Book, Treasure Map, Affirmations and Visualizations.
6) Keep monitoring your self-talk and using your affirmations.
7) Call the PepTalk Hotline.
8) Write to us with any comments or questions that you have.
9) Give yourself a nice, reinforcing reward.

On your second pass through the book, did you learn anything new? How do you like your new style of eating? Hopefully the grocery store looks like a whole new place for you. Is your Dream Book full yet? Where did you put your Treasure Map? Remember, these are not toys ... they're tools that can help you dig up and polish the diamonds right under your feet.

Week 8
1) Weigh and measure yourself and write down your figures.
2) Sit down with your Personal Journal and review your progress.
3) Focus on the positive things that you've accomplished. If you're losing weight, GREAT! If not, why not? You should have some clues into your attitudes, behaviors, eating and exercise habits by this point. Identify your personal "weasels". (See Chapter 37 "Accelerated Plan".)

4) If you're encountering specific problems, review the materials that cover those areas. Work at improving your behaviors so they work for you and not against you. (See Chapter 13 "Troubleshooting Guide").

5) Commit to long-term success. Put it in writing! Gradual changes will lead you to positive results.

6) Write to us with any comments or questions that you have. We want to know how you're doing, and we want to help you in any way that we can.

7 Give yourself a nice, big reinforcing reward!

8 Review your progress with your support person and celebrate your success!

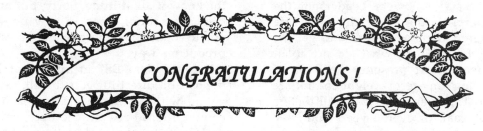

CONGRATULATIONS !

After 8 weeks on the THINNER WINNERS Start-up Plan you have accomplished the following:

1) You've learned the nutritional importance and weight control significance of eating less fat, less sodium and less sugar. And you've learned that even without these diet and health hazards you can still eat pretty darn well.

2) You've learned the importance of eating more fiber and drinking more water.

3) You've learned how to convert some of your favorite recipes into healthier versions.

4) You've become aware of the extensive variety of healthful foods and low and non-fat substitutes that are available in the supermarket.

5) You've learned how to enjoy eating away from home without jeopardizing the effectiveness of your weight control plans.

6) You've become aware of the importance of exercise and have made the crucial step of incorporating activity into your life.

7) You're exercising, at the minimum level recommended by the American Heart Association.

8) You've learned a lot more about how your mind and thought processes function ... and the fact that your thoughts and emotions are under your own control.

9) You've learned about powerful motivational techniques such as goal setting, Dream Books, Treasure Maps, Visualizations and Affirmations.

10) You've learned about the attitudes of winners and why positive attitudes are critical to success in any endeavor.

11) You've learned how to breathe properly and meditate, and in doing so you've gained insight into your personal energy source and reduced stress in your life.

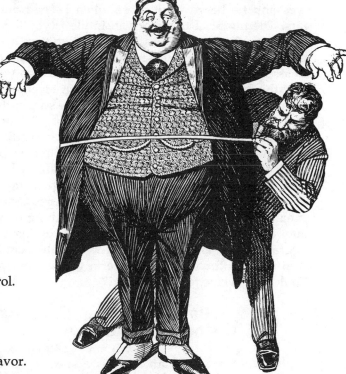

Losing inches is quite the joyous event!

12) You've learned about the importance of rewards and reinforcement.

13) You've increased your confidence and self-esteem. You know that you've done something great for yourself.

14) You have no doubt lost some weight and inches! And you know why.

When you feel confident that you have learned the basic principles of the THINNER WINNERS program and you can consistently apply them to your life, it's time to do just that. Now you've got a stable framework to build upon. Use this program as a reference and resource as you develop and fine-tune your own personalized program.

Reaching peak potential in any field rarely comes to those who stay followers. Leaders are the people who accomplish the great things in life through knowledge and perseverance and get the rewards and glory for it. That's what you are about to become ... a leader. At present, the odds of successfully achieving long-term weight control are greater than 20 to 1. Fewer than 5% of all dieters are able to stay at goal for even a year. You have the opportunity to enter the winner's circle.

Maybe you've seen this classic comedy routine in one form or another: "Missing! One old dog. Blind in one eye. One ear chewed off. Only has three legs. Answers to the name of Lucky". Old Lucky obviously wasn't so lucky. If that old dog could talk he'd probably tell you that he stumbles and falls a lot on only three legs, he could see a lot more with two eyes and he heard a lot more when he had both ears. The moral of this story is simple ... you'll get the best weight control results if you keep your eyes and ears open to all four sections of this program to create a balance instead of just the one or two you may think you need. All the concepts fit together in such a way as to create more than just the sum of the individual parts. The total synergy of the four sections creates another level of understanding about how they work and can propel you to the next level of mastery of this challenge you are facing. Like a great marriage, the relationship is more than Howard and Roseanne. It is a merging and enhancing of all we both are into something more than each of us is separately. That's a key insight to grasp if you are to go beyond 95% of the people who attempt the goal of long term weight control. Could it be a clue to "The Secret"?

Same old stuff ...
I've heard it all before

In the Start-Up Plan there is a specific set of guidelines that you're asked to follow. Now I know that realistically people are going to make their own way through the program. They'll say, "Oh, I want to see what she says about eating fat". And they'll turn to the chapter on "Fat and Cholesterol". Keep in mind the concept of "beginners luck". Very often beginners are "lucky", which means successful, simply because they don't "know it all". They're hopeful, optimistic and trusting, so they follow the directions and it works

for them. While you may feel yourself to be an "experienced dieter", something obviously has been missing from your approach in the past ... otherwise you wouldn't have felt the need to purchase this book. You may believe you know it all already ... but somehow you've left out critical pieces of knowledge or action. This has held you back from the success you're looking for. The solution is to lose the know-it-all attitude. Sorry, but nobody knows it "all". Remaining open to new possibilities allows you to continue learning in an unbiased, flexible and productive way.

If this "no BS" attitude that I'm conveying seems a bit direct for you ... well, that's because I'm trying with all my heart to reach you where it counts. Right between the eyes, smack dab in the middle of your brain. I never cease to be amazed at how many good people I meet who "sincerely" want to lose weight, know as much about nutrition as a registered dietitian, as much about exercise as the average pro coach and still just can't seem to motivate themselves off that squishy old couch.

What THINNER WINNERS is really all about is change. Anyone who expects their life to change for the better while they keep on doing the same old things is missing the point and deluding themselves. This is not an insult ... it's a wake up call. If you mix flour, milk and eggs together and cook it on a griddle ... you get pancakes. Every time. You never get lasagna. If you want to get positive, long-term weight control results you will have to change what you've been putting into it. It's that simple. So far you've gotten temporary results at best. Begin to change what you think, do and believe with the help of THINNER WINNERS and you can get the result of permanent weight control instead. Change is hard, yes. But so is living with an overweight body. (Harder than a microwaved bagel left out on the counter overnight!) Do you see this?

Realize that there is more to controlling your weight than what you already "know". If you think about it, you'll realize your knowledge and perceptions are colored by your past experiences. They are biased as a result. You may be holding yourself back from achieving your goal of being thin even though you "know" a lot about the process. Your flexibility tends to become more limited if efforts you've made in the past did not succeed. Without positive results it's possible to lose sight of hope, and to shorten your horizons. This form of discouragement can feed upon itself, and it's hard to maintain a positive outlook in the face of "failure". But you have not failed. You have simply taken more of the necessary steps towards success. Open yourself to the possibility of taking another direction. This doesn't mean you're wrong or have done anything less than your very best. After all, your efforts have lead you right here, where you are right now entertaining the thought of an even broader perspective. You're on the right track.

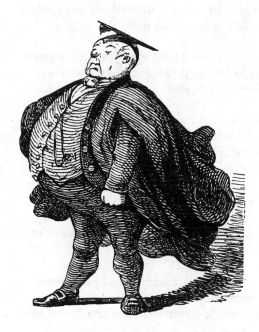

"I have a degree in Dietology, of course, but I'm a special case you see ..."

This is certainly not to demean anything that you've done so far. It's all good work. You've built part of your dream castle already and I congratulate you! Now use the tools outlined in the THINNER WINNERS program to learn how to put on the roof, wire up the lights and raise the banners to fly high on the turrets!

The real winners, those 5% who ultimately get to their goal weight and stay there, will remain open to even more ways to solve their weight problem once and for all, because they realize there

is always more to learn. Believe me, your solution exists. It just takes a little more than you have learned already. Not to worry though! The answers are here and they are learnable and available to you right now! Maybe it's time for you to go back to the drawing board. And so: I strongly recommend that you set aside your all-knowing, "this is old hat" attitude, acknowledge that you haven't had complete success in the past, and put yourself through the Start-Up Plan gladly and eagerly searching for even more answers. I say this in the most loving way possible. Your goal is to successfully and permanently control your weight and to improve your health. The goal of THINNER WINNERS is to help you accomplish those specific objectives. We're on the same team, and we have the same goal.

Leaving the Nest

What follows is going to take some real courage on your part. Having watched a lot of young birds hatch and grow over the years, I know that leaving the nest can be terrifying. I also know that unless a young bird reaches that decision, and takes that big jump, it will usually die. Making a real commitment to long-term weight control is like leaving the nest. And that's what I'm asking you to do.

Below you'll find a commitment contract that you need to copy and sign. It's a commitment to yourself. By signing this commitment you're putting in writing the fact that you care enough about yourself to make some real efforts to improve your life. When you fulfill the commitment you will get positive results. Please note however that like any contract, if you don't like the way it's worded you're welcome to make changes ... cross out what you don't like and write in what works for you. But whatever you do, make the commitment and then stick to it!

THINNER WINNERS Lifetime Weight Control Commitment

I am embarking on a self-improvement adventure. In the process of my journey I will transform myself both physically and mentally. My old, unhealthy habits will be left behind.

I will learn many new skills and the reasons for their importance. I will apply what I learn in a positive, optimistic manner. When I reach my goal weight I will have developed the lifestyle changes necessary to maintain my new, improved levels of health ... and I will continue to use my new skills.

I commit to following the THINNER WINNERS Weight Control Program for at least the next six months. I understand that long-term weight control means developing a true long-term perspective. I will read the entire text at least two times.

I will diligently employ the techniques described in the THINNER WINNERS program to improve my attitude towards myself. I will pursue the goal of loving self-acceptance. Self-acceptance will lead to peace of mind and increased happiness in my life. I can't change the past, but I can make better choices starting now for a better future.

I will honestly monitor my thoughts and behaviors regarding food, exercise and health so that I can gain the insights I need to improve my lifestyle. I will increase positive health behaviors in my life. My overall goal is to improve my health and, in the process, learn to control my weight. I will learn to eat a health-promoting diet. I will drink 8 glasses of water every day.

I am committed to exercising, healthy eating and developing a healthy attitude. I will participate in physical exercise at the minimum recommended levels or beyond. My body is my vehicle in this life and I will maintain it at the highest levels of which I am capable. I commit to adding muscle for increasing my metabolic rate.

I will make no excuses. I will do it! I know that unless I improve my attitude and the way I think I risk reverting back to non-productive habits. So I will guard my attitude as if it were the most valuable thing that I have in life ... which it is! I commit to becoming a healthier, happier and more aware person who is optimistic about what life is and what is to come. I will paint my life as a great masterpiece.

I am taking the steps listed above to improve my health, improve my attitude and to lose excess weight. I am the one who is responsible for following the steps contained in the THINNER WINNERS program. I am the one who must do the necessary work. I will do the work!

_____   Your Name, Date   _____

Before you do another thing, make a copy of the above contract. Then sign and date it.

Self-Assessment

4

"Here's looking at you, kid."
Humphrey Bogart

Looking at Yourself from the Inside Out

All of the world's successful expeditions begin with one thing in common ... preparation! Thinking about your challenges before you meet them face to face, and evaluating your strengths to meet those challenges is the mark of a true winner. If you want to make this journey successful it's a good idea to first find out what resources you have, and what skills you may still need. With intelligent preparation you'll reach your goal safe and sound, and you'll enjoy the trip a whole lot more along the way. You won't waste a lot of energy floundering about without any focus.

Changing the way that you eat, act and think sends many weight loss "wannabees" back to a soft couch with a sack of chips. That's why many dieters never experience the joys of being at goal ... and fewer still know the joys of multi-year success. If you haven't been able to get a handle on your weight before now it might be because you weren't sure what it really would take to get you there, or you may have lacked the willingness to do the things you did know about. That's like the pioneer who headed west with nothing more than his favorite old horse, a few days worth of supplies and his fingers crossed. It's important for you to have a realistic understanding of your strengths and your needs. Then you can focus on developing those skills that will help you the most. You'll be able to get there more easily, without all the molehills becoming mountains.

As you know by now, THINNER WINNERS is a balanced program with four pillars ... attitudes, behavior, exercise and nutrition. I know from experience that you will need adequate knowledge and skills in all four areas to be able to reach, and certainly to maintain, your goal weight. This chapter contains assessment exercises to help you better understand what you already know and identify what you still need to learn in each of the four areas. In order to do this:

1. First, take the **100 question (true/false) survey** to test your general knowledge about attitudes, behavior, exercise and nutrition. Your scores from this survey will then be used to determine your current balance of skills in the four areas on a pie-chart. The chart will show you which areas you should emphasize to improve your balance in the four areas as you work through the program.

2. Second, complete the **Personal Health and Weight History** questionnaire designed to give you a real sense of your attitudes and behavior patterns in terms of your weight. In order to succeed at this noteworthy weight control project you have to really understand your motivations and the obstacles you need to overcome. Think carefully about your answers and you will gain valuable insight into your personal bugaboos needing attention. Do this exercise with your support person, or review it with them later.

3. Third, complete the **Nutritional Assessment**. You're going to take a good close look at what you're eating ... and how it may be affecting your weight and your health. You may be surprised.

4. Fourth, you are going to put it all together and clearly **identify your strengths, your needs and your goals**. This information will all be used to help clarify your weight control issues and help you get to your goal smoothly and steadily. It will reveal the stumbling blocks that may have held you back previously, so you can focus on strengthening them.

100 Things You Need to Know

One of the factors that makes THINNER WINNERS unique is the balanced approach used to cover all four essential areas of weight control: Attitude, Behavior, Exercise and Nutrition. In order to help you get a sense of how your personal weight control style is presently balanced in the four areas, take the following simple test ...

There are 100 true/false questions, 25 from each area. The idea is to help you get a sense of your strengths and needs. Ideally you will have a balanced set of quadrants on the pie chart (later in this chapter). Realistically, you'll probably have some areas that are much stronger than others. The answers are found at the end of the 100 questions.

Attitudes

1) Expecting to succeed will improve your chances at weight control.
2) What you think about expands and grows in your life.
3) If you do what successful people do you can learn to become successful too.
4) You don't need a strategy to succeed, you only need a dream and guts.
5) Persistence is an obnoxious quality that only annoying sales people have.
6) You should avoid dieting mistakes at all costs ... they mean you have failed.
7) Goals are like daydreams.
8) You can retrain your mind by changing your mental pictures.
9) All winners visualize themselves winning in advance.
10) You can create your future by choosing thoughts that picture the future you want.
11) Goals should have deadlines for accomplishment.
12) Ninety-five percent of Americans regularly set goals.
13) Both good and bad habits get stronger with practice.
14) Anybody who admits to talking to themselves is crazy.
15) An Affirmation is a legal contract.
16) If you think you can, or think you can't, you're right since thoughts come before results.
17) You are responsible for your own health, behavior and well-being.
18) Self-Love is vanity.
19) Only new-agers, mystics and kooks practice meditation.
20) Meditation takes special equipment and usually lasts all day.
21) Meditation can heal old pain by putting you in touch with "The Force".
22) Weight control has nothing to do with self-awareness, only food intake and exercise.
23) Denying that you're fat is an effective weight loss technique.
24) It's impossible to find your own solutions to weight control because it's too complicated.
25) A Personal Journal reveals issues over time that you might just forget if you didn't write them down.

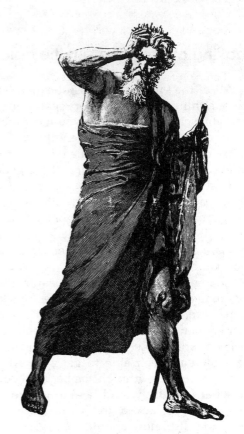

"Hmmm ... I thought I knew that!"

Behavior Changes

26) Learning to handle your stress without overeating is a habit and a skill.
27) It's possible to live a stress-free life.
28) Tickling is a way to reduce negative stress because it makes you laugh.
29) Making funny faces can help you control your fears.
30) Childhood memories connected to certain foods are bad, and you should try to erase them.
31) To stop the craving for fatty food you should eat vegetables and fruit or drink water.
32) You can never eat bad foods like chocolate or pizza on a true long-term weight control program.
33) When you're really hungry, eating is the only thing you should do.
34) Don't share your weight loss plan with anyone. Then, if you fail, no one can make you feel bad.
35) Never join a weight loss group when you're doing your own plan at home.
36) You don't really need to do anything to lose weight but eat less fat and exercise more.
37) Never buy new clothes when you're overweight. Wait until you're at your goal.
38) The only reward that works is money.

39) The better you feel about the way you look, the easier it is to treat yourself with respect by making healthy choices during the day.
40) You should never reward yourself more than once a week.
41) Every step of your weight control program should have a predetermined reward.
42) You should save up your rewards until you reach your goal.
43) For a reward to work it should cost at least $20.
44) For rewards to be most effective they should have special meaning for you.
45) Long-term weight control means never having to weigh yourself again. Only fat percentage is valid.
46) The faster you lose weight the more likely it is to stay off because you will stay motivated.
47) If your weight loss hits a plateau it means that your set point has been reached.
48) Ten to twelve pounds a month is a reasonable weight loss expectation.
49) It is possible for you to determine your personal weight loss pattern by charting your weight weekly.
50) Women should be about 22% body fat and men about 15%.

Exercise

51) Your metabolism slows as you get older because you lose muscle if you don't build it up by exercise, especially by lifting weights.
52) You lose $1/2$ pound of muscle and gain $1^{1/2}$ pounds of fat every year after age 25.
53) You can get in all your exercise for the week in one long day, or on the weekend if you are pressed for time.
54) Regular exercise can reduce the risk of heart disease and depression.
55) Muscle is active tissue that burns calories, whereas fat is inactive.
56) "Aerobic" means "with oxygen". This means you will breathe more heavily while doing aerobic exercise.
57) Lifting weights gives women big, bulky muscles, so they should avoid it in order to appear slender.
58) You should reward yourself for exercising.
59) You have to exercise for at least an hour to do any real good.
60) Our cave dwelling ancestors rarely walked so it's natural to be a "sofa spud".
61) To determine your aerobic level, double your resting pulse rate.
62) A warm-up, cool-down and stretching are critical even if you choose walking as your exercise because lactic acid builds up in your muscles after any exercise.
63) If you sweat a lot, you may be exercising too hard.
64) If you work out at 80% of your maximum pulse, you will burn fat faster.
65) While exercising, all movements should be crisp and precise.
66) Running or jogging is the best exercise for losing weight.
67) Light weights and lots of repetitions will trim and tone muscles.
68) Heavy weights and a few repetitions will build muscle size fastest.
69) Always doing the same exercise insures balanced muscle development.
70) "No pain, no gain" means exercise should hurt to be effective; push yourself until you feel the burn.
71) Some exercises cause sleep disorders.
72) Thin people are more fidgety and active than fat people.
73) A 10 minute walk to the mailbox doesn't do much good to burn fat.
74) You should try to keep your physical activities, like walking, from interfering with your family obligations which are more important than just you.
75) Playing with your kids on the beach doesn't count as real exercise.

Nutrition

76) It's possible to stuff yourself with food and still be starving for nutrients.
77) Processed food with added supplements is just as good for you as whole foods.
78) Most of the 12 zillion cereals in the market are really good for you because they are mostly grains and therefore complex carbohydrates.
79) The more protein you can eat, the stronger and healthier you will be.
80) You need to eat dairy products to get vitamin D and calcium.
81) One tablespoon of fat is one serving.
82) You should drink as much water as you possibly can every day.
83) It's good to fry your food because it kills germs and seals in juices.
84) During your weight loss phase you should plan and eat 3 meals a day, plus a snack.

85) It's okay to go as long as 8 hours without eating to save calories.
86) It's okay to skip breakfast as long as you have a big dinner.
87) Margarine has less calories and fat than butter.
88) The average American eats 120 pounds of sugar a year. In 1900 it was 35 pounds.
89) Mistakes that many fat people make are shopping without a list and going up and down all the grocery store aisles.
90) Half of all the deaths in the U.S. are caused by coronary artery disease related to diet.
91) The average American diet is now 42% fat ... mostly saturated or hydrogenated.
92) LDL cholesterol stands for Lighter Dietary Lipoprotein ... it's the good kind.
93) There are 9 calories in one gram of fat.
94) You should try to eat as much fiber as possible every day.
95) A high sodium diet can cause you to retain large amounts of water and can elevate your blood pressure.
96) A safe guideline for sodium is to have 1 mg for every calorie you eat.
97) Restaurants and food manufacturers add salt to food because the government mandates it as a nutritional supplement.
98) Our bodies only need about 220 milligrams of sodium daily to be healthy.
99) One out of every four Americans has high blood pressure.
100) To lose excess water from your body you must stop drinking extra water.

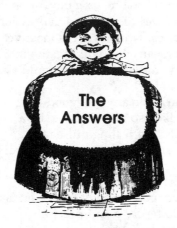

The
Answers

Okay, now it's time to find out what you know. I'm sure you noticed that these weren't real hard technical questions ... just a tad tricky, that's all. The answers are listed under the sections where you'll find the information. All you have to do is count the number of correct answers you got in each section. When you're done, turn to the pie chart later in this chapter.

Attitudes

1) T	2) T	3) T	4) F	5) F	6) F	7) F	8) T	9) T	10) T
11) T	12) F	13) T	14) F	15) F	16) T	17) T	18) F	19) F	20) F
21) T	22) F	23) F	24) F	25) T					

Behaviors

26) T	27) F	28) T	29) T	30) F	31) F	32) F	33) T	34) F	35) F
36) F	37) F	38) F	39) T	40) F	41) T	42) F	43) F	44) T	45) F
46) F	47) F	48) F	49) T	50) T					

Exercise

51) T	52) F	53) F	54) T	55) T	56) T	57) F	58) T	59) F	60) F
61) F	62) T	63) T	64) F	65) F	66) F	67) T	68) T	69) F	70) F
71) F	72) T	73) F	74) F	75) F					

Nutrition

76) T	77) F	78) F	79) F	80) F	81) F	82) F	83) F	84) T	85) F
86) F	87) F	88) T	89) T	90) T	91) T	92) F	93) T	94) F	95) T
96) T	97) F	98) T	99) T	100) F					

Your Personal Health and Weight History

This self-evaluation Health and Weight History questionnaire is designed specifically to help you "see the light" ... and gain insight into your personal attitudes and behavior patterns regarding your weight. Answer the questions as honestly as you can. In addition to helping you gain awareness about your general health the questions are separated into the four THINNER WINNERS program categories so you'll know where to look for a higher watt bulb ... the better to see your enlightenment by.

To maximize the value of this information, I'm going to ask you to do something that will take guts and a really good attitude. Share your responses with your support person (see Chapter 16 "Creating a Powerful Support System"). It's very important that you trust your supporter and feel that they have your best interest at heart. In other words, that they love you and sincerely want to help you gain insight. And that they are not out to merely criticize you, but to help you grow. Explain to them that this is not a need-to-change session. It's a shared exploration that could give you new insights and direction in order to break the grip that being overweight has on you. What they say is not necessarily "right", but at least consider their comments before deciding that. Discuss your answers thoroughly with them. Let them ask questions to clarify what your answers mean and keep an open mind. Sometimes it's amazing how clear your needs are to others. You can learn a lot by making an effort to listen carefully. If they point out things that you don't see or agree with, it doesn't mean you're "bad" or "wrong". It just means that they might see certain aspects of your personality that you may be too close to emotionally to see objectively. They can offer helpful options that you may not have considered. Yes, this can be really tough to do, but it can also be an opportunity to let another person in, open your heart and begin the healing process. The more you allow yourself to learn from the feedback, the faster you will be able to solve the weight problems you have been experiencing. So let go and trust yourself to focus on your needs. Write the answers in your workbook or Personal Journal.

Your General Health

1) How would you describe your general health?
2) Are you under a physicians care?
3) Do you have any specific health problems?
4) What is your average blood pressure?
5) What is your cholesterol reading?   HDL   LDL   HDL/LDL Ratio
6) What is your blood sugar?
7) Are you taking any medications?   What specific problems?
8) Do you take any vitamins or supplements?   Which ones and why?
9) Are you allergic to anything? (including food allergies)
10) Do you smoke?   How much and for how long?
11) Do you drink alcohol?   How much?   How often?
12) Do you drink coffee, tea, or soda?   How much?
13) Are you pregnant or lactating?
14) Do you take birth control pills?

Attitudes and Personal Development

15) Rate your ability to successfully control and maintain your weight over the last 5 years.
        Poor   -   Fair   -   Good
16) Do you expect to be successful on this weight control program?
17) Why or why not?
18) Did you stop going to other weight loss programs? Which ones? Why didn't they work?
19) What is your motivation for using the THINNER WINNERS program?
20) Why do you think you are overweight?
21) How motivated are you to lose your excess weight? (Not Very -- I'll try it -- I'm very motivated!)
22) Who do you feel is responsible for your being overweight? (Your mother? Your spouse? Your friends? Your job? You?)
23) Have you ever lost weight successfully and in a healthy manner?
24) How did you do it?
25) Why did you do it?
26) Does your family want you to lose weight?

27) Why? / Why not?
28) What is your"self talk" (or internal dialogue) regarding your weight?
29) What did you say to yourself at your last weigh-in?
30) Are you honest with yourself regarding your weight?
31) When did you first become overweight?
32) Why?
33) What do you think makes up a successful weight control program?
34) How long do you think it will take to get to your desired weight?
35) Do you ever "see" yourself as thin?
36) Who is responsible for your successful weight control?
37) Is being overweight your #1 problem?
38) Would you do anything to be thin?
39) What changes are you willing to make to become thin?
       (Exercise regularly? Give up your very favorite food?)
40) I want to lose weight, but I am unwilling to:
41) Answer the following question: Sally Forth has finally decided that she wants to get thin for good!
       If she really wants to lose weight and keep it off forever, what should she do?

Behavior Changes

42) What weight loss programs or techniques have you used before?
43) How much weight did you lose?/ For how long?
44) What is your goal weight?
45) Why?
46) Have you ever reached your goal weight?
47) How long have you successfully maintained a goal weight in the past?
48) What is the lowest weight you have maintained for at least one full year as an adult during the last
       ten years?
49) How did you most successfully control your weight?
50) Are any other members of your family overweight?
51) Why?
52) Do you become uncomfortable if you miss a meal?
53) How uncomfortable? Physical or emotional discomfort?
54) Do you plan your meals in advance or eat impulsively?
55) What times of day do you usually eat?
56) Do you eat at regular meal times or do your meal times vary?
57) Does your family eat meals together?
58) Who cooks?
59) If you cook, do you cook for them by request, or do they eat what you serve?
60) How would they feel about trying healthier versions of their favorite foods if it helped you with
       your weight?
61) Do you ever binge?
62) When was the last time you had an eating binge?
63) How long did the binge last?
64) What did you eat during the binge?
65) What triggered the binge? (lonely, bored, angry, stressed, hidden food, etc.?)
66) How did you stop the binge?
67) How often do you weigh yourself?
68) How often do you take your measurements? When was the last time?

Activity and Exercise

69) What physical activities do you enjoy?
70) What physical activities do you participate in?
71) Do you ever sweat during your exercise?
72) Do you consider yourself active and healthy?
73) Do other members of your family have an exercise program?

74) Do you (or can you) exercise together?
75) How often do you think you'll need to exercise to maintain your weight loss and stay healthy?
76) Are you willing to commit to weight control for the rest of your life?
77) Why or why not?

Nutrition and Food

78) Do you use a shopping list?
79) Do you read the labels on the foods you buy?
80) If you read labels, what do you look for?
81) What foods do the other members of your family like ?
82) How often do you eat in restaurants?
83) What type of restaurants?
84) When you eat out do you take steps to eat healthier or do you "go along" with the crowd and eat whatever is served?
85) How often do you eat "fast food"?
86) What foods do you like?
87) What foods do you love?
88) What foods do you crave?
89) Do you know how many calories you eat on an average day?
90) Do you know how many grams of fat you eat on an average day?
91) What is your "style" of eating? (nibbler, 3 meals, night eater, etc.)
**) Any other questions that you feel are significant regarding your health and weight.

Now you should have a clearer picture of who you really are in terms of your relationship with your health and weight. You have a better sense of some of your strengths and needs in terms of weight control. Hopefully there's a big light bulb shining over your head right now because of all the insights you're getting. Good work! I know this was tough and I really admire your courage.

Use this information about yourself to complete the Needs and Strengths section of Your Personal Profile at the end of this chapter.

Nutritional Assessment

Now for the real fun. The third self-assessment tool that you will complete is your Nutritional Assessment. You're going to write down everything you ate in the last three days and then find out what you're putting into that body of yours. In this way you'll see where you need to start making some changes.

This will take a bit of effort on your part, but your food analysis may well prove to be the most enlightening thing you've done in a long time. Many of my clients tell me that they really understand all about nutrition and food. They've read lots of books and know that they're supposed to watch their fats and should try to eat less of it among other things. But when they actually look at what they've been eating, boy, are they ever surprised!

Let me tell you a little story. I used to have a serious problem with water retention. For those of you who aren't familiar with this particular inconvenience it means that from time to time I would start swelling up like a water balloon. From my head to my toes. My eyes would disappear in a bloated face and my calves and ankles would swell up to twice their usual size. Even my shoes would get tight because my feet swelled up. When this happened I always felt like the proverbial "lead balloon". I would have to stop what I was doing and put my feet up or lie down to ease the swelling and throbbing. I never wore skirts just in case this happened during the day.

I had this problem for many years. But now that I have an understanding of the nutritional components of food I know that I was eating way too much salty food and causing my cells to retain water (I was very partial to eating potato chips by the bag). I also know that to get rid of excess salt and eliminate water retention it's necessary to flush out my body with ... that's right, lots and lots of water. Once I learned how this process works I reduced my sodium intake, increased my water and I haven't had any water retention in over eight years. This is just one simple example of how what you eat can directly affect the way you look and feel. Nutrition is vitally important for your health, as you will learn in the Nutrition and Food section of the program. So take this Nutritional Evaluation seriously! Don't cheat. You'll just be cheating yourself.

Write down everything (yes, everything!) you ate today, yesterday and the day before in your workbook or journal. The reason I chose those three days is very simple. Most people can't remember much further back than that with any accuracy. And if I had asked you to do it for the next three days, there would be a tendency to "be good", and the figures just would not reflect what you normally consume. If one of the last three days was really unusual for you (or you just can't remember), substitute a typical day's food instead. The object here is for you to get a clear idea of your average intake.

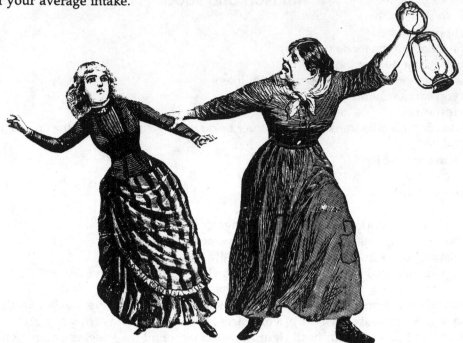

"Come on, it's time for your Nutritional Assessment!"

Now get out your "food analysis handbook" and look up all the figures on what you ate. That's right ... protein grams, carbohydrate grams, fat grams, number of calories, fiber grams and milligrams of sodium. Record the foods you ate and the nutritional breakdowns for each item. Make up a chart similar to the format below. After you have done that for the three days, continue reading to learn how to calculate your nutritional percentage for each category of food.

Nutritional Assessment Format

	Protein	Carbohydrates	Fat	Calories	Fiber	Sodium
Breakfast						
Lunch						
Dinner						
Snacks						
Totals	grams	grams	grams	calories	grams	milligrams

Calculating Your Nutritional Percentages
(how much fat, protein & carbs you're eating simplified for math phobics)

The average American now consumes 42% fat in their daily diet ... and the average American is fat! If you're planning on losing weight you've got to get your daily intake of fat down to 10%-20% and the other components of your food intake such as carbohydrates and protein to fit within healthy guidelines. So how can you do that? Let's start with the ideal percentages which are 65-75% carbohydrates, 15-20% protein and 10-20% fat (and not more than ⅓ of that as saturated or hydrogenated fat). Of course these are general guidelines and can change for individuals with different needs. For example, athletes may need more carbohydrates for fuel or protein to replace muscle break-down and those needing to lose fat will need the low end of the range of fat. That's you. Don't make the mistake of replacing your fat with protein, however. You'd do better to have a higher carbohydrate percentage instead and keep your protein in the lower range also. I now eat high carbs, low protein and fat percentages.

Here is a simple formula (relatively) for figuring out your total nutritional percentages (information that you definitely want to know):

To calculate your own percentages you need to know just three things:

1) The **number of calories in each gram of food**
(Stay with me now. You can do this!)

Protein	= 4 calories per gram
Carbohydrate	= 4 calories per gram
Fat	= 9 calories per gram
Alcohol	= 7 calories per gram

2) The **total number of grams of each type of food**
you ate (protein, carbohydrate, fat).
These are the totals you looked up and recorded on your Nutritional Assessment so you've already done that. Check.

3) The **total number of calories you ate for the day**.
You have that, too. See? Simple.

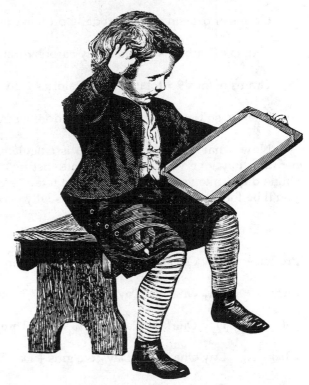

"How many calories in a gram of fat?"

Now let's use Pete Sake's totals as an example to find out what percentage of protein he ate today:

Totals = 90 g   195 g   31 g   1411 cals   16g   2800 mg
        PRO   CARB FAT   CALS   FIBER SODIUM

Pete ate 90 grams of protein. He knows that each gram of protein has 4 calories, right? So he multiplies 90 X 4 = 360 total calories from protein. Next he divides that 360 by 1411 total calories eaten for the day to get the percentage of protein he ate for this day:

360/1411 = 25% (you can round off to the nearest whole number). So Pete ate 25% protein today.

That's the formula. Divide your total calories in each food category by your total calories for the day. Simple, right? Now let's do the same thing to see what percentage of carbs and fat he ate:

Pete ate 195 grams of carbohydrates:195 X 4 = 780/ 1411 = 55%   Pete ate 55% carbohydrates today.

Pete ate 31 grams of fat: 31 X 9 = 279 total fat calories. 279/ 1411 = 20%   Pete ate 20% fat today.

Pete's totals are 25% protein, 55% carbohydrate and 20% fat.

The three categories should total 100% or pretty darn close. Compare his totals with the "ideal range" of 15-20% protein, 65-75% carbohydrate and 10-20% fat. Pete can stand to make some slight adjustments in his food balance (a little less protein and fat, a little more carbs), but all together he's doing pretty well.

Your Food Journal Analysis

Now let's calculate your nutritional percentages just like we did for Pete Sake on the previous page. First, write down your totals for each day on the top line of the Nutritional Assessment chart you made in your workbook. Then follow the instructions to get your percentages. You'll probably find a pocket calculator useful.

Day One Totals   gm   gm   gm   mg   gm   cal   cups
                  Pro   Carbs   Fat   Sodium   Fiber   Calories   Water

Grams of protein x 4 = total daily protein calories / divided by your total daily calories   = % protein

Grams of carbs x 4 = total daily carbohydrate calories / divided by your total daily calories = % carbs

Grams of fat x 9 = total daily fat calories / divided by your total calories   = % fat

That wasn't so hard, was it? Now do the same thing for the other two days.

Now what you're going to do is calculate your three day percentage averages. Averages are valuable because they give you a more accurate picture of your general eating lifestyle than you can get by looking at a single day. Take your daily percentage totals in each category of food, add them together and divide by 3. Then you'll be looking at the averages you usually eat.

Three Day Averages:

Protein -   Day One % + Day Two % + Day Three % = 3 day total   / divided by 3 = ave. daily pro %

Carbs -   Day One % + Day Two % + Day Three % = 3 day total   / divided by 3 = ave. daily carb %

Fat -   Day One % + Day Two % + Day Three % = 3 day total   / divided by 3 = ave. daily fat %

Fiber -   Day One gms + Day Two gms + Day Three gms = 3 day total   / divided by 3 = average daily gms

Sodium -   Day One mg + Day Two mg + Day Three mg = 3 day total   / divided by 3 = average daily mg

Calories -   Day One total + Day Two total + Day Three total = 3 day total / divided by 3 = ave. daily cals

Water -   Day One total + Day Two total + Day Three total = 3 day total / divided by 3 = average daily cups
(8 ounce cup)

Are you surprised? Most people are when they find out how much fat and protein they are eating on a regular basis. No matter what your averages are, if you have been honest, they are what have gotten you into the shape you are presently in. Changing your percentages by applying the principles you will learn in the THINNER WINNERS program will help move you towards your goals of improved health and weight loss.

The number of total calories you should eat is affected by many variables (including your sex, weight, exercise level and whether you're trying to lose or maintain your weight). Number of calories is really not as vital as the type of calories you eat. However, this is not a free ticket to eat as much as you can hold, contrary to recent dietary sensationalisms. Sorry, but calories still do count, just not quite as much as previously believed. Since fat has over twice as many calories as either carbs or protein, when you cut back on it, you can eat more carbs and protein and still stay within a certain calorie range. That should be your goal. Change the types of foods you are eating first, then you can adjust the calories if you need to in order to lose weight.

You should try to eat 25-35 grams of fiber every day (see Chapter 33 "Fiber is Your Friend" for full details), keep your sodium intake to about one milligram for every calorie you eat (see Chapter 34 "Sodium and Salt vs.

Herbs and Spices"), especially if water retention or high blood pressure are a problem for you, and drink at least 8 glasses of water every day (see Chapter 35 "Water — The Magic Potion").

I know this will take a bit of effort, but it's time for you to smarten up about your health, and this is a critical step in pointing out where your trouble spots are, and most importantly, just how far out of line you've been. That way you'll see just exactly what you have to do to correct the situation and start concentrating on how to get to your clearly pictured goals.

Do a food analysis again in 6 months and I'm sure you will have a very pleasant surprise in store!

Your Personal Profile

Now we're getting down to it! You've completed all three of your self-assessments and it's time to put them to work. Refer back to your scores on the true/false test, the answers you gave on your Personal Health and Weight History and your Nutritional Assessment. This profile is the place where you get to make some conclusions on what you have learned about yourself. Then you'll design a Personal Program for yourself that really targets your special areas to work on and recognizes your strong points, too.

#1 - Your Strengths and Needs

You have a number of strengths that are your resource base. You also have some definite needs. Your needs are what have held you back in the past ... so consider them carefully and honestly. List all your major strengths and needs that you've identified with the three assessment tools. This is a good time to ask your support person for some input.

Strengths
List at least 10 skills and strengths that you already have and can readily use in your weight control efforts. Then rate them according to their usefulness to you. An example of a skill: you already check food labels because you know that when you eat too much sodium you retain water and your blood pressure goes up.

Needs
List at least 10 problem areas that you know you really need to work on in order to make weight control progress. Pick out the trouble spots that you feel will be to your highest benefit to deal with first and get started. An example of a need: whenever the subject of weight loss comes up, you have at least three ready excuses for being overweight that you've been using for so long that you almost believe them. What you need are solutions, not excuses.

#2 - The Pie Chart

The pie chart is a way for you to visualize the balance of your overall knowledge regarding your health and weight. Use the sample pie chart on the next page as your guide. The center of the chart is zero and where the lines meet the circle is 25. Put a dot in each quarter of the pie where your score on the true/false test is for that area. Then connect the dots so that you create a box shape. This box is a representation of your current weight control skills. The bigger the box, the more skills you have. If your box is a perfect square, with the corners at the edge of the circle, you're an ace. Chances are, however, that you've got some work left to do. That's okay. That's what this program is for. Now turn back to the answers for the true/false test and transfer your scores to the pie-chart in your workbook or one that you draw in your journal.

Obviously, this is only a reference tool to get you started. But at this point that's just what you need ... to see where you are and get started towards where you want to go!

Sample Chart

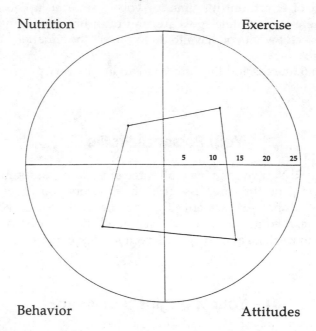

On the sample chart above the scores are: Nutrition=10, Exercise=13, Behavior=14, Attitudes=19

This person needs to focus first and foremost on their nutrition because that is their lowest score. The lower the score, the more work you need to create a balanced lifestyle. They shouldn't skip the other areas, but need to emphasize nutrition first.

Your Current Goals

Now you have a much better idea of what you need to improve and where you might have been overlooking some needs. Let's pinpoint them even further by setting specific goals.

Examples of measurable goals would be: changing the percentage of a certain type of food such as fats, exercising a certain amount of time and a certain number of times during the week or drinking a certain amount of water for the day.

Examples of a subjective goal would be: increasing your positive attitude with the use of affirmations, using a system of rewards for getting and staying motivated or building self-esteem by visualizing yourself being a total THINNER WINNER for 20 minutes each day.

Start with individual goals that will bring you the most personal satisfaction. Make sure you include a deadline for the completion of each goal item and a short strategy for getting there. Your goal might read: "I will reduce my daily fat intake to 15% by eating 20 grams of fat a day or less by (date) and keeping track on my Daily Success Planner". See Chapter 8 "Goal Setting and Treasure Maps" for further details and suggestions for making your goals super strong and mucho motivating.

Measurable Goals
List at least 5 in order of your personal priority.

Subjective Goals
List at least 5 in order of your personal priority.

The next step is to take your newly enlightened self and get started on your personal THINNER WINNERS weight control program by following the graduated Start-up Plan in Chapter 3. In order to stay in touch with your progress it's a good idea to refer back to these evaluations from time to time to see what kind of positive changes you're making. If you check back in six months or a year, I'll bet my last jelly-belly that you'll see a world of difference ... and that difference will show up in your mirror and on your scale, as well as in your doctor's office! Congratulations on a job well done!

In A Nutshell

1) Prepare for your journey of weight loss and maintenance by identifying your strengths and needs. This maximizes your success possibilities.

2) Three tools for doing this are:
    a) 100 question true/false survey
    b) Personal Health & Weight History questionnaire
    c) 3-day Nutritional Assessment

3) Discuss your findings about yourself with your support person to get another perspective and increase your insight.

4) Fill in your Personal Profile with the results of these three tools.

5) Write out your current goals (see Chapter 8 "Goal Setting and Treasure Maps" for more details).

6) Give yourself a big reward, plus a big hug, for all this work and take a day off. Whew!

Part II

Attitudes
and
Personal Development

Motivation and the Success Mindset   5

"Eureka!" (I've got it!)
Archimedes

You know you can lose weight when you make up your mind to do it. The big question is how do you go about making up your mind ... and then keeping it made up?

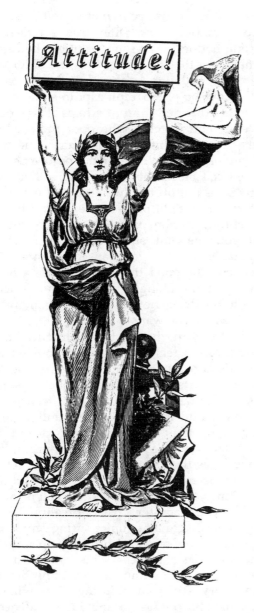

Let's take a look at how weight control winners get motivated and stay motivated by developing ...

The Success Mindset

Amazingly, according to the American Heart Association, more than 47 million Americans over the age of eighteen are 20% or more overweight, and therefore at risk for significant health problems. This is one-fourth of the entire U.S. adult population. To clarify the issue even further, this means that if you are a woman with a normal weight of 135 pounds, you would need to weigh 162 pounds before you even showed up in that 47 million figure. Estimates indicate that an additional large percentage, possibly another 20% of the population are between 10% and 20% overweight. That's nearly 100 million Americans, or half the adult population of the country, who are overweight by 10% or more!

On any given day there are 50 million people actively on diets, and over 95% of them fail in their efforts to keep off any weight that they may lose. That's nineteen out of twenty. Grim. But what about that magic 5%? What do these winners know that the rest of those dieters would give their last bagel to know?

I wanted to identify that knowledge and put it into practice. So, in order to become a "Thin", I studied this successful group to see what traits I needed to develop in order to be successful, too. What I found was there are specific attitudes common to people who have successfully taken charge of their weight and health.

This was great news! And it turned out that I even had a few of these attitudes already, and you probably do, too. So why was I still overweight? Because I failed to take the next essential step that winners take: systematically mastering all these attitudes thus developing a "success mindset" encompassing them. That was the key that I had been missing. I had to "get it all together" with this success mindset.

This was an enlightening time for me. I finally understood that it wasn't a new food, a new herb, a new exercise, a new diet plan or a new doctor (all the things I usually went for) ... but simply thoughts embracing certain essential attitudes and incorporating specific principles. The food, exercise and behavior changes came later, the attitude came first, and was the one and only thing these winners all had in common.

This is the very starting point for all success in weight control. You have to really understand each of these attitudes and principles and get them all to the point where they merge into a total personal philosophy. Like threads woven into a fabric. Without this essential success mindset, we are doomed to fail, or at least to suffer a lot. I didn't want to do either, and I'm sure the same is true for you. So now I'll share with you the ingredients for the success mindset ... how and what winners think, and how you can learn to make these powerful thoughts work to motivate you and keep you on track through all the inevitable ups and downs.

3 Stages of Developing a Winning Attitude

Altogether there are 15 principles in the Success Mindset which will determine your attitude, level of motivation ... and ultimately the degree of success you will have at controlling your weight. These attitudinal principles fall into three stages: 1) Preparation 2) Action 3) Follow- through.

In the **Preparation Stage**:
1) You hit bottom. Thunk.
2) You decide that you deserve success for yourself.
3) You develop a strong desire to succeed by choice.
4) You develop belief in your ability to succeed.
5) You accept personal responsibility.

In the **Action Stage**:
6) You develop clear, focused goals and step-by-step plans for their achievement.
7) You seek out highly motivating personal benefits.
8) You use realistic thinking and common sense.
9) You use balance and moderation to cope with your natural resistance to changes.
10) You learn to gradually ease into your changing habits.
11) You learn that mistakes are necessary learning tools.

In the **Follow-through Stage**:
12) You make a long-term commitment.
13) You forgive yourself for forgetting the principles occasionally.
14) You persist and never give up.
15) You share your success with others.

Stage One: Preparation

The five steps in this first stage of developing a Success Mindset set you up for the action you must take to reach your goal. This is the "psyche you up" stage. When you get your head in the right place, the rest is easy and you won't suffer at all. All the choices you make will just be a natural part of choosing health for yourself. You'll know you're there when you're doing this because you choose to gladly, not because you have to. Keep working on this stage until you get to that place. Unless you do, any following work will only be "castles built on sand" and will only be temporary.

1. Hitting Bottom

In order to get your motivation fired up you need an initial spark. Often this is referred to as "hitting bottom". For some, it might be catching a glimpse of "that fat person" in the shop window and then realizing with a start, "Whoa, that's me!". Maybe a photograph captures the real you in all your expanded glory. Perhaps it's stepping on the scale and watching the poor thing whirl past every previous number like mercury gone mad on a hot summer day. Whatever the occurrence, hitting bottom can be mighty depressing. That's why so many of us put off the "weigh-in" or trying on that certain pair of tight pants in the back of the closet.

Hitting bottom frees you. When you realize that your current state of being is no longer acceptable to you, you can focus in a different direction. The good thing about hitting bottom is that you start looking forward again. It's actually a relief to finally acknowledge where you are, even if it's not where you want to be.

Until you have this "hitting bottom" experience it's really hard to get yourself in gear. The "it's-not-so-bad" attitude dooms you to half-hearted efforts. That's one of the reasons why people who have "only" five to fifteen pounds to lose often find it difficult to commit to losing it. They figure they don't look so bad and nobody notices anyway. The navy skirt and burgundy blazer camouflages the extra, right? Wel-l-l ... let me tell you, the person in the mirror knows, and it colors everything you do when you know you're faking it.

Are you ready for a blast of reality? The sooner you acknowledge that you're sitting on the bottom, the sooner you can start heading up towards the clear blue skies of success. Winners only look in one direction ... up! It's time for you to hit bottom! Off with every stitch of clothing. Say what!? You heard me. Strip. Now examine the evidence in the largest full-length mirror you have ... under bright lights. No sucking it in or posing to best advantage.

Just stand there and take a good honest, objective look at yourself. Then ask, "Do I need to lose weight?". Now, have you hit bottom yet? Yes, this can be a difficult and unpleasant exercise but it's important that you do it, because until you do you may rationalize and compromise away your chances for success. Acknowledge that you need to lose your excess weight to look better, for health reasons, and also to feel better about yourself.

For me the decision was a lot more clear cut. My bottom came one bleak winter day when I heard my Stanford-trained doctor say, "You'll be dead in six months if you don't take off the weight". Period. The end. I was 24 years old and I weighed 272 pounds ... twice my normal body weight. This was the low-point of my life. And the turning point of decision. There was no question that something needed to be done. I was depressed and scared and I simply couldn't put it off any longer. The problem could no longer be hidden by dark pants and a long jacket.

From that pit of despair, I began to climb slowly upward, one step at a time. The first, all-important step had been taken ... hitting bottom. Something opened up inside and I became ready to receive whatever was necessary. I surrendered to the inevitable ... I had to do something NOW.

There is an ancient Zen saying, "When the student is ready, the teacher will appear". At that moment I became ready. I started paying more attention to the available teachers. No more "trying" to lose weight. No more "I know I should but ... ". In short, no more excuses. Winners don't make excuses, they just do what it takes. When you're ready to give up your personal myths and excuses you'll be ready to learn what you need to know to win. Hitting bottom is an eye-opener. THINNER WINNERS Attitude: Honestly acknowledge that you have Hit Bottom and are ready and willing to gladly do whatever it takes to restore your health.

2. You Deserve Success Because You're Worth It!

You can win an occasional game for the Gipper, but the only way to win at long-term weight control is to do it for yourself. No self-improvement program can be done with any real chance of success if it's only to fill someone else's needs (your spouse, family or doctor) or some short-lived event (an upcoming reunion or [gasp!] bathing suit season). As soon as the event is here and gone, well, time to let go and return to the "real you". You're not going to be a winner at something that you have to be dragged into kicking and screaming. It's got to be your choice.

You must decide, before going any further, that you really want to lose all the extra weight forever ... for yourself! Because you're worth it! Look yourself in the eye while you're still in front of that mirror and ask yourself right now, "Am I worth it?". Here's a hint: winners always say YES!

If you're not positive, let me be the first to tell you "You are worth it!" ... and don't you ever forget that. I know that self-esteem can be a fragile issue when you spend your life walking on eggshells. But it can also be a powerful driving force when you realize that you're just as valuable as everybody else ... and just as deserving of success. See Chapter 10, "Self-Acceptance and Self-Esteem", for more on this very important topic.

Winners are confident enough to be willing to change their ways to get the results they want. They know they're worth it! When you're ready to start getting those positive results, and you're willing to make the necessary changes to do it, it's only a matter of time before you're crossing the finish line. THINNER WINNERS Attitude: Make the "Decision" (with a capital D) to do it for yourself because you're worth it!

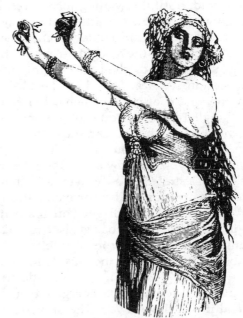

"Something just clicked!"

3. Developing a Strong Desire

Just how do you jump start your motivation? Sometimes a trigger situation like the ones mentioned earlier will simply "click" something in your head and you're off and running. We've all experienced that "something just clicked" feeling, but why do some clicks stay clicked and others fade away? Let's take a closer look at this "magic" occurrence.

Psychologically, there are two basic

motivators ... just two reasons why anybody ever does anything. Desire or fear. Both are powerful driving forces, but each has a very different effect on your life. That's because of an astounding fact: what you think about tends to expand and show up in your life. You get more of it everywhere, like rabbits on holiday.

Consequently, people motivated by fear find that fear pervades their lives. They're afraid of criticism and ridicule. They're afraid of failing or maybe even of succeeding. They develop negative, paranoid outlooks in nearly every situation they encounter. They're timid about weight control, afraid to really all-out commit, holding back their efforts. Their world closes in around them in what they perceive as "safety". They put up lots of walls in the name of protection, but end up also shutting out any help they could receive by being more open and risking a little.

Fearful dieters are afraid not to be "good" or follow their diet to the letter. They're afraid to question or change anything for fear they'll disturb whatever magic formula they're currently dependent upon. They plug away, joylessly doing what they're told, dutifully waiting for the results, grimly hanging on. But their hearts aren't really in it because their motivation comes from outside themselves. Eventually they begin to resent that controlling source and then to flaunt their "disobedience" in its face. "Ha, ha! There ... I'm having another piece of cake ... ha,ha, I'm eating the whole thing!! Take that, you can't tell me what to do!" Driven by the whip of fear, they rebel.

Okay ... fear may get you started, like me, but over the long haul you can now see it doesn't work. So what's left? Desire! That's the winner's choice. An intense desire for self-improvement, and especially vibrant health, will get you motivated positively in the direction of your goals ... and keep you moving. Desire comes from inside yourself, instead of being dictated from the outside like fear.

If you are "for" something, if you desire a positive outcome, you will be energized in that direction and it will flow to you. The universe will seem to line up on your side. Support will come to you in ways that you can't even anticipate. Everything will begin to work for you. In contrast, if you are against something, if you are afraid of a negative outcome, your energy will be drained by trying to fight it. So be "for" your own positive health, instead of being against your fat. Love of your destination works. Hate for your condition is self-defeating and doesn't work.

THINNER WINNERS Attitude: Have a strong DESIRE for a positive outcome, instead of fear of a negative consequence.

4. Believe and Achieve

By firmly believing in your ability to succeed at controlling your weight, by knowing that you can, you'll find it much easier to power through any obstacles. There is a fundamental principle at work here. Remember, what you think about tends to expand and take over your life.

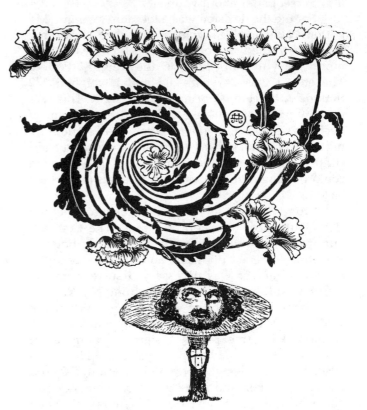

What you think about EXPANDS ...

If you think of yourself as fat, that is what will expand in your life, and you will ultimately fulfill that belief. This is one of the major boo-boos that holds overweight people back from success. They believe they are fat. So they do the things that fat people do and they stay fat. Even if they manage to get thin, they feel like fakes who just somehow beat the system. And because of that attitude they eventually lose their grip on thinness and return to being fat. A self-fulfilling prophecy. What they see and believe in their minds is what they get.

When you begin to realize this truth and experience it for yourself, you'll start to get ver-r-y careful about what kinds of thoughts you allow into your mind! Hedged bet statements like "I'll give it a try" or "Maybe I can" just don't make it. You must develop a deep conviction that successful weight control is possible for you and since it is possible, you are going to make it happen. You'll see, as you read through this book, that if I could do it then certainly you can, too. Why not you? I have no special powers ... I'm just someone who learned how to get and stay thin by first believing I could. I overcame a lifetime of chronic obesity by using these very principles. Once I truly began to believe in all the concepts in this program and began applying them to my life I started getting results after years of ups and downs. The same will be true for you. You can learn the same techniques and you can become thin, too. Dare to believe this. Think health and thinness. Each thought that you create develops a line of future growth. It magnifies the future for you. I call these lines of magnification MAG lines ... lines of Movement, Action and Growth. Your thoughts are like wires stretched out on a garden wall. Ivy will follow the lines and grow into a pattern mapped out by the wires. Your life and all its circumstances, fat or thin, will follow the thought lines you establish. Think struggle, deprivation and failure ... your future will follow those lines and grow into that pattern. Think thoughts only of success, learning, glowing health and thinness ... your future experiences will be thus mapped out and manifested. This cannot be overstated or overestimated in importance. Without this understanding of the power of your thoughts, you will miss the key to the laws of health. Know what you want; see what you want in your mind as if you already had it.

How do you develop this unshakable belief in your ability to get and stay thin? Since faith and belief start in your mind, there really is only one way. Go to the source and direct your thoughts. The most effective way to begin to change your thinking is to talk to yourself (see Chapter 9 "Self-Talk and Affirmations"). Not just loosely have a little conversation once in awhile. But deliberately placing your desired attitudes and beliefs in your mind, so they are picked up and used to shape your thoughts, actions and future. You need to take charge of your mind.

One method for doing this is to use affirmations. All winners use affirmations. It's almost a trademark for them. You might recognize affirmations as sayings or truisms. They're extremely powerful when used correctly. Affirmations are an effective way to induce the characteristic of faith needed to bring on the total belief and conviction of a weight control winner.

Your dominant thoughts determine what you believe, and your beliefs determine your success. To put it another way: "If you believe you can, or believe you can't, you're right!". Your thoughts bring about real things and real situations. You can use this principle to reach your goal by persistently telling yourself that you're getting healthier and

thinner day by day, and that's what you deserve. Winners know this and guard their thinking carefully.

As soon as you understand that belief is not an optional feature, and you begin to take your beliefs seriously, you'll start seeing positive changes taking place in your life. Firmly, and with great conviction, believe it can be done and you can do it. If you still have any doubts , look at my before and after pictures for a few minutes. Similar results are waiting for you! You must know this. If you still don't believe you can, try suspending your disbelief and just fake it until you do.

THINNER WINNERS Attitude: Believe in yourself with all your heart. Know that success is possible, and have no doubts that you can lose your excess weight for good. Nothing can stop a powerful belief ... a belief so strong that it becomes an indisputable knowing. It is destined to become reality.

5. Winners Accept Personal Responsibility

I listed some common excuses that dieters use in Chapter 2 "Myths That Keep You Fat". Did I get any of the ones that keep coming up for you? Or is there something else that you use as a "reason" why you're overweight and can't get thin?

Blaming outside forces for your lack of success just dilutes your power. It really isn't someone else who is making your decisions to eat more than you need. It's not your mother, your less-than-supportive spouse or your skinny friends. Neither is it your slow metabolism or other health problems that you may be hiding behind. As master motivator Zig Ziglar says, "I never ate anything accidentally". And blaming, rationalizing and denying are sure ways to stay fat. Saying that another person or situation has responsibility for your being fat does not make it so.

Uh,oh. There, I went and said it. Responsibility. And I'll go even one further ... personal responsibility. That's what it takes to win at the losing game, or really at anything. Dr. Wayne Dyer said it well, "If it's to be, it's up to me". Developing the discipline and willingness to start and complete this program successfully is your responsibility.

This book offers guidelines, techniques and suggestions and shows you what worked for me and others, but you must make it work for you. Winners take the time to develop their own food and exercise plans, mental strategies and behavioral controls. Self-made plans have been shown to be a key factor in successful weight control. Winners design and produce their own Dream Books and

Affirmations. No one can do this but you. Deciding that you will continue to increase your knowledge and awareness to a level beyond your previous weight loss roadblocks is totally up to you. You must commit to increasing your awareness ... to read, study and learn.

When you truly understand that there is no knight in shining armor coming to your rescue, you will have the power necessary to call your own shots and hit your own targets when and how you want and need to. Yes, it can be scary in the beginning. Just like starting any new, unfamiliar activity that challenges and stretches your level of comfort. They don't call it the "comfort zone" for nothing. But there is no other way. (Believe me, I tried to find one!) Besides, you can also take all the credit for a job well done! THINNER WINNERS Attitude: Winners personally accept all the responsibility for their success. No one else can do it.

Stage Two: Action

Good job! Stage One was definitely a Biggie. But now that you've got a good handle on that all-important attitude, you can get on with the actual work of getting to goal. In this stage, you develop a "mode of operation" ... an ethic for dealing with the work at hand. Be true to these guiding standards and you will have a ready answer for any questions or choices that come up.

6. Winners Use Goals and Plans

Winners know that in order to get from here to there in the least amount of time it's necessary to have written goals and to follow step-by-step plans. One reason many people don't succeed in their weight control efforts is because they don't keep their eye on the ball. They lose focus easily and only put out effort when it seems easy or convenient. A lackadaisical approach only brings marginal results. You've got to stay focused on your target.

Having written goals and plans keeps you focused because you can refer to them along the way. Like a heat-seeking missile, you'll be pulled back on course by a clear goal. You've made a commitment to yourself, and you know in advance how you're going to fulfill it. Goals are like magnifying glasses that cause you to look at your wishes and dreams in greater detail. Instead of saying, "I want to look good" you determine more precisely what you consider looking good to be ... "size 8 looks good on me!". You'll know exactly where you're heading. When you break down the ultimate goal into smaller steps along the way you make it easier to succeed. How do you walk around the world? One step at a time!

THINNER WINNERS Attitude: Winners use goals like the bull's eye on a target. When you've got something definite to aim for you're more likely to hit it. Refer to Chapter 8 "Goal Setting and Treasure Maps" for specifics on using this important principle.

7. Benefits Strengthen Motivation

The golden key to keeping your desire high and motivation strong is having powerful personal benefits. If you have just one reason for wanting to get control of your weight, then your desire will be one benefit strong. However, if you have 100 benefits, and something happens to one or two of them, you will still have plenty of reasons to keep going. I would go so far as to say that benefits equal motivation. They are that important!

So right now, get out your journal and start your own personal "benefits list". Write down all the positive reasons you have for getting thin. Everything! More energy, perfect size wardrobe, looking good at family affairs, feeling good about yourself, confidence to do more, finally ridding yourself of this nagging problem, energetic health, helping others and being able to "strut your stuff" ... anything and everything that signifies to you a benefit for getting thin.

Strong emotions will strengthen the pull of these benefits. The stronger you feel about your benefits the more effective they will be. "Looking better" sounds okay, but "looking like a model in my leopard-skin bodysuit" ... now, that's emotion! (Yes, I do have one!) So really see and feel your benefits and charge them with emotion! See yourself strong, fit and slender. (See Chapter 7 "Visualization and Dream Books".)

Keep your benefits list handy and read it often. Add new benefits as you discover more. The more reasons you have for controlling your weight, the stronger your motivation will be. THINNER WINNERS Attitude: Strongly emotionalized and visualized benefits strengthen motivation.

8. Realistic Thinking

Realistic thinking, being totally honest and based in reality, is another essential key for keeping your motivation running deep and strong. Many dieters fall into the "magic diet pill" trap. They just know that somewhere out there is a miracle pill that will burn off all their extra fat and allow them to eat whatever they want without lifting a finger in exertion (also known as "peel me a grape" syndrome). Science hasn't found it yet, but it's out there, so they keep searching. The diet hucksters prey on this false hope, making fortunes on the unrealistic thinking and lottery mentality of those who haven't yet faced the facts. These are the also-rans ... the poor unfortunates who bounce from this herb to that tea to another combination of foods or drugs that will "melt off the fat".

Winners know better. They realize that they are special people, but they aren't special cases when it comes to controlling weight. They know that in order to be successful they have to diligently follow a logical strategy ... not a mad hatter. If you haven't come to grips with this yet, then chances are you have a flabby motivation and get pulled off track by every sales pitch with a halfway plausible sounding promise of instantly solving your fat problem.

Another common error of the unrealistic dieter is thinking that following someone else's plan to the letter should work for them, too. Sorry, there's that reality again. If eating 1400 calories with 20% fat and exercising for 30 minutes 3 times a week is not getting you as thin as you'd like, then guess what? You're going to have to do more. And furthermore, you are going to have to find out what that "more" is by experimenting until you get the results you are after. Only you can determine your personal success pattern by using realistic thinking.

In the beginning my metabolism was so slow and unresponsive that I needed to exercise at maximum levels and eat the most well-planned food just to lose a pound or two a month! It was when I realized and accepted this about my metabolism that I began to be in control of my weight future. That's just the way it was for me. I believed there was a way for me to get healthfully thin and I was going to find it. I didn't care if I exercised 24 hours a day and ate vitamin pills and water, I would do it! (Fortunately it didn't come to that.) You have to do whatever it takes. As Sylvester Stallone said in the movie Rocky IV, "Ya gotta do what ya gotta do!"

Your needs are unique. It's not realistic to think that you can follow a one-size-fits-all diet and expect cookie-cutter results. A reality-based program offers guidelines and you have to tailor those guidelines into a workable and livable plan for yourself. If it's not working the way you want, make adjustments until it does. Your own informed choices, not somebody else's rules, will lead you to your success.

Once you begin thinking realistically and honestly, your time and energy will be directed towards the real solutions to your unique weight control challenges. There will be plenty of them and you'll need all the energy and brain-power you can muster. Don't hamper yourself with the fluffy hopes of an also-ran. Be honest with yourself, be realistic and focus on finding solutions that work for

you. You're just wasting your time if you don't. THINNER WINNERS Attitude: Use realistic, honest thinking to accept your own needs, craft your own solutions and set your own direction.

9. Master the Arts of Balance and Flexibility

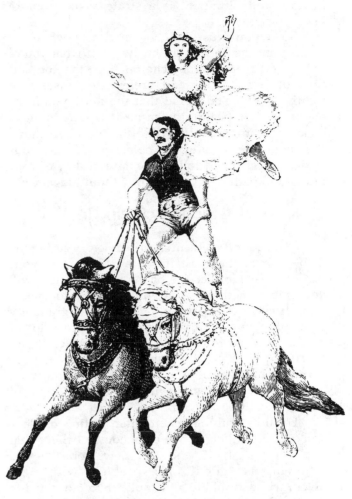

"How high did you say that hurdle is?"

Perfectionistic thinking is a paradoxical trap. It would seem that being "perfect" guarantees perfection. Instead it usually guarantees frustration because perfection is an impossible standard. In reality there is no "perfect way" to control your weight, except the very way that unfolds for you. And you can't determine that ahead of time ... it evolves as you learn and grow. If you are locked into the way you "should" lose weight and that way doesn't work out exactly according to your hopes (and let me clue you in, it almost certainly will not!) then when you go off your perfect path, you will be knocked off balance and fall on your nose.

Instead, developing the qualities of flexibility and balance will allow you to successfully bend with circumstances as they inevitably change.

Weight control sometimes seems like a high-wire act. You keep your balance by learning to make more healthy choices than unhealthy ones (which wiggle the wire and try to knock you off). When you make a poor choice, just counter-balance it with a better one. Feeling like you have to be "perfect" is rigid and self-destructive. Allowing yourself to be flexible and "human" is a strategy much more likely to succeed.

So if you must indulge once in a while, be flexible and go ahead. But be aware of what you're doing and balance your choices. Use the ebb and flow of your moods and preferences, instead of fighting them. You'll find that the more you learn about positive health, the easier it will be to make balanced choices. THINNER WINNERS Attitude: Be flexible and maintain balance with all your choices. Accept and follow the natural flow of your individual path to good health without judgement.

10. Gracefully Easing In

I consider the essential principle of "easing in" to be one of the most important factors in your success! The correct use of the ease principle will determine whether or not you'll be able to change your lifestyle permanently. You must gradually ease into your changes. Trying to force a lot of changes all at once will inevitably send you scurrying back to the unhealthy habits of your current comfort zone. Abrupt changes go along with "instant weight loss" thinking ... the kind of strategy that doesn't work.

Unsuccessful dieters are often victims of black and white thinking. They erroneously believe that one way is "bad" and the new hope they're following is "good". The problem with rigid black/white thinking is simply that most of life takes place in the "Gray Zone". On a scale of 1 to 100, there are 98 numbers in between and that's where you spend most of your time.

The secret is to give yourself enough time to acclimate and to get used to new ways gradually. You're not racing anyone to change your habits. If you're in reasonably good health, there is no reason why you can't allow your tastes and habits to acclimate over a year or so. Yes, I know that sounds unbearably long! And your big reunion is only two months away. Well, now is a good time to start some realistic thinking. By limiting yourself to thinking only in terms of instant results you are, in effect, doomed to repeat your old habit patterns ... the ones that didn't work. It's time to ease into some new habit patterns.

It took me six full years to be able to make my particular claim of success. If I had allowed the need for instant change to rule my life, I would have ended up with nothing but another string of yo-yo diets during that time. It may take some major attitude and strategy changes on your part to apply the "ease" philosophy, but I can sincerely tell you that it's well worth the effort.

Your goal is to implement permanent change, not just to get quick results. Instead of abruptly yanking out all the "bad" stuff and facing unfamiliar foods and habits, ease yourself into lifestyle changes and your goals will be much more readily attainable. Easing in is recommended for increasing fiber in your diet, increasing your water intake, increasing exercise, increasing positive thoughts ... all sorts of great, healthy things that you just may have had a bit of trouble dealing with in the past.

THINNER WINNERS Attitude: Ease into your new, improved habits. Make it a priority for your diet and lifestyle changes. Give yourself time and don't force rapid, uncomfortable changes. Allow yourself to make gradual, long-range changes that will be easy to maintain over your whole, happy, healthy lifetime!

11. See Opportunities, Not Failures

One of the unmistakable characteristics of weight control winners is the ability to see that an unsuccessful attempt is not a failure. It is merely an opportunity to identify what did not work, and to correct the situation by trying something else. The also-ran will "try" this diet or that, and when the weight doesn't come tumbling off immediately they'll scrap that one and label the attempt another failure.

Thomas Edison, perhaps the greatest inventor of our age, said it perfectly and exemplified the true winners attitude. In his attempts to perfect the incandescent light bulb, he had conducted over 5,000 unsuccessful experiments. A reporter asked him why he persisted in this venture when he had "failed" so many times. Edison replied, "You don't understand how the world works. I have not failed at all. I have successfully identified 5,000 ways not to make a light bulb." Edison went on to conduct over 10,000 experiments before finally producing the electric light bulb!

Like Edison, if you are to succeed, failure cannot be in your vocabulary. In the same vein, I personally have identified hundreds, if not thousands, of ways to remain fat! (Just think how useful that information would be to Sumo wrestlers!) But there was never any question in my mind about giving up. Being fat was a temporary condition for me. My birthright is good health, and that includes a normal body weight. The same is true for you. So instead of "failure", substitute the word "opportunity". Or you can say "challenge". Even "glitch" or "hurdle" will do. I like to call them "bumps in the road".

Every time you think you've blown it, look for the lesson to be learned from your experience. Seize the opportunity to learn from your mistakes. It may possibly take you many years, like me, to really understand all the lessons needed to fully succeed. But hopefully not, now that you know how to profit from these challenges. You may get discouraged at times ... it happens. Take a rest if you must, but always see the resting place as just that, a temporary pit stop. Turn your lemons into lemonade. THINNER WINNERS Attitude: Always see your setbacks as opportunities for learning and seeds of growth towards your inevitable success.

Stage Three: Follow-through

Congratulations! You're moving along strong and sure now. You're developing the confidence of a weight-control winner because you know what you need to do and how to do it. You've picked the right racket, learned how to hold it and hit that ball. Now, to complete the Success Mindset, you need to develop Follow-through. This stage will assure that your work will continue to bring you the health and thinness that you desire for a lifetime.

12. Commitment to a "Lifelong Lifestyle"

I used to think that a "diet" was a weight loss strategy that you followed until the weight was gone (or as long as you could stand it), and then you went off the program. The notion of a diet as simply a way of eating did not emerge until the realization came that I was not eating differently for the sole purpose of losing weight. I was changing my eating patterns for a healthier, higher quality (and hopefully longer) lifetime.

So, here's the good news! You never have to go on a "diet" again! The pressure that this attitude relieves has often been enough for me to make a healthier choice in foods at the moment. It's a whole different perspective.

One of my favorite sayings when I used to "diet" was, "The condemned man ate a hearty meal". And, boy, I could really eat a hearty meal the night and day (sometimes the whole week!) before I condemned myself to yet another "diet"! My revised attitude towards food has released me from the binge style eating that kept me glued to the "diet" cycle for years. For me it was "binge and do penance by dieting, starving and denial". So, no more "diets"! Just a style of eating where choices for healthy foods are made more often, and choices for unhealthful foods are made less often. Simply

because you deserve good health.

Gradually, the new, healthier foods became fixtures in my regular eating patterns. And still more gradually, the healthy foods began to outnumber the nutritional duds. To ensure a smooth transition you need to begin thinking differently about your concept of losing weight.

First, you must eradicate the notion that a weight control program is an on-again/off-again project. Once you learn the reasons that one food is unhealthy for your body and another is healthful, the notion of "dieting" will begin to fade. You'll realize that maintaining positive health is an ongoing project. Eventually the benefits of success will outweigh the appeal of your old habits. Once that happens you're home free.

To fully succeed at weight control you must continue to be able to eat out at restaurants and parties, to entertain and travel and still maintain a level of good health. The world goes on, and special situations are part of that world. Learning to live with them in a healthy manner is essential to your success. As you learned from the earlier section on "balance", if you make a poor choice, you can still balance that with a better choice. The average of those choices equals your improved diet and lifestyle.

Second, you must make the commitment to change permanently to a healthier lifestyle. It sounds like a lot to ask, but when you consider the negative side effects of an unhealthy lifestyle you'll realize it's not.

In my case I was able to turn food from a challenging adversary into a friend again and I now enjoy shopping, cooking, and being around food all day. This is a miracle in itself, because before my commitment to a healthy lifestyle I was riddled with guilt even at the moment of dearest taste bud ecstasy. I was eating all the time but enjoying it very little, since I knew that the food was killing me and squashing the dreams out of my life. Today, with my commitment to health, I can revel in the joyful experience of eating without guilt or worry about tomorrow! The time for your commitment to health is now!

One of my favorite refrigerator door quotes is this:

"Until one is committed, there is hesitancy, the chance to draw back, always ineffectiveness ... Whatever you can do, or dream you can, begin it. Boldness has genius, power and magic in it. Begin it now."

Johann Goethe was the author of this beauty. I might add, "Then keep at it until you succeed".

Begin where you are. Commit now to discovering the ideas in this book that will help you on your weight control quest. Take those concepts and run with them. More solutions will grow from these, and you will soon snowball your health into the positive dream you deserve.

Join the growing ranks of healthy men and women who know that they can have it all! You can free yourself and become the person of your dreams: joyful, energetic and healthy! You can also spread this wonderful tradition of positive health to others in your life. There is no better legacy than passing along good health and joy to show that you are an aware, balanced person. Truly, when you have your health, you have everything. Your commitment to self-improvement and personal growth for a lifetime will allow you to experience the potential you are capable of. Once you commit, it immediately begins to work! Make the commitment and watch it work in your life. THINNER WINNERS Attitude: Develop a Lifelong Lifestyle! Commit to seeking health, instead of just trying to lose weight. See positive health as a lifelong journey, not merely an "on again/off again" project.

13. Forgive Yourself for Forgetting

Babe Ruth, baseball's legendary home-run hitter, struck out 60% of the time he stood at bat. But that's not what we remember about him. He gets due credit for what he did right. You need to use the same philosophy when it comes to your weight control efforts. Look at what you're doing right. There will be plenty of times in the future when you lose your edge or even fall off the wagon. When cowboys get bucked off a horse they know the wisest thing to do is get right back on. The longer they stand around rubbing their fannies the more time fear and doubt have to take hold.

Learn to forgive yourself. When you lose focus and slack off your program, which happens to everyone on occasion, you have to understand that you haven't failed. You haven't become a worthless slacker overnight. You're a winner! But even winners have peaks and valleys. Relax, lighten up and forgive yourself for forgetting your goals for a while. Your goals are still there waiting for you ... and you're still on your way towards achieving them. THINNER WINNERS Attitude: Whenever you get off-track, just gently guide yourself back. No blame and no wasted guilt time either.

14. Be Persistent

Eliminating the concept of failure leads to another important, and related, characteristic needed for success: persistence. No matter how tough it gets, remember there is no such thing as quitting for a winner. "Winners never quit, and quitters never win". It's an old saying, but still holds true. Pull back, re-evaluate, set your course again and continue working at the possible solutions until they yield the answers. Try again. That's what it means to make things happen.

Many dieters make the mistake of seeing themselves as failures because they've tried so many times without success. But as Napoleon Hill wisely pointed out, "Each obstacle carries with it the seed of an equivalent benefit". Those obstacles are out there to test your persistence! And I know you're persistent because you're reading this book looking for answers. Your persistence will fuel your forward motion just like the gas in your car keeps it going. As long as you keep moving forward you'll eventually reach your goal.

People who give up, stop learning, and abandon hope are admitting that they're not strong enough to even question their own actions anymore. Their actions, accordingly, get out of their control. If you can acknowledge your feelings and behaviors, even after stumbling badly, then at least you have not totally given up. You're still accepting the responsibility for your own actions. That's the seed of a future benefit. You have not quit, because you know this obstacle is just one of the experiments needed to get to your success. You are in the process of growth.

I always knew that I was just temporarily fat and someday I would truly be thin (even though for a while there temporary seemed to be measured in decades). I never gave up. All I needed was the right formula to follow. My persistence paid off and I found it! And as long as you cultivate your persistence you will end up thin, also. No one can make you quit except yourself. Keep up the pressure instead of buckling in. So never give up on yourself. Winners know they are worth the persistence ... and you are, too. THINNER WINNERS Attitude: "Never give up, never give up, never give up" (a quote by Winston Churchill).

15. Sharing Your Success With Others

As I began to learn how to take off weight safely, and understand why I had remained fat for so long, I gradually developed a burning desire to rush out and tell other overweight people about my discoveries. I hope this happens to you, too, because it's the most wonderful feeling to be able to share ideas that help others, in your old position, to improve their lives and climb out of that horrible whirlpool of fat. Feeling good about yourself gives you the energy to help others. It's as if you can't really help, love or share with others unless you first have it inside to give.

Indeed, it is one of the steps of 12-step programs, such as Overeater's Anonymous, to help others with the same addiction from which you are recovering. It's a very healing, energizing experience and an incredibly effective way to keep yourself thin for the rest of your life. I hope, as you become a successful THINNER WINNER, that you spread the word to all who are still searching for the answers. The world will be a better place when we all start helping each other! You're on your way to making that happen for yourself and other people who need to hear what you know.

Well, there they are. The commonly held attitudes and principles of weight control winners. Now that you have them isolated you can work to adopt these concepts into your life, build them up and strengthen them. Use these principles as the basis of your motivational efforts. With these strong convictions you'll be able to address any situations that come up with answers based on the belief that you can and will succeed. By practicing these principles you will bring about a paradigm shift in your perception. You won't be suffering through another "diet", but instead you'll be sailing smoothly on the river of true health ... right where you want to be.

The remainder of this chapter offers an overview of specific techniques you can use to build and strengthen your motivation. And, perhaps even more importantly, provides you with a look at the skills which will help you maintain your motivation.

But first, as a way to help you determine where you stand with each of these essential attitudes, take the following self-evaluation.

Rating Your Attitudes

Incorporating the Success Mindset into your lifestyle is essential for your success. In order to get a sense of where you are right now, please rate yourself on the following attitudes. Give yourself a score on each item ... 1 is the lowest level and 10 is the highest. Be honest with yourself. Your ultimate objective, of course, is to get to the highest levels that you can. It's a good idea to re-evaluate yourself every six months to check your progress. Discuss your results with your support person for maximum benefit.

1) I have had the experience of hitting bottom and I'm ready for positive change in my life ... with no more excuses.
2) I am losing weight for myself, not for any external events or to please other people.
3) I am motivated by a strong desire to succeed, not the fear of failing. I'm aware that what I think about expands in my life.
4) I have a strong belief in my ability to succeed.
5) I accept personal responsibility to do whatever it takes to succeed, with no exceptions.
6) I have clear, focused goals and step-by-step plans for their achievement.
7) I understand that my personal benefits strengthen my motivation.
8) I use realistic thinking and common sense.
9) I use balance and flexibility to cope with my resistance to changes.
10) I gracefully and gradually ease my way into lifestyle changes, giving myself time to adjust.
11) I see mistakes as opportunities for learning, not as failures or reasons for quitting.
12) I realize that I am pursuing lifelong lifestyle changes, not a temporary fix. I am seeking positive health, instead of simply weight loss.
13) I forgive myself when I occasionally forget the success principles.
14) I am persistent! I never give up!
15) I share my success with others.

Staying Motivated

So far you've learned that there is a core of critical attitudes and principles that stimulate motivation. Getting motivated is essential for success in any endeavor. Obviously, if you don't get up and moving it's going to be awfully hard to finish the job. But as Zig Ziglar wisely pointed out, "Motivation is like bathing, you need to do it every day". You wouldn't be reading this book at all if you weren't already motivated to some degree ... and that's great news! Unfortunately, at times the whole issue of weight control tends to be a very draining experience ... especially if you're fighting it. It's all too easy to lose your momentum. The most heart-rending and typical stories I have heard from my weight loss clients over the years started out:

"I was doing just fine, and then ... " (Take your pick of the following or write down your own.)

My husband came home with a 10-pound pizza.
I hurt my hip (my lip, my bippy).
I got a 5-pound box of candy for my birthday.
We had visitors for 2 weeks and it threw my routine off.
My son's little league team had a celebration down at Greaso's Eatery.
I ate 4 pounds of chocolate-chip cookies at the mall.
I forgot, and ordered a large, buttered popcorn at the movies ... plus 2 candy bars.
Etc., etc. ...

These things will always be there. What has to change is YOU!

The pitfalls to weight control are potentially beyond count. But that's what success at weight control is really all about ... OVERCOMING OBSTACLES! The most dangerous obstacle of all is the one who stares back at you from the mirror each morning. You and your attitudes. In order to maintain your attitude and motivation at positive levels there are a variety of skills and resources that you can learn, develop and draw upon. The more work you do on building powerful supportive resources and skills in yourself the more they will be there to assist you during those critical trying times.

Specific Techniques for Maintaining Motivation

What follows is an overview of the realistic, practical and proven success tools you will learn more about in following chapters. When your tool box is full of shiny, well-oiled tools you'll be able to maintain your motivation and your weight by knowing how to use them.

Written Goals

There is no greater way that you can express your commitment than to put your weight control goals in writing. Putting your dreams and desires into writing sends a powerful, reinforcing message to your subconscious mind. During those tough times when doubt is nipping at your heels make it a point to rewrite your goals every morning and say them out loud at least twice a day. See Chapter 8 "Goal Setting and Treasure Maps".

Treasure Maps

A picture is worth a thousand words and more. A Treasure Map is a device for drawing your goals towards you almost like a magnet. Take a poster-sized piece of cardboard and put your own photo in the middle. Then surround your image with pictures of the way you want to become and the things you want to have. If you gaze upon your Treasure Map often, it will have the same effect as looking at a billboard of your own design. It will propel you into buying what YOU are selling. This is a proven technique for getting results and staying motivated.

Positive Self-Talk

Self-talk is the running dialogue that goes on in your head all day long. In case you ever wondered who was doing the talking and who was listening, the answer is: it's you! You're the boss! What most people neglect to do is take charge of this internal conversation. Psychologists have found that it tends towards the negative over 80% of the time. By taking command of your own internal communications and making sure to trash the negativity you can make amazing changes in your life. See Chapter 9 "Self-Talk and Affirmations".

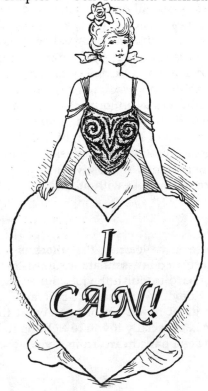

Affirmations

Affirmations are condensed, positive statements which support what you are trying to accomplish for yourself. You can read them, write them and state them aloud. Rather than leaving your self-talk to chance, you provide exactly what you want to hear yourself saying. They put a present tense, action-oriented thought straight into your mind. State your affirmations out loud and with conviction. These proven motivators are in the tool box of every winner.

Dream Books

Dream Books are a cross between Affirmations and Treasure Maps. They combine carefully chosen images with powerful, positive statements. Look at your Dream Book often ... especially first thing in the morning, last thing before going to sleep or right after you meditate. Let the first thoughts coming into your cleared mind be powerful and positive. See Chapter 7 "Visualization and Dream Books".

Meditation

For thousands of years people have known that to attain peace of mind you must go to the quiet place within your inner being. Happiness is not an external event or possession ... it is simply a state of mind. When you learn to meditate you will be able to silence any negative self-talk and replace it with a peaceful calm. When you're feeling positive it will be a lot easier to stay motivated. See Chapter 11 "Breathing and Meditation".

Exercise

It's a funny thing about exercise, but you always feel better for having done it. That's true even if you can think of a thousand excuses to avoid it beforehand. Your body loves it when you work up a good sweat. That's what it was designed for. When you're up and moving the negative thinking tends to get swept aside. When the endorphins start flowing you really feel on top of the world. Refer to the section on Activity and Exercise.

Stress Reduction Techniques

When you lose your motivation you nearly always gain some stress in its place. Have you noticed that when you're motivated and focused on your goals you always seem very clear-headed? And when you're stressed-out and feeling defeated it's hard to think clearly. So take a break. Give yourself a chance to unwind and see things more clearly. There are a hundred ways to relax. Pick one. See Chapter 14 "Taming Your Stress".

Benefits List

If you have a nice, long list of all the reasons why it's important for you to lose weight, and the benefits you'll derive for succeeding, you've got the carrot to dangle in front of your nose. If you ever forget why you're working so hard to lose weight and get healthy, look here first.

Personal Journal

One of the most crucial factors regarding weight control is that you must come to understand that mistakes are not failures, they are merely opportunities for learning. Be keeping track of your weight-related experiences, both good and bad, you get a strong sense of what specific techniques work best for you. By keeping a journal of your own solutions you will gain the confidence necessary to keep going even when life seems bleak. See Chapter 12 "Your Personal Journal".

Support People

Whether it's a weight loss group, your spouse, or your sister in Chicago it's important to develop a support net for yourself. Sometimes you just have to talk about your experiences with a person who understands what you're trying to accomplish. A truly helpful supporter will lend you a shoulder to cry on and give you a good kick in the seat of the pants when you need it. See Chapter 16 "Creating a Powerful Support System".

Rewards and Reinforcement

When you've accomplished something make sure you get the big payoff for it. From a behavioral perspective, actions that are followed by reinforcement become more prevalent. That's what you want! More of the healthy and less of the unhealthy. The best technique is to plan your program and rewards in advance. When you achieve your goal give yourself the reward immediately. See Chapter 17 "Rewards".

Daily Success Planner

Here's where you keep track of what you're eating and how much exercise you're getting (among other things). As long as you're honest with yourself, this tool can provide you with the hard evidence necessary to make intelligent decisions and adjustments to your weight control program. Whenever I'm in danger of slipping I turn to diligent record-keeping. It works. When you tighten up your program, your body will respond by tightening up. See Chapter 18 "Daily Success Planner".

Charts and graphs

There is nothing that hits home in the weight control world quite as intensely as seeing the line on your weight graph going down. It's the thrill to beat all thrills. That's why you should make it a regular practice to weigh and measure yourself, keep up your Daily Success Planners and stay on top of your game in general. Controlling your weight is a fine-tuning process. Sometimes you'll have better results than at other times. There will even be times when you just won't know why your body seems to have a sense of complete independence. That's where record keeping really helps. If you put on your Sherlock Holmes hat and look for clues you will find the culprits. Look at all your records and your Personal Journal notes and find out what's going on in your life. You might just find that a slight attitude adjustment or other change is in order. See Chapter 19 "Keeping Track of Your Progress".

Eat Healthy Food

The reason reading labels on food is such a big deal is because the nutrients you put into your body directly affect every aspect of your health. The government acknowledges this ... and thus we have food labeling. By coming to understand what you eat and how it affects you, you are taking a powerful step towards self-empowerment. By eliminating the "junk" in your diet, you take the grand leap to good health. This knowledge will eventually outweigh any sense of loss over your old favorite goodies. You won't even want these unhealthy substances in your body, even if attempts have been made to make them palatable by Chef Delusion. He's taken advantage of your senses ... usually smell, sight and taste. See past this "low-blow" approach and demand good health as well as good smell, sight and taste. It can be done and it actually takes skill to do it ... not just more butter, salt or sugar.

There are many more positive, active steps which you can take to maintain your motivation, stay on program and reach your weight control goals. Positive health is a lifetime process, not an event or short-term cure-all. By following your weight control goals and developing the constructive habits that support them, you are taking the true path to the light of good health.

In A Nutshell

1) Motivational skills can be developed and strengthened.

2) At the present time, less than 1 out of 20 dieters succeed in maintaining their weight losses.

3) The successful 5% have developed a Success Mindset ... a complex of attitudes that determines their success. You can predict anyone's success at losing weight permanently by how many of these attitudes they master.

4) This essential "Success Mindset" comes first ... before diet, exercise or behavior changes.

5) The 15 principles of the "SUCCESS MINDSET":
   In the **Preparation Stage**:
   1) You hit bottom.
   2) You decide that you deserve success for yourself.
   3) You develop a strong desire to succeed by choice.
   4) You develop belief in your ability to succeed.
   5) You accept personal responsibility.

   In the **Action Stage**:
   6) You develop clear, focused goals and step-by-step plans for their achievement.
   7) You seek out highly motivating personal benefits.
   8) You use realistic thinking and common sense.
   9) You use balance and moderation to cope with your natural resistance to changes.
   10) You learn to gradually ease into your changing habits.
   11) You learn that mistakes are necessary learning tools.

   In the **Follow-through Stage**:
   12) You make a long-term commitment.
   13) You forgive yourself for forgetting the principles occasionally.
   14) You persist and never give up.
   15) You share your success with others.

6) A variety of specific methods for getting and staying motivated were briefly listed. Use them!

Great Expectations   6

"If you think you can, or think you can't, you're right."
Brian Tracy

Attitude Adjustments

The above quotation is both philosophical and intensely practical. From an intellectual standpoint it reminds us that we very often accomplish those things in life which we believe we can. If we expect to succeed, we do. If we don't happen to succeed on this round, we go back and try again because we expect to succeed, after all. Soon enough we're holding the prize. From the practical point of view, you usually expect to succeed when you've gone to the trouble of some preparation or training. Expectation involves a sense of "knowing" in advance. "I knew I was going to succeed ... there was never any doubt in my mind" is the typical statement of someone who has prepared in advance for success. They weren't counting on luck or heavenly intervention. They were thinking "I can" and "I will"... or in some cases, as you will see, they simply avoided thinking the ever-deadly "I can't".

Perhaps the greatest mental gift we're given is the ability to daydream on a lazy, sunny afternoon. I remember being transported to places of wonder and happiness in many a youthful daydream. Unfortunately, my teachers often failed to note the benefits being derived from this activity, and they would transport me down to the principal's office. Oh, those poor unenlightened people. In the 1950's they just didn't know the power of the mind. After all, it took them until 1957 to get the design right on Chevys and T-Birds.

But even as a child I knew that imagination was a storehouse of incredible creations, wonderful sensations and endless power. Now, nearly forty years later, science is finally catching on.

Expect the Best

One of the things that all winners do is apply the concept of "positive self-expectancy". What's that? It's a pretty simple concept. Expect the best things to happen and they very often will. Expect less than the best and that's all you'll ever get.

The following story gives a powerful example of the amazing influence that expectations can have upon performance. Dr. David McClelland has done much research on the way in which expectations influence outcomes. One controlled study he designed involved school children and their teachers and shows the clear benefits and real power of positive expectations. A small group of teachers were chosen at random and told (falsely) that they had been specially selected to teach classes of "highly gifted" children (also false information). In fact, the teachers were average and chosen at random, and so were the students. The only specific instructions that the teachers were given was that they couldn't tell the children or the parents of these students that they were in special classes for "gifted students" (the experimenters didn't want the parents to bias the study). The students didn't know they were supposed to be gifted and the teachers didn't know they were simply chosen at random. This is referred to as a "double-blind" study. The study was designed to test the power of expectations. It turned out that these average students being taught by average teachers got better test performance results than any other students in that entire school district. The reason was simply that the teachers expected more from the students and the children met the higher expectations. The moral: expect the best and maybe you'll even surprise yourself.

Don't Waste Your Time

Each thought that passes through your mind uses up some time, so it's important to understand the relationship between time and your thoughts. Positive expectations are great examples of the productive use of your "mental time". The only "time" we really have control over, in any way, is the present moment. In this moment we can "be here now", focused on what we're presently doing, or we can use the time to dwell on some past event or a possible future occurrence (such as an expectation). These thoughts can be either positive or negative.

The least productive thinking involves either worrying about the future or feeling guilty about the past. The past is gone, done, kaput ... there's nothing you can do to change it. However, you can choose to recall good things that happened to you. This will certainly make you feel better than wallowing in the misery of guilt over something negative you may have done yesterday, or even twenty years ago. Try and stick with productive thinking if you're concerned with the past at all.

The future presents a more interesting dilemma. It's not here yet, but it will be. It's inevitable ...you can be sure that the future is heading your way. This provides you with a great opportunity to plan your outcome in advance. Pretend for a moment that you're driving your car on the freeway. Everything behind you is in the past. You'll never have to deal with that exact same traffic again. The future looms ahead however. You know that you want to get off the freeway in $3\frac{1}{2}$ miles. A sign just told you so. At this point you expect to get off the freeway at your proper off ramp. Expectations often lead to actions. After all, you expect to get off so why not act? You figure that in about two miles you'll ease your way over from the fast lane to the slow lane and then cruise down your off ramp. This is known as planning. You expect to get off at your exit with no problem, right? Do you waste a lot of time clouding your judgment by worrying about possible alien attacks or earthquakes between here and your off ramp? Probably not. You follow your plan and expect to succeed.

That's what winners do. They know where they're headed. They expect to get there. They plan a logical course of action. They aim for the destination offramp. They don't spend a lot of time immobilized, worrying about what might go wrong, whether it's flat tires or traffic jams. Certainly, they prepare for the obvious contingencies, but they aren't afraid to get out on the highway either. When obstacles do come up (which they inevitably do) they deal with them in the best possible way, and then keep going towards their objective. If you're not sure about what's going to happen in the future, you may as well expect the best. That's what you'll get.

Your Powerful Mind

Countless stories have been told about people who performed amazing physical feats while under great stress. A woman who single-handedly lifts a car off her trapped husband. A man who jumped over an eight-foot fence when chased by a bull. How is it possible that "impossible" events like these can take place? Part of the explanation may be due to the huge jolt of adrenaline that a fearful situation can cause. But that's only part of the explanation. The other, and more important part, is that in those instances when emotions completely override reason, we simply don't know that we can't do something. It then becomes possible to perform any action, even one that is "impossible".

You've certainly heard of "beginner's luck", but have you ever stopped to think about what it really is? Beginner's luck happens to people who simply don't know that they can't do something. So they go ahead and do it.

Consider this story for example. Athletes are specialists. They train hard for years to be successful at their chosen sport. The number of athletes who excel in more than one event are rare indeed. I remember attending a UCLA vs. USC track meet about 25 years ago that I have never forgotten. That was back in the days before triathlons by the way. There was a pole-vaulter named Bob Seagren who had achieved national recognition for his ability. However, at this particular meet he decided to add a new, slightly offbeat event ... the steeplechase. Now this is an event that requires a whole new batch of skills. Pole vaulting is based on a sprint. The steeplechase is a long, cross country event with hurdles and water hazards thrown in for interest. Completely different skills and talents were called for, and he had never participated in this event before. But Bob Seagren literally left the field behind. He finished a full half lap ahead of the favored runner. He was certainly a talented athlete to begin with. But what really made the difference was that nobody told him that he couldn't win the steeplechase. Nobody told him how hard it was, and that he didn't have the necessary skills. So he won.

When Opportunity Meets Preparation

Everybody loves a good rags to riches story. America is filled with them. It's what our country is known for the world over, and the reason why so many people want to immigrate here. We're also very much attuned to what is referred to as the "overnight sensation". We idolize people like Elvis Presley who have certain talents and gifts and who seem to rise to stardom from the time they first open their mouths in song. What we tend to forget is the humble beginnings from which so many of our idols rose and all of the obstacles they had to overcome. We see the star, and conveniently forget about the years of toil, training and paying those hard dues.

Abraham Lincoln struggled unsuccessfully through careers as a storekeeper, lawyer, soldier and politician before he was elected President. His persistence and understanding, developed over long, seemingly fruitless years, gave him the wisdom to excel as one of our greatest leaders.

Thomas Edison had to conduct over *ten thousand* experiments before he was finally able to design a functional electric light bulb. In the process, he also invented the vacuum tube which allowed for the development of later inventions such as radio, television and computers. If this one man had given up on his vision and expectation for success imagine how much different our lives would be today. Yet during the period prior to perfecting the light bulb, Edison was ridiculed by the scientific community and derided in the press as a lunatic. The general opinion was that it was mankind's destiny to read by gas lights. It's a good thing old Tom Edison expected to succeed, and knew how to ignore the critics.

The truth of the matter is that "luck" happens when opportunity meets preparation. You have a tremendous opportunity ahead of you to improve your health, your appearance, the way you feel and very possibly your life span. To reap these rewards you will have to "pay some dues" in the form of preparation. In order to lose weight, wear smaller clothing sizes and look better in general you will have to change some of your habits. You will also have to change some of your attitudes and expectations.

Expect to succeed and you will greatly increase your odds of losing your excess weight forever. You will find that positive expectation of almost anything brings connected energy, people, events, TV shows, articles, books and other "coincidental happenings" into your life in an initially unbelievable stream. This is what is meant by getting into "the flow". But be sure the flow you're in is the one you want. That's why so many overweight people stay fat. They're in the "fat flow", not the "thin flow". The energies they are drawing in act to keep them fat. If you can only see yourself as fat, struggling and unable to cope, that's the flow you will remain caught up in. Events and people around you will tend to verify your beliefs.

In order to break this cycle of negativity you need to begin to see the world through "rose-colored glasses" and expect different and more positive things to happen in your life. When you can visualize yourself as thin and healthy these qualities will begin to manifest in your life in different ways. You still have to do the work, of course. The children in the school study succeeded because they worked harder in response to their teachers' expectations. Just as an A+ student studies, and an athlete trains many hours every day, a THINNER WINNER knows and practices winning attitudes, including positive expectancy, that lead to being slim and healthy ... naturally.

What are your expectations for yourself? Do you expect to be thin for good? You'd better. Because what you expect is what you'll get. It's that simple.

Neuro-Linguistic Programming

Expecting the best for yourself is easier if you have a method. Neuro-Linguistic programming or NLP is one of the more focused "success philosophies" that have emerged in recent years. This approach to changing behavior uses the direct connection between your mind and your body.

A large part of the NLP approach is the concept of "modeling" the behavior of successful individuals. Depending upon what you want to accomplish, modeling can include posture, tone of voice or attitudes among other behaviors. Anthony Robbins, one of the most publicized NLP proponents, helped the army cut 50% off the training time required for its sharp-shooting program and improved performance as well. He studied the finest marksmen in the country, analyzed their behavior down to thirty postures and attitudes regarding target shooting and then trained new recruits using the behaviors he observed. The performance results showed dramatic improvements.

NLP uses a combination of modeling behaviors, positive attitudes and expectations, careful planning and persistent action on your plans. One of the most direct statements on the subject of success was made by motivational trainer Brian Tracy and summarizes NLP's philosophy. To paraphrase his quote "If you want to succeed, find out what successful people do and then copy their methods. Find out what failures do ... and don't do it".

NLP uses a highly directed approach to get results. Here are five basic steps that you can apply to your life to get successful results with any worthwhile project, including weight control.

1) **Know what you want to accomplish, and why.** You want to lose weight and improve your health, right? Why is this important to you? You need to know the answer to this critical question. Controlling your weight needs to be a burning desire for you. You have to really believe that it's important to control your weight and that you can accomplish your goal.

2) **You have to take action according to a particular strategy.** You need to have a weight control plan that works, makes sense to you and that you have faith in and then use this as your model. Find out what successful weight control experts have done to control their weight and do the same things. By following the four balanced sections of the THINNER WINNERS program (behavior, exercise, attitude and nutrition) you can control your weight and improve your health. You need to believe it, too. The answers are right in your hand. You need to follow the program, learn the concepts and master the principles. If you don't know all the details of the program you need to learn them. If you need assistance from others to help you succeed, then you need to seek them out. You need to put all your resources to work and act on your plan. This is

not a passive approach to achieving your goal. If you want to get the job done of controlling your weight, then follow a proven strategy and be confident it will work for you, too.

3) You have to be persistent. Winning those big victories takes more than wishful thinking and pushing the buttons on your remote control. In the process of learning to control your weight once and for all there will be inevitable setbacks. If you fall off the wagon, what do you do? That's right, you get right back on and keep going. My weight control success came because I knew I would eventually succeed and because I believed in what I was doing. That didn't guarantee a perfectly smooth trip, by the way. I had many a tough day to power through. Be realistic and persistent ... and you will get positive results.

Here are a few noteworthy examples of the rewards of persistence. Ross Perot, billionaire and presidential contender, was turned down on his first 78 sales calls when he first started his company, Electronic Data Systems. Through his persistence and determination he built a multi-billion dollar corporation. You can't just take action once and expect it to last a lifetime. You have to keep at it. That's what separates the winners from the also-rans. Colonel Sanders of Kentucky Fried Chicken fame was 65 years old and living on social security. He realized that life had to have more to offer than that, so he evaluated his assets and decided to get out and sell his not-yet-famous favorite fried chicken recipe ... the one thing he had which he believed to be of real value. He spent two years trying to find a restaurant owner who would pay him a small royalty in exchange for the use of that recipe. He made over *one thousand* sales calls before anybody took him seriously. The rest is restaurant history. The Colonel's face is now all over the place. Giving up is always the easy way out in the short term, and the hardest thing to live with in the long run. (Please note that while we admire the Colonel's persistence and success, we don't endorse fried foods on the THINNER WINNERS program).

4) You have to learn from your mistakes. That's what mistakes are for. They show you where to correct your course. Winners learn from their mistakes and head back to the drawing board. They don't quit. In fact, they never give up. They do make corrections when the plan they were following wasn't giving them the results they wanted. They look closely at what is working and what isn't. Then they make adjustments and get back into action again. They keep following this corrective procedure until they get the results they want. That's what you need to do with your weight

control program ... you will have to personalize it until it works your way.

5) You have to do whatever it takes to get the job done. If that means giving up your favorite triple-scoop ice cream cones, then you do it. If it means exercising every day, then you do that. Everything worth having has a price, and a trade off. You have to create a state of balance and then work to maintain that balance. You can't realistically expect to keep your old bad habits and get good health and weight control results. It won't happen. So you give up the old habits. And you reap the benefits of good health and good looks.

I recently saw a movie called "Rudy" that expresses these principles wonderfully. This was the amazing, true story about a young man who set as his life's goal the unlikely prospect of playing football for Notre Dame. It was an unlikely prospect for Rudy Ruettiger because of several factors. He was too small. Nobody in his family had ever gone to college before. His family members ridiculed his dream and tried to discourage him from stepping outside of "family expectations". He wasn't a very good student ... he was prone to daydreaming in class. But Rudy had a fire in his belly. From the time he was quite young he had been preparing himself mentally for being on the team. He had a recording of inspiring speeches by the legendary Notre Dame coach, Knute Rockne. Rudy memorized those speeches, word for word. Finally, he saved up enough money to leave his little town. He also had to leave behind his fiancée who had expected the money to be used as the down payment on their honeymoon cottage. So Rudy headed out alone.

The first thing he found out was that he didn't have the grades to qualify for Notre Dame. But a sympathetic priest helped him get into the local junior college. Then he went to see Ara Parsegian, the Notre Dame football coach. He told the coach that he was going to be on the team. To say the least, Parsegian didn't take him seriously. He wasn't a great student, so he found a tutor. He didn't have much money, so he got a job as a groundskeeper at the university football stadium ... at least he was in the stadium and on the field! He persisted through several years of difficult, trying times until he was finally accepted into Notre Dame. Then he showed up for "open tryouts" for the football team, where hopefuls get put through their paces. He had such spirit and tenacity that he made the cut. He was now on the team. The "second" team. These are the players who the starters practice against. In other words Rudy became a walking, talking tackling dummy. He spent day after day, month after month, year after year being pummeled by men who were twice his size. But he never gave up and he never backed down. His dream now was to play "officially" in a game. All this time, his family didn't even believe that he was even on the football team. But Rudy persisted ... he wanted to share his accomplishment with his father. So the big day finally came (you knew it would). But of course there were more obstacles to overcome. There was a new coach, who had just started and who could care less about Rudy. It was the last game Rudy could ever possibly play in, because he was scheduled to graduate. It was down to the last five minutes. And then something magical happened. The players on the Notre Dame team believed in Rudy's positive spirit so much that they started to chant his name. They really wanted the coach to put him in. Then the cheerleaders picked up the chant. Soon the entire crowd of tens of thousands was chanting "Rudy, Rudy, Rudy". What was the poor coach going to do? He put Rudy into the game. Of course Notre Dame won and the team carried Rudy out of the stadium on their shoulders. It was a wonderful, heartwarming tale filled with important messages about belief, expectations, overcoming obstacles and persistence. Trust me, when you've stayed at your goal weight for a whole year you'll know the crowd is chanting your name, too!

Find heroes and heroines of your own. They're all over the place. In the papers, the movies, on television. Libraries are filled with biographies of famous people. And plenty of them had to overcome horrendous obstacles ... but they weren't quitters. If they had been you never would have heard their names. Make a list of these winners and observe their attitudes. The winning qualities that they all share is what you're learning about in this book. You can learn so much and be greatly inspired by high-caliber role models.

Walk in the footsteps of Buddha and Jesus, rise above the challenges of Everest, determine to win the Olympics. Others have done these things and more. I'm thin now and so are plenty of other former heavy-weight champs. It's not a fluke ... it's attitude, beliefs and a good plan to follow. You can do it, too!

NLP is a practical, no-nonsense approach to accomplishing your goals. It may have a bit less appeal for you than some other approaches that sound easier, but if you really plan on being successful at controlling your weight for an extended period these are basic strategies that you'll incorporate into your program.

With the right frame of mind, belief in yourself and a driving, non-stop persistence you will succeed.

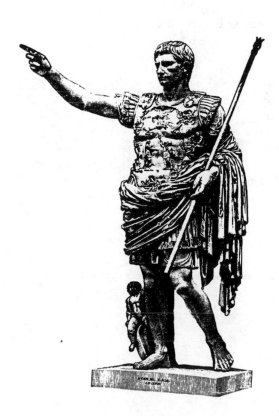

"Hey, isn't that Clint Eastwood over there?"

In A Nutshell

1) Allow your imagination to stretch your dreams, and allow your heart the expectation of fulfilling them. Expect greatness!

2) Expect the best for yourself. The results can be surprisingly good. Expect to be successful.

3) Don't waste your time ... use it constructively and fill it with positive, present moment thoughts or positive, expectant future thoughts.

4) Winners aim for the openings. They know where they're headed. They plan, take action and don't let obstacles get them down.

5) Beginner's Luck happens when you don't know that you can't do something ... so you do it.

6) Luck happens when opportunity meets preparation. "There ain't no free lunch".

7) Neuro-Linguistic Programming (NLP) techniques get you positive results by modeling the behaviors and attitudes of winners. Act like a slim person and you will become one.

8) Find heroes and heroines you identify with and emulate their winning qualities.

9) There are five key NLP steps to ultimate success:
   a) Know what you want, and expect to accomplish it.
   b) Take action according to a proven strategy or plan.
   c) Be persistent.
   d) Learn from your mistakes. Take corrective measures, and then try it again.
   e) Do whatever you have to do to get the job done.

10) Remember Rudy!

Visualization and Dream Books   7

"What is life without a dream?"
Edmond Rostand

Creating a New Self-Image

All animal life on Earth has some sort of brain. Birds, bees, dogs and frogs all have brains. As a general rule, the larger the brain, the more you can do with it. Note that your brain (hardware or "wetware" as computer buffs call it) is not the same as your mind (which can be considered similar in ways to the software or operating instructions). The human brain and mind differ from those of other animals through our large capacity to manipulate the information that we take in. During thousands of years of careful observation we have learned quite a few things about the incredible way our brains and minds work. Here are some of the highlights:

1) Your brain and mind have a virtually unlimited capacity to store and manipulate information.
2) Your brain and mind, in combination, store every thought, feeling and perception you have ever had, often through the use of complex visual images.
3) In general, you tend to store new information in a haphazard manner, but you can train your mind to store information in ways that are more effective in achieving your desires.
4) Your conscious mind, which you can directly influence, can only concentrate on one thought at a time.
5) Your conscious mind often "thinks" and learns through pictures or visualizations. These are incredibly complex combinations of thoughts.
6) You often "remember" by recalling mental pictures. Remember, one picture is worth a thousand words.
7) You "imagine" by creating mental pictures.
8) You react physically and emotionally to the images in your mind.
9) Your subconscious mind functions with computer-like precision in a non-evaluative fashion. It processes information according to instructions you have provided ... whether you're aware of doing this or not. It takes in, and takes seriously, everything you think about. Through repetitious thinking you are continually reprogramming your subconscious mind to fulfill your most prevalent thought instructions. What you think about, good or bad, tends to manifest in your life.
10) You can control the images in your mind through certain easy-to-learn techniques.
11) By planning and deliberately programming the images in your mind you can influence your actions and the resulting outcomes.
12) By predetermining your desired actions and outcomes you can effectively control and engineer your future.

What is the conclusion this leads to? Incredibly, that it is possible for you to effectively control and predict your own future. Impossible, you say! Only if you think so. Through the efforts of vast numbers of people studying many different groups of successful "winners" and "losers" for decades, it can now be stated with some assurance that the primary perception or image you have of yourself is where you will most likely end up. Or as Earl Nightingale said, "You become what you think about".

How does this work? Let's use a hypothetical example. Barbie Ballet always wanted to be a ballerina. From the time she was a little girl, and saw her first ballet, she surrounded herself with the trappings of dancing. She put up ballet posters in her bedroom. She listened to ballet themes on the stereo. She read books about famous ballerinas. She started taking dancing lessons as soon as she could. In her mind, she danced the most famous ballets on the stages of the great theaters of the world. Because Barbie was such a devotee of dancing, she never missed a lesson. Not only that ... she always practiced diligently, and was well prepared for her next class. Eventually, and to no one's particular surprise, she became the lead dancer in her school. Soon, she was helping the instructors give classes. When a traveling ballet company came to her town, she bought front row tickets. When ballet auditions were held, Barbie was the first in line. Guess what? Today, Barbie is a ballerina on tour around the world.

"Well, that's great for Barbie", you're saying, "but what about me?" Let's take another look. It all started in Barbie's mind. When she was so little that she could barely skip across a room without tripping, she could dance the lead role of a complex ballet in her mind. All she had to do was close her eyes, the music in her head started up ... and she was dancing. Now obviously there's more to it than that. It takes more than mental pictures viewed once or twice to bring actual physical results. Otherwise, everybody would be thin, drive a Rolls Royce and live in a castle. Imagination is only the beginning. But it is critical.

It took creative imagination for Barbie to activate the visualization process. Actively imagining allowed her to go from merely watching a mental ballet to being able to dance the lead role on stage. She had plenty of work to do, but first she had to dream it. You've got to have a dream to make a dream come true. Without the vividly visualized images she never would have been motivated enough to get the job done. Getting the job done is what counts. And that is exactly what you are going to do. In your mind, you are going to put yourself in the starring role. Then you're going to get the job done!

Front Row Center ... You!

Picture this clearly in your mind: You're at a giant three-ring circus with a huge red and white canvas tent. There are thousands of people in the bleachers and tons of people milling around. You're swept along by the crowd. It smells like popcorn and fresh straw ... and animals. There are cages lined up full of lions, tigers and bears. You hear some growling and turn to look! A clown walks by and honks his nose at you. All of a sudden you're sitting in the best seat in the house, front row center, looking up at Lilly Lollapalooza the flying trapeze artist as she does a series of three triple back flips ... and then miraculously lands in the seat right next to you! She smiles and then says, "Thanks for saving my spot".

Chances are good that, as you read the descriptive scene above, your creative imagination generated a mental picture to go along with the words. Did you see it? Were you there? What color was Lilly's outfit in your vision? What color was her hair? How were you able to "see" all this?

Your Mind's Eye

We are born with three eyes. Two eyes are designed to see the physical world, plus a very special third eye whose purpose is to see inside our own minds. This special internal vision is often called our "Mind's Eye". With your mind's eye you can read the words on this page and, if they describe objects and events, actually see the action in your mind. It is possible for you to get so caught up

in a story that you can get "lost in the pages of a good book". You can fall in love with the main characters and hate the villains. You can travel on great journeys and even escape the bounds of time ... all in your mind. Quick ... what did Rhett Butler say to Scarlet O'Hara as he walked out of her life in "Gone With the Wind"? Was he wearing a hat when he said it? It's amazing what little tidbits of information you have stored away in your mind.

In your mind it's possible for you to do almost anything and become almost anyone, anywhere, anytime. Think of the comic strip "Calvin and Hobbes" ... Calvin truly has a boundless imagination. And so do you. Your thoughts are not limited in any way by time or space. You can relive your favorite movie scenes over and over if you wish. You can hold conversations with people who are far away and out of touch, or even dead.

You can also get very emotionally involved in your internal dialogues. Conversations often continue when people part company ... sometimes they can go on for years in the minds of the participants. Our minds are amazing storehouses of information. They hold everything that we have ever seen, smelled, tasted, heard, touched and done in our entire lives. It's all in there.

Picture Yourself as a Winner

Now you are about to learn one of the fastest and easiest ways available for you to preprogram your mind for success. The people who win at the game of weight control are the people who choose to win. They do what it takes! Whatever it takes. They "make up their minds" to win! They don't quit and won't even consider giving up. The reason that they keep persisting is because they have such a clear picture of success in their mind's eye that they are compelled to keep going until they do succeed. Pictures ... it all comes back to pictures. With a clear enough visualization it almost becomes automatic to fulfill the picture you have created for yourself in your mind. All of this information has been building up to a specific conclusion. It's time for you to start visualizing yourself as a winner, too.

It is possible for you to reprogram your mind. The issue now becomes ... what are you going to put in there? It's no coincidence that all popular fast food restaurant chains repeatedly advertise that their food is fun, "hip", inexpensive, convenient and tasty and that they never, ever say that their foods are high in fat, cholesterol, salt and sugar, low in fiber and vitamins, and ultimately a fast trip to high blood pressure and other obesity-related illnesses. They deliberately attempt to program your mind with what they want you to believe. Whether it's good for your health or not. And it generally isn't. The finest advertising minds in history have been paid billions of dollars to plug these messages into your mind. And guess what? Those messages are in there! I'll bet you can hum at least two burger jingles right now without thinking much about it. Your brain is filled with messages put there by other people. Don't you think it might be a good idea to plant some ideas of your own?

Winners visualize themselves winning in advance. We know that the people who own "Big Belly Burgers" are winning. People flock in droves to eat those greasy burgers and fries. Their definition of winning is to make a lot of money by selling low-cost food at a nice high mark-up. Your definition of winning is to be slim and healthy ... there is a serious conflict here. It boils down to one simple question ... who do you want to win?

Assuming, at this point, that you want to be the winner, you must learn to fight fire with fire. The advertisers do not pull punches ... they continually tell you to buy another greasy burger or bucket of fried chicken, and they're not going to stop until pigs can fly ... if they ever do. To counteract this advertising onslaught you must substitute your own positive messages into your mind. The following technique can help you do just that.

Your Dream Book

A Dream Book is basically a book of pictures with accompanying affirmations (see Chapter 9 "Self-Talk and Affirmations"). Just like one of those little kid's picture books. However, from an adult perspective, you can think of your pictures as the keys to reprogramming your thoughts. By carefully selecting the images for your Dream Book based on your current desires, you are pointing your mind in the direction that you want to go. Where your mind goes, you will surely follow.

The visualization concept is simple, but the power of a Dream Book is tremendous. This is due to the way our minds use images to process information. Our minds have evolved in such a way as to maximize the usage of our brain's capacity. The merest glimpse of a mental picture is enough to bring back a flood of memories and life experiences. So there is great truth in the expression, "One picture is worth a thousand words". However, simply using words falls far short in terms of the information they can provide.

Do you know why we have come to use picture books for little children? For starters, if they're young enough, they can't read yet. But their minds are still processing new information at an incredible volume and rate of speed. They are learning how to think. And they are learning how to think in pictures. They can't talk and they can't read, but

they are developing concepts and learning to understand the world around them. Sights, sounds, tastes, smells, touches ... all swirling around in their rapidly developing minds. All being processed with the aid of mental images. Information is entering the child's mind in vast, immeasurable quantities. The combinations are virtually endless.

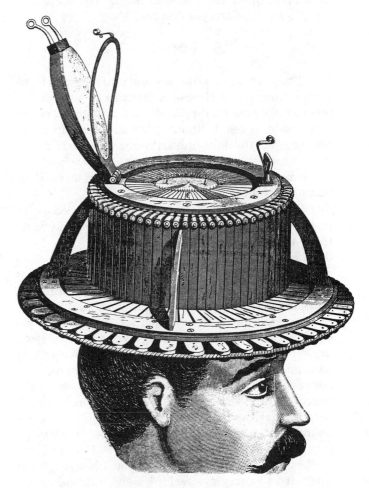

Most minds aren't this well organized.

Eventually all this input begins to gel. The child begins to make sense of her world. She begins to crawl, speak and test the world by interacting with it. There isn't a day that goes by without at least a zillion new pieces of information being processed by that young mind. She continues to store and process the incredible volume of information by using pictures in her mind. And that's what you've been doing with all the information that's been going into your mind ... for your entire life! How many days have you been alive? Multiply that number by a zillion and it will give you some idea of how much information is floating around in your head. It's quite a bit, isn't it?

Now consider the fact that you never did file all that stuff in any particular order. Whoops. But still it's all in there. It keeps popping up, sort of at random. Well, no wonder you can never remember where you left your glasses. And no wonder when you start getting hungry you think about those "supremely tasty, amazingly cheap and ever so convenient" fast food grease-burgers. The odds are good that you have far more grease-burger and cheese-slathered pizza ads circulating in your mind than most other food-related input. There aren't a lot of asparagus ads playing on TV.

Focus

The purpose of a dream book is to help you focus on the things you choose to happen in your life ... instead of being manipulated and influenced solely by outside forces. Without this focus you can easily fall prey to the swirling info-mass of your mind. With focus you can target your thoughts where you want them to go. And where your mind leads, your body will follow.

Since your goal is to lose weight you need to put messages and images in your mind of yourself being thin and healthy. As this chapter has been describing, the reason for this is so your subconscious mind can develop an internal "program" that defines you as slim and trim. You want your mind to work in ways that will get you to your goal faster.

In large measure, your actual, current physical body was shaped by the image your subconscious mind pictured. All those internalized messages that have been randomly popping into your head for your entire life have created the person you see in the mirror today. Messages such as: "Food is love", "I hate food without sauce", "Mexican food is always festive and happy", "You have to be crazy to go jogging at six in the morning", "If I wear loose clothes nobody will see my stomach hanging over my belt", "I carry my weight well", "Grandma ate anything she wanted, lived to be ninety-nine, and was never sick a day in her life", "Exercise is for jocks and mindless cheerleaders", "I can't help it, I was born fat", "I'm large-boned".

The tendency is for your subconscious mind, which is nothing less than the "program" for your life, to generate a lifestyle which is a self-fulfilling prophecy of the picture it has of you. This is important ... you will inevitably act to conform with your own internalized, subconscious view of yourself. In order to effect permanent changes in your life it is necessary to reprogram your own mind for positive results. The results you want.

Words and Pictures

The next time you're flipping through a newspaper or magazine and you see one of those all-too-prevalent diet pill ads with a size 3 girl holding out, at arm's length, the waistline of a pair of size 58 pants, cut out the picture and then cut off the girl's head. Show no mercy. Then take a photo of yourself and cut off your body. (For men use a picture of your favorite athlete). What happens next is a combination of Frankenstein, art director and applied psychology. Get a piece of heavy paper and paste your head on your "new body". Then get a wide-tipped marker and underneath the picture write "I feel great in my new size eight ... and I'm really glad I lost the weight" (or the affirmation of your choice). The "magic" of this process is that your computer-like subconscious mind will input this picture and caption of the "new you" under the general category of "This is how I am". Then your subconscious mind will begin to shape you into the person that fits the new internal model. And you now have the first entry in your Dream Book. If you want to change your body, you need to give your mind a new picture of what you want. So it can go to work to bring that to you.

From now on, every time you find a picture of a person who looks the way you would like to look, or is engaged in an activity that you would like to be doing (such as line-dancing or playing tennis), cut it out and put it in your Dream Book. Try to have a hundred pages or more if you can. The more images, the stronger your mind's understanding will be of what you want. Write a caption or affirmation for every picture, and keep in mind that everything you say will be used by your subconscious mind to begin generating the "new you". You are beginning to take control of your own mind.

Spend some time every day slowly taking a mental journey on your new life path, by savoring the pictures and reading each caption carefully. Allow the messages to burn into your subconscious mind: "It feels wonderful being in control of my weight", "I never felt so self-assured as I do now that I'm thin", "I enjoy feeling healthy", "I enjoy exercising ... I always feel strong and energized when I work-out".

Keep in mind that this is no childish pipe-dream into never-never land. What you are doing is deliberately counteracting a lifetime of negative self-images and replacing them with positive ones. You are specifically taking processing time away from the negative advertising morass and your own negative, destructive internal images. You are putting into your mind exactly what you want to go into your mind.

There are a few more guidelines by which our minds operate that you should know about. One is called the Primacy Effect. So called because we tend to remember very clearly the first "facts" we learned about a subject. That's why George Washington's most noteworthy accomplishment always seems to be cutting down that cherry tree. We learned it from a picture-book or story when we were three years old. We could picture it clearly, and still can. The other very important mental operating principle is called the Recency Effect ... we remember very clearly the things we put into our minds most recently. You are about to take full advantage of the recency effect by making sure that the last thing you put into your mind is always something positive about your self-image.

That's why your Dream Book will become a very powerful and important tool for you. Its purpose is to replace the images that may have been holding you back with ones that will drive you forward. It provides you with a ready, organized and focused source of positive images and statements for you to feed your ever-hungry brain.

Overcome Resistance with Persistence

If you run into feelings of resistance as you are working on your first few pictures and captions, pay special attention to the "self-talk" that pops into your head (see Chapter 9 "Self-Talk and Affirmations"). Be ever vigilant to the words used by "Mr. Counter-Productivity" who lives inside your brain. When "Mr. Counter-Productivity" says "This is stupid, everybody eats at Greaso's", what you're hearing is a lifetime's worth of negative programming.

For a while there may be a battle between your conscious mind, with your stated goal of getting thin, and your subconscious (computer/robot) mind with it's objective of maintaining equilibrium. "Mr. Counter-Productivity" wants to keep you where you are. He lives in your comfort zone, and isn't the least bit interested in leaving. Right now your counter-productive, robot mind has more messages describing you as fat than your "Ms. Thinbody" has thin images of you. "Mr. Counter-Productivity" has been known to be so resistant to change that even with a physician's warning of impending death it will sometimes continue on its merry way. The way to beat him is with persistence. You must empower your personal "Ms. Thinbody". She will grow stronger through repetition.

For a while you may feel like you're in one of those cartoons with an angel on one shoulder and a little devil on the other. If you look carefully, you'll see that the angel (Ms. Thinbody) is thin and healthy and the devil (Mr. Counter-Productivity) is fat and has food dribbling down his chin.

As mentioned earlier, your conscious mind can only hold or process one thought at a time. It is your sworn duty as an aspiring Thinbody to make sure that the current thought in your mind is a positive, thin thought. It may take some serious work,

focused energy and skill development on your part. "Mr. Counter-Productivity" may fight you every step of the way for quite a while. But eventually, if you are persistent and consistent with your positive inputs, you will find that it gets progressively easier to hold those positive thoughts. Keep at it, it's worth it!

Actions Speak Louder than Words

Getting those positive thoughts to stick in your mind is a tremendous accomplishment. Not only will you have succeeded in overcoming negative self-talk but you get a spectacular added benefit: *positive thoughts feel good!*

But the best is yet to come. Your positive thoughts will energize you and empower you to take further control of your life. Positive thoughts will drive you to action. When you read "I enjoy exercising regularly to stay slim and healthy" beneath the athletic picture in your Dream Book, you'll find yourself saying, "Yeah, and it's time for me to exercise". And you will exercise. Your new self-image will encourage, and nearly demand it. You'll feel energized and proud of yourself when you're done. And your subconscious mind will get hit with a double whammy. The combination of the image, the affirmation and the activity will program your robot brain into a positive feedback loop. Instead of thinking "Exercise ... Yuck ... Better get a donut ... I'm fat ... I hate myself", you'll start thinking "Exercise ... firm muscles ... self control ... confidence ... good health ... I feel great" (see Chapter 15 "Managing The Food-Mood Connection").

It's the actions and results that you are really after. All the good intentions in the world will not add a single ounce of muscle or lose a pound of fat. But with the right internal messages and attitudes, your new activity levels will help you conquer the world. And you can do it much more easily than you may think (see Chapter 23 "Creating An Active Lifestyle").

See Your Future, Be Your Future

The stronger you picture the benefits that await you, and the more you practice taking control of your thoughts with images, the easier it will become. Ultimately, you will think like a thin person and therefore have the actions and results of a thin person automatically. If you practice your mental reprogramming techniques enough (regularly for at least a month or two) they will gradually become habits. After that it will be automatic and natural for your mind to begin generating positive thoughts. You won't have to consciously think about replacing fat images with thin ones. Just like riding a bike, learning to type or preparing a new recipe, acting thin and thinking thin will become "normal" and natural for you over time.

For right now, PRACTICE, PRACTICE, PRACTICE your new, positive agenda. This will move you towards being thin much faster than spending your precious time battling negative "old" thoughts of difficulty and failure. What you tell yourself about this journey to Thinland will be what you experience. Choose the route that you prefer: "A long hard row to hoe" or "an enlightening, empowering, exciting adventure ... filled with discovery and positive personal choices". You can lose the weight and become permanently thin by choice, and enjoy the trip along the way.

Now you have some powerful tools ... practice with them until you develop strong skills and you will succeed. You will inevitably bring into being what you see in your mind. Picture success!

In A Nutshell

1) Your brain is designed to maximize the use of your creative intelligence.

2) You can retrain your mind by changing the pictures and messages you send your mind.

3) You can control and predict your future by pre-selecting the thoughts and actions of your choice. If you don't fill your mind by choice, others (such as advertisers) will anyway.

4) Winners visualize themselves winning in advance. In order to effect permanent changes it is necessary for you to reprogram your own mind so you visualize yourself thinner and healthier.

5) With the right internal pictures you can compel yourself to win, and automatically fulfill your specific goals.

6) A Dream Book helps you visualize and control your internalized pictures.

7) Start your Dream Book now, and fill it with the images and messages you want for your future.

8) Be persistent ... PRACTICE DAILY. Due to the Recency Effect you will remember most clearly the most recent thoughts you allow into your mind.

9) Your Dream Book helps develop your positive images into positive thoughts and actions.

10) Positive thoughts feel good and positive actions look good on you.

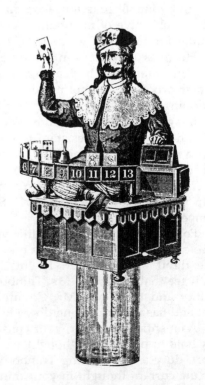

"I see a healthier heart in your future."

Goal Setting and Treasure Maps   8

"Oh yet we trust that somehow good will be the final goal ..."
Alfred Lord Tennyson

Have you ever wondered what the future will bring? Most people wonder about their futures. But only a select few actually have a realistic idea about what their futures hold for them. How do these fortunate individuals know where they will be and what they will accomplish in the months and years to come? They set goals and follow a plan! If you want to accomplish the big things in your life, too, you need to have goals.

Your Road Map to Success

If you were in Los Angeles and wanted to drive to New York, and you didn't have a map, how would you get there? You could rely on general knowledge. Everyone you ask says that New York is east of Los Angeles. So you head east. And before you know it you're in Wilmington, South Carolina ... which is directly east of Los Angeles.

This is actually closer than most people get to planning their futures. It's more typical to find people with only the vaguest idea about where they would like to end up. And due to the lack of a specific destination, plan or detailed strategy they are more likely to find themselves in places they never intended to go. Like a guided missile without a gyroscope, many people go through life without ever being sure where they are really headed. They get blown along with the ever-shifting winds of change. Instead of making conscious adjustments to keep on a chosen course they continually react to unrelated information which sends them off in new and different directions.

But no more of that for you! In order to get to a specific destination, whether it's a city , a well-filled bank account or a particular goal weight, you can improve your ability to get there by setting a specific goal, writing down a step-by-step strategy to reach that goal and then making appropriate corrections along the way. Now it's time to draw a map for your goal of weight control.

Setting Your Subconscious Mind on Course

Your subconscious mind acts like an internal guidance system. When you set it to go in a specific direction it will keep you moving that way. It is a highly refined, almost magical, part of your mental equipment, constantly monitoring your thoughts and readjusting your direction toward your goals. Whether you realize it or not, your subconscious mind is continually listening to your self-talk (see Chapter 9 "Self-Talk and Affirmations"). The secret to ultimate success is to make sure that the information you feed your subconscious mind is crystal clear regarding your goals because that is what it will act upon.

To illustrate, let's take the ever-popular "Tropical Dream" that many people have. You're basking on a secluded beach, with palm trees swaying and gentle music playing. A tuxedoed waiter walks up with a tall frosty drink on a silver tray. He hands you the drink and then disappears, mysteriously. Ah, paradise! It's a great vision. Advertising firms use it liberally. Can you see yourself in this dream? Do you want this glorious event to become a reality in your life? Then really concentrate on that vision in your mind's eye. Get a clear picture of the scene, including the smallest details. For instance, see the condensation running down the sides of the glass. Try to use all five senses when creating this multi-sense image. Then get out a piece of paper and write down exactly how you want your perfect tropical dream to materialize in your life. These are the first steps ... getting a clear, precise and sense-laden visualization and then writing it down. This process energizes and focuses your subconscious mind. It begins to steer you in the direction of this target visualization.

The Chain of Events

One event always follows another and there is a specific sequence of events that leads towards any goal. In the Tropical Dream, you ate lunch at the hotel's patio restaurant shortly before walking out to your lounge chair on the beach. Before that you were checking into your hotel room. Before that the hotel limousine picked you up at the airport. Before that you were taking a first class plane flight. Before that you called your travel agent to arrange for the trip to the tropics. Before that you decided when you would take your vacation. Before that you were arranging for the money to pay for your trip. Before that you were sitting in your lounge chair at home doodling palm trees and the names of tropical islands on a pad of paper. Each step leads logically to the next. When you write down the individual steps to achieve your goal in a logical order, and can see that each step is attainable, you are well on your way towards accomplishing your goals. The more details that you account for in your goal planning the easier it will be for you to see success as attainable. These same principles apply to planning a vacation or enjoying the benefits of a successful weight control program.

What still remains, of course, is developing the necessary motivation that will drive you into action to achieve your goals. You have to do the work required by each step along the way. Each step that you complete brings you closer to your final goal. There are several techniques that can help you. Treasure Mapping is coming up. (See Chapter 7 "Visualization and Dream Books" and Chapter 9 "Self-Talk and Affirmations".)

Which brings us back to the important question: Where do you want to go? And, of course, the all-important supplemental questions: When do you plan to have your goal accomplished and what do you need to do to get there?

Progressive Goals :
The Carrot on the Stick

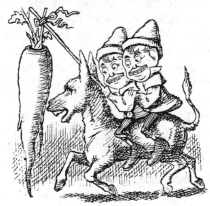

*A well-placed carrot
does wonders for motivation.*

First of all you should have a clear idea of where you want to end up (your goal weight), and when. You must first select a goal weight that is both attainable and highly rewarding to you. Generally, this will be the lowest weight that you have maintained for at least one year during the past five to ten years. It's very important however that you set a realistic goal. If you are 100 pounds overweight and wear size 20 clothes, it is not realistic to set a goal of losing 100 pounds and wearing size 8 within six months. While it might be physically possible to do so, by using diet pills and fasting, you would be seriously compromising your

health. You are far more likely to end up discouraged and unfulfilled ... and back at your starting weight like a yo-yo.

A far more sensible approach would be to set a goal of dropping 25 pounds over the next six months. One pound a week on the average would be your short-term goal. This is realistic, attainable and healthier. What's more, that 25 pounds will probably be lost permanently.

In order to accomplish this you will have to change both your eating, thinking and activity habits. You will have to ease up on certain high fat foods and replace them with healthier substitutes. You will have to exchange several hours a week of sofa-spud time and for aerobic activities. You will have to substitute positive self-talk for the negative, circular mental conversations that keep you overweight. During the first few months you will be finding out how your body actually responds to your new routine. It may turn out that you lose 20 pounds in the first three months, or it may be difficult for you to make the transition to a more active lifestyle ... so you may lose five pounds.

After three months, take the time for a review session. Ask yourself if you are on track towards your six month goal. Are you averaging 1 pound per week? Base your next 3 months of eating and activity behaviors on your results so far and your level of motivation. It's important to stay enthusiastic, and you can maintain your motivation by achieving your short term goals. If the goals you set were unrealistic and you didn't achieve them, it will be easy to get discouraged and sidetracked from the program.

Take a close look at your behavior and your results. If you have been comfortably eating 1200 calories a day and exercising 6 hours a week and you lost 15 pounds in the last three months, this may also be a realistic goal for your next three months. In order to achieve consistent results you need to be able to maintain consistent habits. Sorry, that's just the way it is ... hit or miss won't get you there. Keep your long term weight goal in mind, but fine-tune your objectives and make bite-sized, short-term goals you can achieve along the way to keep your motivation up.

For example, if your regular exercise routine (after 3 months) consists of briskly walking 2 miles, four times a week, you might decide to increase your activity additionally by joining a softball league. You reset your exercise goal by committing to have 5 days of exercise each week. You decide to re-evaluate your status after 3 more months. After a total of six months on your program you may well find that you are deriving additional benefits from your increased activity levels: (1) You are burning up more calories (2) You feel better because you're moving around more (3) You're making friends with "active" people, which is a very important factor for your success because there is a strong tendency for people to pick up the habit patterns of the people around them. Having active friends will help you with your weight control program far more than hanging out with "munching buddies".

As a reward for the extra activity you're now doing you decide to go to a professional baseball game with one of your new softball pals. To conclude this example: You're feeling better about yourself, you're more active, and you found out it wasn't all that bad to get moving. It's hard to believe that just six months ago you were a card-carrying couch potato.

Your overall objective on the THINNER WINNERS program is to not only lose weight but to develop the skills necessary to maintain your healthy new lifestyle. Just like a guided missile, you will have to continually watch the variables and make adjustments to stay on course. You might decide to change your primary form of exercise, only to discover that you aren't burning as many calories as before. You may have to deal with food cravings and emotional conflicts related to your lifestyle change. Remain on your toes and be flexible. By keeping your goals in mind you will come closer and closer to achieving them.

A simple, straight-forward goal might read: I enjoy weighing $\underline{X}$ pounds and wearing my size $\underline{X}$ clothes. (You fill in the X's of your choice.)

For your goals to have maximum effectiveness:

1) **Put them in writing.** And sign them! It's a sign of commitment.
2) **Have a clear understanding of why you want to achieve the goal.** Is it a burning desire of yours? Does the goal excite you? If it does, nothing will stop you from reaching your goal. If it doesn't excite you, adjust it until it does.
3) **Be very specific** as to the details. The more details you can describe and envision the easier it will be to actually see the goal as already accomplished in your mind.
4) **Have a step-by-step action plan** for accomplishing the goal. Even a simple goal can have many steps. Map them out in the proper sequence so you know what to do, and in what order. You can also tell how close you are to achieving the goal at any given point.
5) **Have a deadline for accomplishment.** Nothing will get you going as well as a good, solid target date.
6) **Set deadlines that are realistic** for the specific goal. Your mind must be able to grasp the concept of your goal and see it as attainable. Losing 50 pounds over a year and learning to maintain that level is realistic. Losing 30 pounds in a month is not. Set goals that drive you to action and are possible to do in the allotted time.
7) **Review your goals often.** Many motivational trainers recommend that you rewrite your goals each morning to set your mind towards finding ways to achieve them daily. Try it!
8) **Get going!** If you expect to achieve your goals the time to start is NOW! This turns a dream or wish into a solid goal and an accomplished project.

By carefully planning your goals and the methods you will use to reach them, you can know, with some assurance, just what your future will bring.

Treasure Mapping

Treasure Mapping is a technique that goes along perfectly with your written goals and plans. You know from other lessons in this program that you can address the issues of mental reprogramming from a number of angles. In addition to goal setting, these include visualization, positive self-talk, affirmations, and meditation. Treasure Mapping is one of the most fun. It is also a very effective visual and affirmation technique. The purpose of Treasure Mapping is to draw specific energies towards you. In a way, the idea is to turn yourself into a magnet for the things you want to be, have or do.

The way to make a Treasure Map is simple and fun. Take a large piece of heavy paper or cardboard. Choose a background color that energizes you, like gold or hot pink. Place a photograph of yourself in the middle of the sheet with a dab of glue or some scotch tape. Then find pictures of people have qualities that you admire and aspire to achieve, and surround your photo with them. These are your role models. Write an affirmation under your picture such as: "I have a slim, healthy body. I weigh X pounds and I love it. I attract good health and well-being to myself." Put your Treasure Map in a place where you will see it often, and imagine that you are drawing the positive energy from your selected goal pictures towards yourself. Draw power from the images.

As you can see, a Treasure Map is a combination of goals, Dream Book visualizations and affirmations. It can be large and conspicuous, or if you like, you can also make a small, wallet-size version to carry around with you. The idea, of course, is to constantly feed positive thoughts to your conscious and subconscious minds. Remember how your conscious mind works ... it can only concentrate on one thought at a time. If you eliminate negative images from your thoughts, everything that's left will be positive. And that's what you want.

Actually, all the positive energy you will ever need is already there in your mind. It may just be obscured by negative thoughts acquired through habit or neglect. Like a beautiful garden overgrown with weeds, you need only to clip back the vines to reveal the innate loveliness.

By the way, Treasure Mapping works equally well for gathering possessions or meaningful relationships to you. You can learn to draw anything to yourself by reaching out with your personal positive energy. Just remember the essentials: firm belief in your abilities, boundless faith in your possibilities, specific written step-be-step goals and a positive, focused mental attitude. When you nurture and develop these qualities, everything you desire will come to you... including being thin!

In A Nutshell

1) You need goals to clearly define, and therefore receive exactly, what you want in life. If you don't have inspiring goals of your own, you will always be acting to fulfill someone else's.

2) Put your goals in writing and make step-by-step plans for their attainment. How did they build the pyramids? One block at a time! Remember to break your goals into bite-sized, do-able chunks. Take a large goal (losing 137 pounds) and make smaller daily goals (I will have 20 grams of fat and exercise 30 30 minutes today). As you make progress every day, before long you will accomplish your goal.

3) Make both short and long-term goals and take regular status checks along the way.

4) By following your plans and making the necessary changes required you must inevitably achieve your goals.

5) Use supplemental motivational tools to help you keep your goals clearly in mind. These include Visualization, Treasure Maps, Dream Books and Affirmations.

6) Treasure Maps are powerful motivational tools which can draw positive energies towards   you. They combine Dream Book visualizations and Affirmations.

7) According to statisticians, only 5% or less of all people actively set goals for themselves. The other 95% lead undirected, less focused lives. Notice too that only 5% or less of the people who try to maintain their weight losses are successful over the long run. Hmm, makes you stop and think, doesn't it?

Self-Talk and Affirmations   9

"These success encourages: they can because they think they can."
                                                        Virgil

Talking to Yourself

The one thing that distinguishes us the most from our early ancestor, Og the hunter, is our use of language. Back in his time, thinking was much more visual and expressive, and communication was much more difficult. If Og wanted to tell Ogette where he caught the food they were in the process of eating, it was necessary for him to act out an elaborate ritualized dance. He simply didn't have the words to say "I spotted the steakasaurus by the south end of the lake, then tracked it for three hours before I got it". He had vivid pictures in his mind of all that he had done, but poor skills for sharing that knowledge with others. He had the concepts but not the language skills.

Modern day humans do have the concepts and the language skills to communicate effectively with peers. Our brains are larger and we can do more with them. We have become creatures of communication. We use pictures extensively, and we also use words. So much so that a complete English dictionary now weighs about fifty pounds! Of course we don't all personally use each and every one of those hundreds of thousands of words. We have our favorites ... a few thousand words that we use most often. Those words tend to define the boundaries of our knowledge. We are constantly checking our borders by using those words. We talk to ourselves.

In fact, this internal dialogue or "self-talk" seems to be an essential part of our thought process. If you question this, just try to stop your inner mental voice from talking for a while. It's doubtful that you'll be able to for very long, unless you go into some form of meditative state (see Chapter 11 "Breathing and Meditation").

This being the case, that you do talk to yourself all day long, doesn't it make sense to use this internal conversation to your benefit? You're darn tootin' it does. If you start seeing your self-talk as one of the most powerful tools you have, which it is, you'll be able to harness that power to propel yourself towards your goals much more rapidly.

Choosing your own self-talk puts you in direct control of your thoughts. If you simply let all your old "mental tapes" run over and over, out of habit, without questioning or being aware of them, you are giving up a huge opportunity to reshape any thoughts that have been holding you back in your weight control progress.

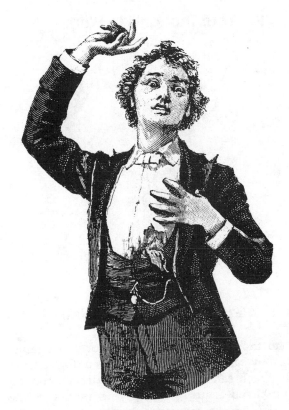

*"Oh no! I just realized
what I've been saying to myself all these years."*

For example, if you tell yourself that you "can't have pizza on a diet", then you might start craving pizza without even knowing why! Plus you are sending yourself the message that you are on a "diet" and therefore if you ever eat pizza again you must go "off" that diet! What a set-up for failure. I personally can't imagine life as I know it without pizza. On the other hand, if you recognize your specific self-talk and change it to: "I can have pizza in many ways, if ... :

1) "I choose lower fat cheeses and toppings, it will be healthier and I'll lose weight faster."

2) "I can learn to order a healthier variety when I eat out".

3) "I can learn to make a healthier version at home".

4) "I can learn to eat pizza and balance it with the rest of my food on a specific day, so I don't over-do it" ... etc.

What have you done? You've changed your own self-defeating self-talk into a message that gives you the choice of multiple options. It puts you in control and doesn't set up feelings of deprivation and possible failure. You have taken back your power to be flexible and successful. That's the power of self-talk.

Put Your Thoughts to Work

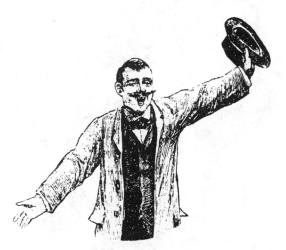

"It's a THINNER WINNERS day!"

Your thoughts can either work for you, against you, or they can spin you around like a dog chasing its tail (which can make you pretty dizzy). Having an internalized argument with your mother while you're driving to the store is probably not the highest and best use of your mind or your time. Getting your thoughts to work for you as much of the time as possible is a skill.

If we know that our internal dialogues run all day long, it makes sense to take charge of these thoughts in any way that we can. A powerful technique you can use to begin guiding your thoughts in your own chosen direction is an affirmation. These are carefully crafted, positive statements that you deliberately present to your mind. The affirmation concept is based on simple repetition. The result, on the other hand, is amazingly powerful, complex and positive.

In some ways our minds function like a vast labyrinth of caves. When a thought enters our conscious awareness it tends to continue on its own ... almost like an echo. Even when the thought is no longer in our awareness it continues to reverberate.

This analogy helps explain how, at times, thoughts "pop into our heads" unexpectedly. They are like echoes that worked their way to the surface of our consciousness. Your goal is to have these "echoing thoughts" be positive and of your own choosing.

Building Your Affirmations

Our thoughts are not limited by time. We can think about past, present or future events with equal ease. However, from a practical standpoint this can be very confusing, since the only "time" we really experience is the present. When you're driving down the freeway thinking about the movie you saw yesterday, you're actually doing it in the present. In effect you are using up your present time on a past event. Knowing that this "time warp" process is going on gives us the insight to construct an affirmation in a specific way. We live in the present. So to give our affirmations the most power we make them in the present tense.

1) An affirmation should be stated in the present tense.
2) It should be worded "as if" the goal has already been accomplished.
3) It should be short and to the point.

In addition, you should be able to see it in your mind, and it should energize and excite you. For example: "I love being at my goal weight of X pounds" is worded appropriately. When this affirmation echoes in your mind it will be positive, in the present tense and will serve to drive you to action relating to your goal. It is visual, briefly worded and exciting.

On the other hand if you say "I want to weigh X pounds" you are using a reference point in the future. This statement has very little lasting motivational power. Wanting to be something and actually being it (in your mind) are miles apart in terms of experience. "Wanting" is nothing but a wish, and it also sends the message to your mind that you are not at X pounds now. And "now" is all you have. In other words, you'll never weigh X pounds if you always see it in the future, instead of right now. Tricky, but true.

Here are some more examples of simple, positive affirmations you can use to boost your attitude:

"I can do it!" (simple, straight-forward and powerful)
"I am the best!"
"I feel wonderful today!"
"I smile at everyone I meet"
"I am a winner!"

Exercise: Now is the perfect time for you start using affirmations. Get your journal, workbook, a 3x5 card, a small piece of paper or your Daily Success Planner and write out an affirmation for yourself. Say your affirmation out loud three times. Say it as if you mean it, too! Don't just repeat the words ... convince yourself!

Exercise: Annie and Fannie are two people you know. Annie is always happy and upbeat, the kind of person who could light up a small town single-handedly. Fannie is just the opposite. She sucks energy out of everyone she gets near. Spend a few minutes imagining the differences in the self-talk between these two people. Fannie may say "I didn't lose weight this week. I'll never get to goal. I might as well give up. Where's the fudge sauce?". But Annie may say "I didn't lose any weight. Hmm, maybe I'm losing inches. I'll measure myself. I feel so much better and in control though. I'm making progress in lots of other ways. I know if I continue, I'll be healthier and I'll start losing again soon. In the meantime I'll try a new, healthy recipe, check to make sure I'm getting all my nutrients and take an extra walk. Wow! I can do this!". Same situation, different outcomes. Why? Different self-talk. Everything Annie thinks is positive and constructive. Everything Fannie thinks is negative and destructive. Now ask yourself which person you would rather spend the day with. And who do you think is going to end up losing weight?

Using Affirmations Effectively

The reasons that affirmations work is because your subconscious mind doesn't know the difference between past, present and future ... it experiences all thoughts in the present. In effect you are tricking your own mind into thinking something has occurred which hasn't taken place yet. Is this an ethical thing to do? It's your mind so you get to decide on questions of personal ethics. What's important is that it works.

It's also important to consider that your mind works in very subtle and complex ways. If it hears your affirmation stated as if you have already achieved your goal, your mind will begin to send out messages to the various parts of your body in such a manner that they will begin to comply with the affirmation. In essence, you are using the approach of "fake it until you make it". Your mind and body begin to act "as if" you are at your goal weight. If you see yourself there, you will get there faster. This is an immutable law of nature.

Your mind then draws on all its hidden resources to help you attain the affirmation. You will find yourself more inclined to exercise and less inclined to eat fatty foods, because this is in harmony with your new self-perception, as defined by your affirmation.

The whole purpose of affirmations is to focus your thinking on what you really want to accomplish. In other words, affirmations are specifically directed towards attaining your goals. Since you know that accomplishing any important goal takes effort, discipline and persistence, it's logical to assume that any thoughts you have that aren't goal oriented and positive are simply holding you back.

This being the case, it's important to repeat your affirmations frequently. Say them out loud when you're at home or in your car. It is also important to state them with strong conviction. Say your affirmations as if you believe them to be true with all your heart.

4)   Repeat your affirmations often during the day.
5)   State them out loud for additional emphasis. Try singing them!
6)   State them with conviction and belief.

The emotional factor is very important. This is what drives you to action. Let's look at a simple example:

Example A: Your self-talk says "I really have to lose weight. I know it's healthier and I have to do something about it. I wish I was thin".

This dialogue is powerless, flat, actually deflating and disheartening! It makes you want to stay in bed and pull the covers over your head.

Example B: Your affirmative self-talk says "I am thin, athletic and feel so energetic! I can wear anything and look great. I'm proud of my accomplishment and I help others when they ask how I did it. Life is great!"

WOW! With thoughts like that running through your mind you'll jump right out of bed fully charged. This dialogue is emotional, visual and energizing. Which do you prefer?

A well-applied affirmation will allow you to develop the power and motivation described in Example B. It is this sense of being pulled towards a desired outcome that will truly allow you to accomplish your goals in the shortest time possible. You'll be focused and alert. You'll be able to power through obstacles and you won't allow them to slow you down or hold you back ... because you can see beyond them now. An affirmation you're almost certainly familiar with is the phrase used in baseball, "Keep your eye on the ball, and put it over the wall". Many a big-name slugger has relied on this simple, powerful affirmation and combined it with visualization to improve their results.

To further increase the effective use of your affirmations you can write them on cards and post them in highly visible places ... like your bathroom mirror, refrigerator door and the dashboard of your car. Repeat them often and you'll be amazed by the results.

For additional self-reinforcing techniques see Chapter 7 "Visualization And Dream Books".

In A Nutshell

1) You are constantly talking to yourself as an essential part of your thought process.

2) Learn to use affirmations to focus your self-talk and thought processes on goals of your own choosing, not "old tapes" of thoughts that may be limiting your success.

3) To be most effective an affirmation should be:
   a) Stated in the present tense.
   b) Worded "as if" the goal has already been accomplished.
   c) Short and to the point.

4) To use an affirmation effectively:
   d) Repeat your affirmations often and consistently during the day.
   e) State them out loud for additional emphasis. Try singing them!
   f) State them with conviction and belief. Emotionalize them for more power.

5) Post affirmation cards where you will see them often. In sight, in mind!

Self-Acceptance and Self-Esteem   10

"Oft times nothing profits more than self-esteem grounded on just and right ..."
John Milton

Self-Acceptance

Peace of mind, and being able to value and love yourself just the way you are means learning to accept yourself "as is" in the present moment. This can be very difficult because the latest media or fashion industry values or our own expectations invite comparison. Even yesterday's stars rarely feel like they meet today's glamour standards. And of course, being fat in the current American culture is not considered the ideal condition. We are continually fed the message that overweight people are "weak-willed", "gluttons" or not too bright because they can't figure out how to stay at a normal weight. Prejudice against corpulence is rampant from the workplace to stand-up comedians. You may have to continually work at developing a positive acceptance of yourself, in the face of all this propaganda.

In the "Wizard of Oz" the scarecrow needed a diploma before he could state his knowledge with confidence. That piece of parchment allowed him to acknowledge and use the skills which he already possessed. The cowardly lion needed a medal to "prove" that he had courage. The tin man needed a symbolic heart before he could truly allow himself to express his feelings openly. They all needed some type of external symbol to show what they, in fact, had inside themselves all along.

How much like them are you? If you take a close look at yourself you'll realize that you have plenty of intelligence to do all the things you need to in your life. You've got courage, too. You keep on trying to control your weight. You're persistent ... and that's one of the most important qualities for accomplishing great deeds. You've got plenty of heart as well. You're probably swamped with feelings the better part of the time. You don't really need anything outside of yourself to affirm your value. In fact, the most important self-acceptance factor of all can only come from within ... believing in yourself.

Self-Esteem

Your self-esteem is the amount of value and respect you have for who you are and what you do. High esteem means high personal value. When you learn to hold yourself in high esteem you will feel stronger, more capable and unstoppable! You'll know you can do whatever you set out to accomplish!

What personal qualities or skills do you have that you consider valuable? Are you a good cook? Are you funny? Are you well-coordinated? Are you a positive thinker? Do you care about other people? Are you a hard worker? There might be a million such qualities. The complex of valuable life skills that you have helps determine your value in your own eyes. Recognize those skills as unique and wonderful and keep developing them.

Exercise: As a simple but important exercise, get out your journal and write down a list of all the things you can do and qualities that you have which you consider to be valuable. They don't have to be big things either. Always remembering to send your grandmother a Valentine's day card is just as important to the universe as winning a Nobel prize.

You are a valuable, completely unique person. There will never be another you! Explore who you are. Recognize the goodness and greatness within yourself. If you have doubts about the value being there, don't worry ... it's in all of us. You just have to be confident enough to bring out your best. Allow yourself the freedom to perceive and develop the unique talents you have been given.

Self-Love

Many people mistakenly think of self-love as an egotistical trait that has no place in the humble, good persons life. But just think about this: If you don't love what you are and who you are, then what do you really have to give all those people who you purportedly want to give your best? Not much, according to you. So loving yourself is actually the beginning of a larger, awakened ability to love and nurture everyone you touch. It's the key to a grander universe, and it all begins with you.

By learning to look within yourself with love you'll begin to recognize the universal qualities that we all share. It will allow you to love the divine presence within yourself and to honor all precious life. You'll develop a wonderful sense of empathy and compassion for others. You'll understand you can never really be alone because we're all part of the same universal source of life.

You'll experience more joy in life because you'll be able to enjoy other people's victories. You will also share in their sorrows when they occur, but these will lead you on to greater insights.

How do you go about developing this self-love? The only thing in life that you truly have complete and total control over is the thoughts and attitudes that you allow into your mind. Early computer programmers came up with an appropriate expression that applies here: "Garbage In, Garbage Out". The opposite is also true ... "Love In, Love Out". If you fill your mind with loving, self-accepting thoughts and ideas, then that's what you will have to give out. The finest thing that you can ever do for yourself and those you love most is to nurture your growth in positive directions that increase your self-esteem.

The Age of Self-Help

Self-acceptance and self-esteem are complex personal issues, and unfortunately there are no quick fixes for low levels of these feelings. You are the only person qualified to determine the acceptable levels for yourself. You are also the only person who can raise yourself into a happier state of being. Nobody can do that for you. It's up to you to care for and nurture yourself! The exciting, practical aspect of this emphasis on personal responsibility is simply that you have the opportunity to become more self-reliant. In doing so you will also come to feel stronger and more self-assured.

The self-help movement has been saying for years that you are responsible for your own health, behavior and mental well-being, as well as for maximizing the quality of your own life. This doesn't mean that you can't turn to others for help, advice or information. Far from it. The wisest approach is to learn all that you can, from as many sources as possible. That way you can make your own intelligent, aware decisions about the factors that affect your attitudes and your health. Take an active role in your own healing and growth process and you'll progress most rapidly ... and also be healthier and happier along the way.

Getting to Know Yourself

In order to maximize your sense of self-acceptance it's important to have a good understanding of your relationship with yourself. That's why it's so important to do a realistic evaluation (Chapter 4 "Self-Assessment"). In order to most effectively grow towards a more loving and beneficial level of self-acceptance, you must first find out your present status by continuing the questioning process. Some of questions you find

yourself asking may seem difficult and uncomfortable, but the answers can help you discover the "real you", so you can build on to your existing strengths.

Many people have a difficult time loving, accepting, liking or even tolerating themselves. Their self-esteem is poor and their self-acceptance level needs real improvement. Oh, they want to feel good about themselves, they really do. And they might too, if only they were better looking, smarter, had more money or better hair. And of course, if they were thin self-esteem would overflow in their lives.

Do you ever find yourself saying "I'd love myself but ... my parents never really loved me ... I'm a victim of child abuse (or spouse abuse, or IRS abuse) ... I'm not as smart as my sister (brother, cousin, friend, boss, coworker, etc.) ... I'm a failure at life ... I'm too fat to love." Sadly, these are issues for many people who feel like they're not worthy of living a wonderful life.

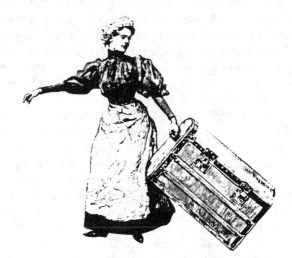

*How much emotional baggage
are you dragging around?*

Many people have a lot of negative emotional baggage to deal with ... plenty of obstacles to face and lots of self-destructive myths surrounding them. These emotional "balloon poppers" or self-criticisms may involve what they consider to be "facts" about themselves but are merely perceptions or often misperceptions. It's their interpretation of these so-called facts that influence their dealings with the rest of the world, and how they feel about themselves.

That's a critical point. If you are busily caught up in emotional nets of your own devise, you may be unable to see those acres of diamonds right under your feet. It's a trap. If you believe you're overweight because you were born with big bones, then you won't even bother to try changing.

Taking Back Control of Your Life

Fortunately, your thinking is under your own control. Unenlightened media and guilt-slinging relatives only play at thought control ... the real power is your ability to make choices. By choosing to take command of your thoughts you can lead a very successful and fulfilling life of your own design. It's a definite choice you must make though. If you continue to allow outside influences to direct your emotions and "pull your strings" you'll spend a lot of time drifting aimlessly like a small boat on a rough sea, looking for any port (or weight loss hope) in a storm.

In order to break the habit of allowing external factors to manipulate your life, you need to begin to question your thoughts and actions ... to start asking "WHY?". Why do you do this or think that? Where do your values and motivations come from? Until you begin to explore these areas much of your life will seem like an unanswered question ... and your self-esteem will suffer accordingly.

The next time you find yourself saying "I really should be thinner, richer, smarter, neater, more loving, etc." ask yourself "WHY?". Why do you need to be thinner, richer or smarter? Why do you feel the need to be anything other than what you are? Do you do things because your parents or others expect it of you? Or do you do them because they make you smile inside? Are you passionate about your life or do feel pushed into it? Who runs your life? If it's not you, it might be a good idea to find out who it is. Then you can ask yourself why you've given away your power of choice.

Once you start asking yourself "WHY?", don't stop until you're convinced that you "know" the real answers. "I need to be smarter because doctors are smart and make lots of money. I should have been a doctor". Aha. Why compare yourself with doctors? "My parents always wanted me to be a doctor". Aha. WHY? Why did they want you to become a doctor? And why didn't you go to medical school? Continue the "WHY?" process until you feel like you're getting to the core of the issue. Be honest with yourself. It's okay to admit that science textbooks always put you to sleep and the sight of blood makes you queasy. If you hate the smell of hospitals, say so. You may find this process difficult, but every significant accomplishment has it's price. By pursuing an honest personal dialogue you may come to realize that you always wanted to be an artist, a tennis pro or a comedy writer. That's why you're not a doctor. It's not because you're not smart enough. Your mother wanted a doctor in the family? Let her go to medical school.

Sometimes you'll come to a conclusion that just "feels right". When you finally get to an answer that rings of the truth, you'll be able to start rewriting the script in your mind based on your own current needs and desires. Then you can say to yourself "I don't need to lose weight because of my mother's unfilled fantasy of being a ballerina. I'm choosing to lose weight because I want to be healthy and to look and feel my best". You can make a true call for action in your own mind. Action, accomplishment and self-acceptance go hand-in-hand.

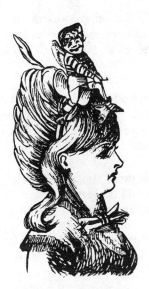

If you're not careful
other people will do your thinking for you.

More Exercises for Boosting Self-Esteem and Self-Acceptance:

1) **Start a daily self-esteem journal** where you write down:
    a) All of the things that you feel you do well.
    b) All of the things that you do to help other people.
    c) All of the worthwhile things you've ever accomplished in your life.
    d) All of the ways in which you are taking self-responsibility in your own life.

2) **Start a "Joy Book"** and write down everything that happens to you that makes you feel good about yourself or your life. Try for at least one highlight every day!

3) **Improve your skills** in the areas that are important to you. There are some things that you already do very well. Take the effort to learn even more about your "passions". Read a new book or take a class in your favorite subject. Share your expertise with other interested people. If your skills are sufficient, start writing the definitive book on your subject.

4) **Share your good times** with your friends. The next time something good happens to you, call up your best friend and tell them about it. Share your positive energy.

5) **Start being a friend to yourself**. Practice smiling when you look in the mirror. A smile always feels good. When you smile at other people they will usually smile back. Sometimes a simple smile from a stranger can make the whole day seem brighter.

6) **Do something every day to nurture yourself**. Loving yourself means taking the extra time to respect your inner spirit. You're not a machine whose purpose is to perform endless tasks. You are a wondrous, unlimited being. Treat yourself with kindness just as you would with someone you really love.

7) **Reward yourself** for being a great person. Buy yourself a gift that you've been wanting. Wrap it up like a present. Open it when you're feeling particularly good about yourself. That way you'll get a double reward. And you deserve it!

8) **Practice positive self-talk.** Many times during the course of the day repeat positive affirmations like: "I'm a good person who's worthy of love", "I'm in charge of my life and I'm accomplishing my goals". "I'm a THINNER WINNER. I'm healthier than ever before". Before long you'll believe even more strongly in what you're saying.

9) **Look at the bright side of life.** Life dishes out both good and bad for everyone. We all get our share of both. When bad things happen it doesn't mean you're a bad person. In fact, sometimes it seems like the people who have to overcome the greatest hardships end up accomplishing the most. See through your obstacles to the solutions beyond.

10) **Take charge of your own thoughts and actions.** The next time someone tries to manipulate you or make you feel guilty, simply call their bluff. Say to them, sweetly and with a smile: "Excuse me, but are you trying to make me feel guilty?". Don't allow other people to take advantage of you. You'll become a stronger person and you'll be respected for it.

11) **Find out what "makes you tick".** Stop doing things because you feel like you "should". When you say "I should do this or that" ... take the time to ask yourself why. The more self-understanding you develop, the more you will be able to appreciate your gifts. Develop the habit of knowing that you choose your actions.

12) **Set goals for yourself.** Develop a purpose and objectives for your life that excite you, and make you want to work towards them. Then make step-by-step plans to accomplish them (see Chapter 8 "Goal Setting"). Accomplishing your goals will make you feel wonderful.

13) **Love YOU!** Start getting a kick out of what you do. Aren't you the friendliest and most lovable person on the face of the planet? Be in love with you for a whole day. Feel the nurturing acceptance, instead of critical self-judgment. You're working so hard and I'm so proud of you. Be proud of yourself, too!

14) **Put a picture up of you as a child**. You still have that child inside. Send love to your inner child and let that love extend to you now. Embrace yourself gently and with great tolerance for all your choices.

Your Body Image

Now I'd like to look at a slightly different aspect of self-acceptance. If you are like most women and many men who have struggled with their weight , your body image, the mental picture you have of your physical self, may not match your true size. For instance, over 50% of all American women overestimate their size, mostly their hips, by up to 25%. (Cheer up! You probably look smaller than you think you do!) In the extreme, anorexics can stand emaciated before a mirror and point to huge fat deposits only they can see. Even after losing all my weight, I still "saw" myself as too big and even kept shopping in the plus size clothes racks! I was a size 8 with a size 24 image! It really felt weird to hold up a teeny, tiny size 8 pair of pants, look in the mirror and see size 24 me, then pull on those pants and have them fit! This is really a fascinating phenomenon.

Living with a distorted image can be unnecessarily painful, causing you to "hate" your body and feel "fat and ugly" when in reality you could be appreciating your progress and accepting your innate form as beautiful. When you feel better about yourself, you will project a more positive attitude and attract like energy. An air of resignation and negativity, resulting from a poor body-image not only feels rotten, but shuts off the flow of energizing support. Oh, sure, we can all see a few changes we would make if we could wave that old magic wand. By understanding where your body image comes from, you can then adopt strategies to boost self-acceptance and help smooth the way towards appreciation of the real you ... make your own magic!

As an overweight child, you may not even realize that you are bigger than others until someone tells you. Your parents or your peers usually clue you in with words or actions. If you were teased about your size or awkwardness in athletics, a poor body image may have started there. Always picking out "slimming" outfits and colors, emphasizing the way you looked instead of the way you felt, and early attempts to help you reduce by limiting food are all ways your early life may have sent the message that you were too big. Unfortunately , these incidents tend to stick like peanut butter on hips ... a long time. The media, especially movies, magazines and television, portray the prettiest and most handsome stars as trim and very slender. Nary a lump or roll in sight for Arnold or Julia. But this unrealistic ideal is so high that few can reach it ... not even the stars that portray it unless they have an army of make-up, hair, wardrobe, lighting and editing professionals plus personal trainers, personal chefs and the carrot of making another million or two if they forego the butter and work out instead.

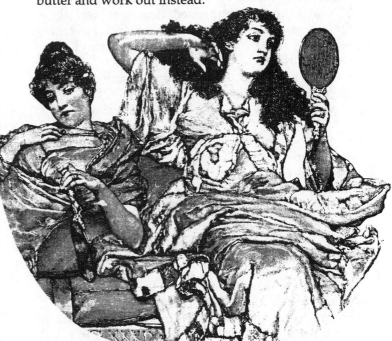

There is more to you than your body image.

Overweight actors are usually a pal or the bad guy, and are often cast in sexless roles. The message is loud and clear: thinner is sexier, prettier, better. This certainly helps shape the way people treat each other in the real world. And in fact, studies show that teachers and nurses attribute higher I.Q.'s to "attractive" babies and children. Juries acquit "beautiful" people more often.

If you are extremely fearful or reluctant to meet people, interview for a job or attend social functions because of the way you look, are preoccupied with your looks or feel guilt or shame because of a perceived imperfection you could have a serious disorder and may need to talk with a therapist. Most people however can benefit from the following exercises designed to help you ...

Feel Better About Your Body

Many of the following suggestions are found in greater detail elsewhere in this book. Check the Index or Table of Contents for lengthier discussions and even more insights.

1) **Focus on the positive** - Instead of zeroing in on that "flaw" every time, choose to focus on a part of your body you love and feel good about. Use your mirror to appreciate your good points, not to obsessively check your rear view and confirm how fat you are.

2) **Exercise** - The #1 body image booster. Take a class, buy an aerobic tape, walk, stretch ... get in touch with your body. According to Rita Freedman, 87% of exercisers improved how they feel about their bodies. Yoga, martial arts and stretching especially help you lengthen, strengthen and get in touch with your deeper physical self. As your posture improves, so will your breathing, spinal alignment and flexibility. You will feel better about your body and your attitude will show it.

3) **Pamper your body** - Find activities and experiences that make your body feel good ... a brisk walk, bubble baths, massage, meditation, silk clothes, sex, fluffy comforters or scented lotion. You deserve to feel sensual and relaxed, so never wear clothes that are too tight or endure an uncomfortable chair. Concentrate on feeling good instead of looking perfect.

4) **Visualize** - Use this powerful technique to see yourself beautiful and perfect just the way you are. See yourself as a five year old child and talk to your inner child about how you look and feel. Nurture yourself, be your own best friend instead of worst critic.

5) **Accept your genetics** - Some of us have pear shapes, some of us have large legs, well-developed muscles, broad backs, or other body types inherited from our ancestors. Make yours the best and fittest you can be and accept the structural features you were given. Same with age. Accept your natural changes and gracefully incorporate them into your look. Maturity means acceptance, wisdom and freedom for many of the beauties of the world ... you, too.

6) **Appreciate your uniqueness** - Look for unique, one-of-a-kind features of famous people ... Sally Field's cheeks, Lauren Hutton's tooth gap, my hair (!). Uniqueness adds appeal. Wouldn't it be boring if we all looked alike? Accept your special features as your trademark and stop comparing yourself to the Beauty Ideal dreamed up by Madison Avenue. You're the best you that ever was.

7) **Flaunt it** - When you get better at appreciating yourself in all your glory, make the most of your best features. Develop flair in dressing by buying a pretty scarf, wearing red or don unique, arty jewelry. Express your deeper self through style.

8) **Focus on others** - Really notice other peoples' best points and strengths. Compliment them and watch your attention spark happiness in them. Appreciation is wonderful for you to give. Come out of your shell and see the difference you can make. It's good practice for spotting your own fine points.

9) **Put it in perspective** - Your body isn't just an object too be judged by yourself or others. It is your vehicle through life. If you are healthy, vital and vigorous and show it in your attitude, you will be beautiful in anyone's book. Live your life with zest.

In A Nutshell

1)   Self-acceptance is being able to value and respect yourself just as you are in the present moment.

2)   You already have all the intelligence, courage and heart you need ... you just have to belief in yourself.

3)   To develop this belief begin by making an honest appraisal of your valuable qualities. Your self-esteem will increase as you realize how many assets you already have.

4)   Self-love is the emotional connection between all people. The more you love yourself, the more love you have to give.

5)   You are responsible for developing your own emotional strength. No one can do it for you.

6)   Learn to question your thoughts and motives. Ask "WHY?". When you truly understand your actions you'll be more in control of your life and better able to pull your own strings.

7)   Several self-esteem and body image boosting exercises are suggested.

8)   Your Body Image is a crucial self-acceptance factor. Avoid judging your body more harshly than it deserves.

Breathing and Meditation   11

"It is a beauteous evening, calm and free, breathless with adoration."
William Wordsworth

Getting Unstuck
on the Way to Self-Discovery

I'd like to share with you one of the finest discoveries I've made on this journey to becoming Thin. It's a wonderful way in which your stress is drained away, leaving you calm, relaxed and quietly energized. Happiness and feeling pleasant will also fill your new awareness. It's simple and easy to learn. The benefits are many, and cumulative, too. Think you might be interested? Let me tell you how I made this wonderful discovery, and why it's so important to me now.

Back when I was fat, I sometimes had a hard time holding on to the feeling of being an okay person. I would look at the world and see so many obstacles that at times I forgot what an incredible wonderland we really live in. I built tall emotional walls around myself, and set impossibly high standards that always left me emotionally drained when I tried to meet them. Then I trapped myself into believing that I was the only person who found it so hard to be "perfect".

My defensiveness and isolation were actually key reasons why I felt so powerless. I stuffed down any real feelings and self-awareness with food at every chance . Why? Because whenever I got in touch with my feelings, it always seemed to lead to an awareness of myself as fat and hopelessly out of control. Life seemed so easy for everyone else. But it was difficult and painful for me. Like the character Joe Banks in the movie "Joe vs. The Volcano", I had a vague dream of being happy some day but seemed instead to be suffering from a "brain cloud". My own negative self-obsession beat up my self-worth and obscured my vision of how the world really is. And I couldn't see a way out. I simply had never really learned to love and accept myself. I hated what I was instead of accepting myself and my condition as part of the whole spectrum of my life journey. Acceptance would have allowed me to learn from my experience of being overweight. Hatred of it stopped anything positive or constructive from happening. I shut off my own opportunity to change by locking myself in with negativity.

No matter how hard I tried over the years, all my searching for approval from someone or something else only led me to unfulfilling relationships. Never to the approval which I sought. If anyone did show signs of friendship I figured they were flawed just for liking me! It was like Groucho Marx used to say, "I wouldn't join a club that would have me as a member". Self-acceptance was just a part of the distant dream. Somehow I needed to get myself on my own side. It took years before I finally realized that there was only one place left to turn for solace: inside myself. It had to begin with me. Of course, I'd heard this before, but I didn't believe it. I said I liked myself, but that was so nobody could question the truth about me. Or could they? I doubt seriously that I ever fooled anybody.

I decided that I needed to begin taking some chances with my life if I was ever to break this negative cycle. The message "you can't expect your life to change for the better if you continue to do things the same old way" finally began to sink in. What I needed was a method to develop some real power and determination to rise above the self-defeating emotional world that I forced myself to live in. I needed to open up to a larger and more loving world. But I was paralyzed by fear of rejection, of my own imperfections, of not being "good enough". I needed to learn how to heal the fear and pain and isolation and accept myself for who I was, right where I was, before I could move on to accomplish my goals. I had to learn to forgive.

I had to find a way to transcend and transform my current perceptions beyond the overwhelming experience of "being fat", and the narrow viewpoint that this was "bad". Only then could I accept what, where and who I was, and begin to get unstuck. What's more, since I was so emotionally isolated, I had to do it alone! Like the blind leading the blind. I was ready to change even though I knew the change would be difficult. The pain was simply no longer acceptable. I knew I deserved something better. So do you!

Techniques to Try When You're Ready
to Change Your Mind

Maybe you're not hurting as much as I was, but none-the-less what I learned was that there are healthier ways to fill your emotional voids, to feel in-touch and whole, other than eating to excess and other self-destructive activities. They only masked the pain anyway ... it was still there. Chapter 16 "Creating a Powerful Support System" should be useful in giving you some ideas to begin ... such as groups, a special friend, books and tapes, etc. But here I would like to talk about getting in touch with yourself ... the inner person. Just you, and who you are when you're alone and learning how to respect and care for yourself.

self-developed form of listening, calming and reflection that grew from my personal need, and any label may bring up preconceived notions that could color your willingness to give it a try. What started as a way to think and get in touch with myself, a retreat, turned out to be an opening and way of reaching beyond myself. It was like tapping into The Force, as Luke Skywalker did in Star Wars.

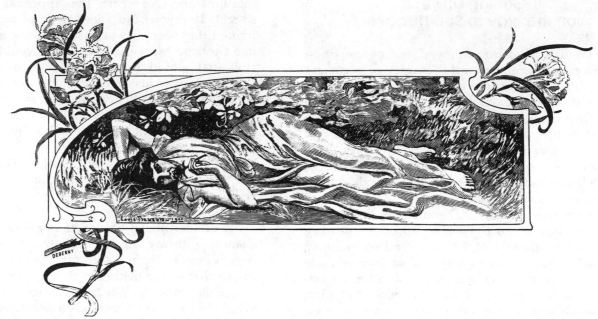

Allowing yourself to relax and open up to your "inner self" will put you in contact with a larger source of energy, healing and assistance. God, The Universal Source, The Force, The Big Bagel, whatever you choose to call it. The name is unimportant. It exists, and is always present. Simply clearing away your own resistance to it will reveal the energy to you. When you focus attention on it you become aware of it. And it's such a wonderful, loving feeling to realize that you are not alone or separate. All life is connected by bonds of energy, thought, consciousness and intelligence.

Techniques such as meditation, massage, Tai Chi or other body work, yoga, prayer, and combinations of these disciplines have been shown to increase self-awareness while beginning to bridge the gap between you and the rest of the world. I began to study various approaches which would allow my mind to experience a release from stress, and also allow me to tap into energy sources beyond myself ... a new concept for me, because my focus had always been so self-contained.

After trying several different methods I came upon a process that I really enjoy. The benefits to me have been immense. I simply sit quietly, listen to the "inner silence" and just be with myself. I call it "listening". This later evolved into what some call meditation. I really hesitate to label it, as it is a

The purpose was to heal, and to come into harmony with this Force, to draw upon the power and release the pain and tension. In the process of quieting my mind and learning to listen, an awakening occurred. An awakening into a more mindful or aware state about eating, relationships and really paying attention to feelings and experiences. Instead of bludgeoning them with brownies.

If all this sounds a little "far out" to you, it may just be your unfamiliarity with the concepts. Or maybe it's your natural resistance to change that's showing. That's okay. If any of this makes you uncomfortable right now, that's okay, too ... it's new. But make sure you come back to the idea periodically and see if it makes any more sense to you. I feel it is essential for permanent weight management, since this requires personal growth, maturity, insight and flexibility towards real changes by breaking the cycle of fear and isolation.

This process all happens so naturally and easily, once you allow yourself to realize how much it can help release you from that emotional pain you may be experiencing. The benefits build on each other as you become more accustomed to the experience, and it becomes part of your regular activities. Eventually there is just a relaxed attitude of acceptance and joyful anticipation.

I really look forward to these quiet times in my day. I feel refreshed and energized after I meditate.

And I've now found that there are many people who "practice" some form of meditation or "listening". A lot of them are older people who, over time, have developed ways of finding inner peace. Many of them devised their own techniques based on their own life experiences. Some may lie quietly resting and allow their minds to go calm, and gradually drift into a light nap. Others may sink into a bubble bath and allow the soothing warmth to take them into this special place. And still others may find this state of awareness while running, playing an instrument or painting.

In the final analysis, life is a meditation. The more mindfully awake you are to each moment in life, the more you realize that the power and belongingness are there for you. The more you allow yourself to be included in this flow of energy, the less isolated you will feel. The meditation process allows you to become aware of and feel the all-pervasive energy in you and around you. It breaks down, or at least softens, the walls that divide you from the world. I was (and maybe you are) like a fragile butterfly who was so afraid of possible pain that she shut herself away in a tiny, dark box ... safe from injury. But also with no chance to see and share beauty, touch others or fly on life's breezes. Locked away, dreaming of the sun. Meditation can open your eyes to life's true wonders. It puts you in touch with an infinite source of power and love and helps you realize you are part of this flow as well.

Beyond these meager words that try to explain this energy expanding process is the experience itself. To benefit, it must be practiced and experienced. Why not give it a try and see for yourself? Who knows, this just might help you move closer to becoming "thin" by allowing you to address your emotional and spiritual needs in a renewing and refreshing way. It can be a powerful tool in helping your dream become a reality, just like it did for me.

Breathe the Right Way

You've been breathing all your life. Why do you have to learn to breathe? It's like learning to eat ... you just know how, right? Well, learning to breathe properly is the key for opening up your body and mind to relaxation and energy flow. Have you ever noticed that when you're under pressure or tense, you hold your breath or breathe shallowly? This in turn tends to make you more tense since shallow chest or upper lung breathing actually changes the acidity of your blood and promotes anxiety. Also, your brain uses fully 20% of your available oxygen and it's simply not there just when you need it the most!

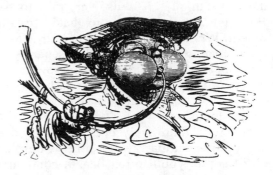

Proper breathing
can change your whole outlook on life.

When you learn to breathe fully with a technique such as the one I will describe here called diaphragmatic or belly breathing, you will trigger your physiology to be on your side when you need it to be. Herbert Bensen described this reaction in a book entitled "The Relaxation Response". He noted that as an antidote to the generally accepted automatic "fight or flight" response to danger or stress that we all exhibit, there was a third learned option. This he called the "relaxation response" which is to calmly assess the situation and consider your choices before responding. It begins with proper breathing and meditation. He also found that how you meditated, mind-stillness oriented or body-active oriented wasn't that important. So sit or walk, but be aware of the process. It seems that just the intention of contacting this inner place of peace and stillness was enough to trigger the positive response. So don't worry that you aren't doing it right. Just trying to open to controlled relaxation will allow you to experience some of the benefits. Besides, you'll get better with practice!

The interaction of the subtle but palpable energy of the air that you breathe as it flows through your body's breathing apparatus is recognized in many ancient cultures as a powerful force. Indeed, breath is life itself. It is called "chi" (chee) in China and "kundalini" in India. This energy is stored in specific places in your body, such as the "chakras" (an east Indian term for the energy nodes in the body) and you can learn to contact and access this energy. Many people with blocked energies could begin to learn to release it through these simple breathing exercises.

Because breathing seems like such a "natural" thing, that we all do, it is easy to overlook it as having much significance and to take it for granted. But that's like saying, "We can all walk, so why bother learning to run or dance?". Belly breathing is a very powerful way of bringing your body into readiness for peaceful "being", anxiety release and meditative techniques. It is also very easy to learn.

First let me describe your basic breathing equipment. What comes to mind initially are your lungs. In breathing these are further separated into the upper part of your lungs and the lower part of your lungs. Most of us use the upper part only, so our upper chest breathing habit has developed this part of our lungs very well. The lower part of your lungs has more than likely been under-used and, like any under-used part, will not be as developed. In older people, you'll often hear a complaint of difficulty in breathing. This may come from a lifetime of shallow chest breathing while the lower lungs have shrunken and diminished. The sooner you begin this lower lung awareness and practice strengthening them, the easier it will be to change this potentially debilitating habit.

Your diaphragm is a sheet of muscle stretched across the bottom of your chest cavity on which your lungs rest. It is the main group of muscles used in breathing. When you breathe in properly, expanding the abdominal, lower back and torso muscles it flexes downward, and the movement and resulting vacuum causes more air to be pulled into your lungs. As we have seen, more air is better since it brings oxygen to your brain and other tissues. As you exhale, your diaphragm bows upward, helping you exhale fully. As you learn and practice "diaphragmatic breathing" you will be able to more fully inhale fresh air and oxygen, and exhale more carbon dioxide and waste products from your body.

All right, it's time to get mellow. To begin, stand or sit erect, or lie on your back. Your shoulders should stay relaxed and down and not move up or down when you breathe. Tuck your tailbone under slightly for stability. Your chin should be level, your head and neck in a straight line with your spine all the way down to your tailbone. Don't allow your head or jaw to jut forward or down. Don't lock your knees if you are standing. Now relax your face and jaw. Your tongue should feel loose and relaxed. Soften your throat and neck. You should feel tall, evenly balanced and aligned, light and strong. This posture alignment alone will help you begin to feel more relaxed and in control as you bring your awareness back into your body, part by part.

Now place your hands on your abdomen, at your belly button, fingers pointing inward but not touching. Breathing in through your nose, take a deep breath. Your hands should move noticeably outward if you are breathing diaphragmatically. Most people will only move outward slightly or even move inward instead. That is because we are used to breathing from the upper chest area only. Okay, breathe out.

With your hands still on your lower abdomen

take another breath, and this time concentrate on pushing against your hands with your breath and abdominal muscles as you breathe in through your nose. Did your hands move more? Congratulations! You have just taken a full, proper breath! As you exhale through your mouth, your hands should move back inward. Practice this 3 or 4 times until you begin to know and remember what it feels like to breathe properly.

Say A-a-a-a-h-h

After you have practiced this technique several times over the next few days, it will be much more natural and automatic for you. Now whenever you feel any negative emotion such as tension, anxiety, fear, worry, anger or depression stop and breathe deeply 3-4 times. Just breathe in fully, then let it all out in a huge sigh of relief. A-a-a-h-h! Doesn't that feel great? This big breath serves to reset the diaphragm for more automatic deep belly breathing, clears your head with more oxygen, relaxes your body with the relaxation response and most importantly helps you to come back into the moment. Realize that any of those negative emotions mentioned are a result of mentally being in an unpleasant past memory or anticipating the future in a negative way. By being aware and mindful in the moment right now, you are contacting the core of your being. A lot of those emotions are put into a broader perspective when you come into the "now". It opens your heart to your real purpose ... to love and learn from all your experiences.

As you begin to practice this technique, you might find it helpful, as I do, to have a positive affirmation to link with the release you feel after your big breath. I often say, "Everything is exactly as it should be right now." Wow! That's a big one to swallow sometimes! But it's amazing how just saying it puts the situation, no matter how extreme, into a completely different light. I begin looking for the lesson and the way to learn it, instead of feeding into the negative energy and falling for that trap again. Find your own affirmation to pair with your big breath and see if it isn't as powerful for you, too.

Basic Meditation

Now that you know how to breathe properly and you see how easy it is, let's get you started on learning how to meditate. Now don't get spooked with this word. It's not just a "60's thing" any more (in fact it's been around for more than 60 centuries!). If this is a completely new experience for you, beginning in a non-stressful way can help to take off any pressure or uncertainty you may be feeling. Just let go of your judgment right now. There's nobody here but you and me. The process shouldn't make you feel uncomfortable. The objective is simply to aim your awareness in a slightly different direction than you're used to. Quietly listening or just being in a calm atmosphere is an easy start ... but very powerful.

Find a quiet, comfortable spot, such as your bedroom chair or favorite lounger, where you won't be disturbed for 15 to 20 minutes (some people set up meditation rooms as private, quiet spots ... "Don't bother me for a while, but if there's an emergency I'll be in the closet"). Sitting up is best. It allows you to breathe easily and fully, and to keep your spine erect (which is important for energy flow). You'll also be less likely to fall asleep. Now just sit quietly with your eyes closed and breathe normally. Don't do anything. Just listen. Listen to what? Well, it's different for everyone. The best description I can give you is to listen to the silence inside yourself. Let your breath be natural. Maybe you'll feel yourself expanding and lifting slightly, or floating with each inhalation. And then drifting down with each exhalation. Chances are good that your mind will be full of self-talk. Random thoughts will drift into your awareness. If they do, give them a gentle mental shove out of your consciousness. This is not the time for thinking. The state you want to achieve is an absence of thought ... only a pleasant, warm, full feeling. Eventually, with practice, you may hear tones or even music, but it's the silence that is calming. At some point you may begin to "sense" a "benevolent presence". Some people use similar techniques to contact "angels" or inner guides. After you sit quietly and relax a few moments and start to feel comfortable, begin to more consciously let go of all your thoughts and emotions. Allow yourself to release all the tension, the thoughts, and any stress you may be holding. They'll be there waiting for you in 20 minutes. This is your special time, so let them go for now.

Become aware of your body feeling so very relaxed, loose, pleasant and warm (a feeling like hot fudge sauce oozing over warm cake). Then begin to focus on relaxing your body, one part at a time, in a progressive relaxation pattern. Start with your toes. Think about your toes, maybe even feel them getting warm or the circulation spiraling through them. These sensations are different for everyone, so do your own thing here. Next move to your feet and again relax them and let all tension drain away. They may begin to feel heavy. Move on progressively to your ankles, calves, knees, thighs, pelvis, buttocks, hips, abdomen, torso, chest, small of your back, up your back, shoulders, upper arms, lower arms, hands and fingers, neck, jaw

(especially), tongue, face and scalp. Spend a few moments on each part of your body. Pay particular attention to where any tension is held, usually the neck or shoulders, face and jaw. Spend a little more time concentrating on relaxing your most tense areas. Breathe normally and evenly while progressively relaxing. This can take anywhere from 30 seconds to 5 minutes depending on your concentration, level of tension and time available.

Now just be quiet and "listen" or simply "be". Picture your mind as the surface of water, such as a pond or lake, and see how calm and still you can make it ... without any ripples at all. Practice resting yourself in this peaceful state, and let the force you will begin to sense flow through you. You might feel yourself floating. As you practice you'll get better ... as with most things.

When you have mastered this method of getting totally relaxed you can experiment with adding a single word to the stillness. This technique helps to focus your mind and keeps it off the random thoughts that will appear in your mind. Various meditative disciplines use words such as "amen" or "om". When I use a word, I prefer to choose one that pictures something to me such as "serenity", "peace", "safe", "tranquillity" or "calm". Simply repeat the word you choose silently in your mind in a pleasant way. Whenever a stray thought drifts into your mind, gently let it go, no forcing or rough stuff, and move back to your chosen word. This whole experience should feel pleasant, peaceful and caring. No need to pay particular attention to your breath. Let it be natural. There may be a tendency to time your word with your breath. This is unnecessary and possibly distracting. Your word should be repeated very softly, randomly and eventually should only be felt ... not even thought "out loud" in your mind. During this state your brain waves change gradually to alpha which is closer to sleeping. Your breath will be slower also, similar to deep rest or sleep. You are still alert but resting deeply. Don't go to sleep! Stay awake.

When you're ready to stop, let your word go and allow your thoughts to gradually return to normal. Try to keep your thoughts positive and happy. This is a good time to picture yourself as successfully moving towards good health at a sure, positive pace, and being happy with your progress. Or you can pose a question to yourself such as "What can I do to move closer to my goals of health and fitness?". Begin to become aware of your breathing and then very slowly open your eyes. Let your focus be soft at first. Get up gradually and smoothly. Take your time. Sometimes I'm so relaxed after my listening session that I grab a little snooze to extend this wonderful feeling.

Stretching Time

It seems like everybody wishes that there were more hours in a day, so they could get more done. Well, I find that 20 minutes of meditation can equal as much as a full hour of deep sleep. It is so refreshing and restful. Two 20 minutes sessions a day have allowed me to reduce my long-standing 8 hours a night to 6 or 7 hours and I have much more energy than ever before. Try to set aside time daily to practice meditating and I'm sure you will find that it more than rewards you for the effort. If you just can't find the time, snatch a few minutes here and there wherever you can. I might just stop for 5 minutes at my desk or 10 minutes while parked in my car.

Daily practice is the key here, just as it is with exercise and so many other positive habits. I think of it as plugging myself in and draining out the tension while gathering in positive energy. It doesn't seem to do half as much good if only done sporadically. Commit yourself to this process for a few months and see if it doesn't make a huge difference in your state of mind and feeling of calm control, happiness and connectedness.

Listen to What You've Been Missin'

As you learn to listen and pay attention to your inner world, you may become more aware of your own intuition or feelings about a situation or relationship. I used to discount these internal cues and rely only on seemingly more logical choices. But the purely logical choices usually turned out to be less beneficial to me than my intuitions. My little voice inside was usually right!

I have come to believe that intuition is really the Force or the Universe or God or your own self-wisdom sending you a message of guidance. It's like an internal guidance system for aligning with the proper course in your life. Now I follow those feelings. Especially after experiencing the more positive results that I obtain by using intuition as the basis of my judgments. Where before I felt so alone and inadequate, I now "know" that there is guidance, acceptance and real wisdom when I go within and just listen for it. The Bible says " ... be ye transformed by the renewing of your mind ... ". For me it was like waking up to find a cold fog lifting away, and a sunny, colorful life opened up before my eyes. But there is a catch ... you cannot hear unless you listen.

As unbelievable as it is to me now, I can see that the pain of my former fat life was for a worthwhile reason. It was really a gift to me (in disguise of course). One I just had to allow myself to see as an opportunity to reach out and push open a door ... instead of beating my head against it. Without the fat and its related traumas, I wouldn't have discovered this "listening" process. And I wouldn't have knowledge of the healing energy that it provides. It makes me happy to be able to share this with you and I'm excited for the changes and growth that you can experience as you discover yourself and a deeper, more joyful and powerful life. As you let your aloneness go, I think you'll be amazed at the wonderful things that begin to happen in your life.

There's More to You than Meets the Eye

Amazing discoveries are being made on a regular basis about our universe . One of the most dramatic conceptual breakthroughs is the connection between our bodies, our minds and quantum physics. This is the realm of thinking where you have to keep an open mind, but some of the finest thinkers in the fields of consciousness and healing are convinced that we are made up of intelligent energy at the sub-atomic levels of our physical beings.

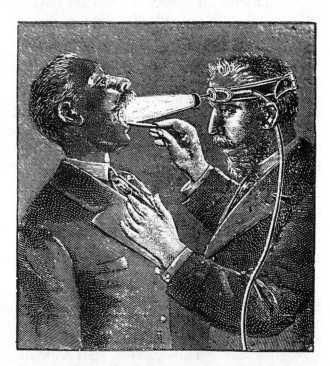

"It looks like the quantum void to me."

The basic theory is that science has broken our component parts down into levels so small that there is virtually nothing left but energy and intelligence. For example, if you take a sample of your skin and put it under a microscope, you will see a collection of cells. Take a single cell and magnify it and you will see thousands of tiny component parts. Take one of these parts and magnify it enough, and you can actually see atoms. Until recently this was a far as scientific technology could go. But now we can even go inside of the atom. Protons, neutrons and electrons (and croutons?) are the basic structural components that you're probably familiar with. But in addition there are hundreds of types of subatomic particles ... so small and fast that the only way to tell that they exist at all is by watching the trails they leave behind. These little bundles of matter/energy are racing around at light speed all day long. They're everywhere, and they're passing through your body right now. They are, in fact, what you are made of. These particles are so small that they are, in essence, nothing but energy. They are something of a cross between matter and light. Pure energy, bonded by an intelligence. Obviously they don't just fly apart, otherwise you wouldn't be reading this now. Everything works just the way it is supposed to. It is very intelligent stuff.

In between all of these indescribably small energy particles is "space". This has been referred to as the quantum field. The quantum field is essentially "intelligent space". This is in effect what the entire universe is ... an intelligent void inhabited by energy. Mostly, there is just a void. A void with a purpose, if you will. As hard as it might be for you or me to conceive of, this is essentially what we are made of. So the next time you hear somebody say, "He's full of hot air", you'll have a whole different picture in mind.

The reason that this discussion is mentioned here is so you will have a better sense of the meditative process. The place you want your awareness to go during meditation is into this quantum field. To the void where there is nothing but intelligent energy. When you bring your awareness into that place you will find that there is unlimited energy and power for you to draw upon. Yes, this a lot to swallow. Believe me, I lived in Missouri for a while and I'm inclined to say "show me". If I didn't think there was value in sharing these concepts with you, I certainly wouldn't. Keep in mind however that less than 100 years ago nobody really believed that man could fly. A mere century ago horses were the prime mode of transportation, there were no electric lights, no telephones or radios and no psychotherapists. Freud hadn't described the workings of our inner minds and Einstein hadn't discovered the equation describing Energy. So try to keep an open mind.

As you can tell I feel very strongly about the process of meditation. I'm not the only one. Meditation techniques of various forms are practiced all over the world and have been for thousands of years, particularly in ancient, Eastern cultures. But, more and more, Western medicine is recommending the use of meditation because of its proven restorative and stress-reducing value. Cardiologist Dean Ornish recommends it as part of his method of actually reversing heart disease. It seems that meditation can heal the heart both emotionally and physically. Worth a try, eh?

Other Meditation Options

Understand that what is important is the result, not the particular technique. So this section describes a few more easy ways for you to access your inner energy source.

A simple way to disengage your busy conscious mind is by mentally performing a repetitive word, phrase or mantra (this was mentioned above). You can get the same effect by using a simple sequence of numbers synchronized with your breathing.

Find a comfortable, sitting up position. Start breathing slowly and deeply for a few minutes until you begin to relax. Then begin to count in time with your breathing. As you inhale count "one and two and", then as you exhale count "three and four and". Repeat this counting process until you can gently allow the numbers to visually drift into your mind. Remember the idea of the meditative process is to guide your awareness to the spaces between thoughts. So if you find stray thoughts sneaking into your mind, gently release them. If this is difficult simply resume counting from one to four.

Another approach to meditation is to listen to calming repetitive music or sounds. Nature audios have become very popular in recent years. You can put on a tape and listen to rainstorms, waterfalls, forest sounds of wind in the trees, birds chirping and even whales singing. These are soothing to the soul and allow your mind to easily drift to that wonderful state of being "between the thoughts".

You don't have to be in a physically immobile state to derive the benefits of meditation. There is a technique called walking meditation which is a way of focusing your awareness on your simple actions in a positive way. Some eastern philosophies express the message that every footstep that you take in life leaves behind it the energy of the emotions you were feeling at the time. Like an endless tapestry of woven emotions. Becoming mindful of this possibility, it makes sense to try and keep your emotions positive. When you find yourself walking somewhere, consider what emotional trails you are leaving behind. This awareness of your connectedness and influence with all things will put you in closer touch with the universal energy that we all share.

The point is to become more mindful or aware of your "now" to really be in the present moment. You can let go of the past and the future, and allow yourself to experience this state of perfect being. Here you can be free of the guilt, anxiety or pain that drives you to eat excessively, to the destruction of your one-and-only body. You can go to the place that houses your true self ... your core being that knows, accepts and loves who and what you are, and is pure and free from judgment. You just are. And you are perfect. From that place of peace and respect for what is, you can see clearly the reason you are here ... which is to love, to learn, to share and to grow in a constructive way. To honor and fulfill the perfect life you are living.

It's your choice. You can follow the old road of struggle and stagnation, or you can learn positive new ways of approaching life. You can learn to forgive, accept, and grow. You now have many techniques to begin opening to your own healing. Love and nourish the beauty that is you, then spread it around. Loving is the mortar that surrounds and connects all us bricks. Be a brick in the solid house of love!

In A Nutshell

1)   You can heal your self-image by looking within yourself, not to outside sources.

2)   Opening yourself up emotionally takes courage, but the benefits outweigh the risks and effort.

3)   Learning to breathe properly with diaphragmatic or belly breathing technique relaxes, centers and brings you back to the present moment.

4)   Many meditative techniques including "listening" put you in touch with a universal energy force, your core.

5)   You can draw upon the powerful healing energy of this force and the power you receive will help you heal.

6)   Powerful insights can come to you in the form of intuition. Learn to listen and respect them.

7)   Practice meditating for 20 minutes, once or twice a day.

8)   Be a brick in the solid house of love! Spread that mortar!

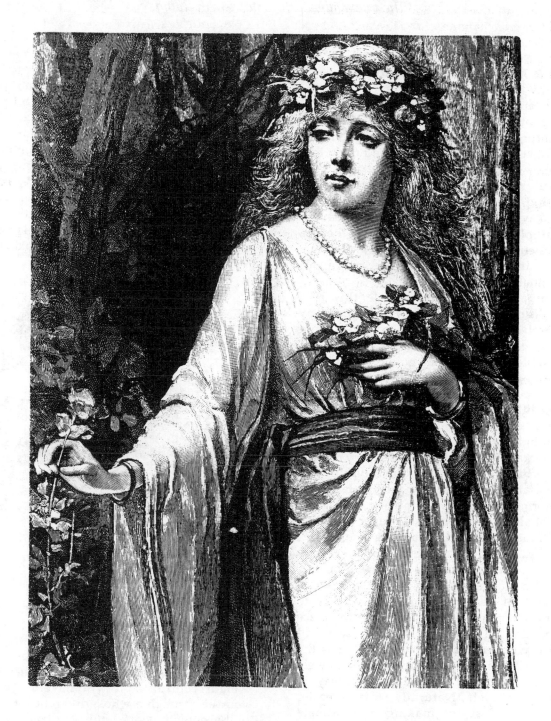

Love everyone and everything unconditionally ... especially yourself.

Your Personal Journal   12

"The unexamined life is not worth living."
Socrates

The Adventure Lies Within

There is an important aspect of weight control that most people don't often take into consideration ... the adventure of self-discovery. Throughout this program I have made references to the notion that you are okay just the way you are. This is a philosophical theme that shows up in a great many sources ... and I believe in my heart that it's true. We are all okay just the way we are. Each of us is in a particular place on his or her path to health, fitness and slenderdom. There is no right or wrong place to be. It is just where we are, given our individual circumstances.

Unfortunately, for many people this is a difficult philosophy to accept. They don't feel okay about themselves, and a catchy slogan is not about to change those feelings. They perceive insurmountable difficulties in going through the process leading to the belief that they are okay (self-acceptance) in their own hearts. This can be particularly difficult when coming from an attitude of self-disgust about weight, which is where I was at one point in my life. As I became more self-aware over the years I realized that so many of the standards which I used to judge myself with unmerciful harshness were my interpretation of society's "norms" and not really my own feelings on the subject at all. I didn't look like a super model, so in my mind I made some very damaging assumptions about myself ... I was fat, and therefore I was bad, wrong, weak or unacceptable somehow. And this viewpoint affected nearly every aspect of my life. It took a lot of research, learning, reflection, spiritual and emotional growth to get to the place where I am today ... I am okay. I accept myself and I am at peace with my level of health. That is the emotional place that I suggest you aim for as well. It's a big improvement over any other way of dealing with yourself. Naturally, this is easier said than done. But by making a legitimate commitment and effort towards self-acceptance you will surely get there sooner than by waiting for some transformational miracle to turn you into Cinderella.

I feel the need to pass along a certain warning to you that may seem a bit paradoxical regarding the "okay" philosophy. There are certain unhealthy physical conditions which have, as an integral symptom, the tendency to deny the problem. These include alcoholism and obesity. You may say that you are "okay" ... but in reality, choosing to remain in a physical state (fat) where you are knowingly damaging your health and emotional well-being is not, in truth, honoring and respecting yourself. It's like choosing to drink a daily quart of gin and saying that it's okay, you've made peace with it. Choosing consciously to damage yourself is not very loving or constructive. In order to grow into a healthier state it really is necessary to get a better sense of how and why you do things.

The Logbook of Your Life

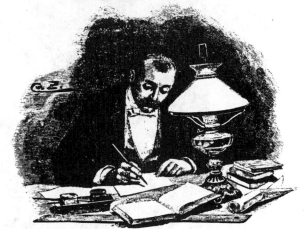

*"I could hardly believe
what I found myself saying..."*

Part of the growth process that can be highly beneficial to you is noting the changes occuring in your life. Change generally takes place slowly. This is especially true of attitudes ... and developing positive, constructive attitudes towards yourself is particularly important when it comes to weight control. You will have to learn to see yourself through a whole different set of eyes. You will eventually work your way from an attitude of harsh self-judgment to a viewpoint of loving acceptance and respect. That's the goal. I found that by keeping a Personal Journal I came to know and understand myself in a way I never had before. In addition, I have never met anyone who kept a journal, however sporadically, who did not dramatically improve their level of self-understanding. This, in turn, led them ultimately to making wiser choices more often.

What does a Personal Journal look like? Anything you want! From a cute little diary with a lock and key, to a pile of plain white typing paper or a computer disk. What it looks like is not nearly as important as what you use it for. One of the skills that successful people in life have in common is that they tend to "think on paper". They write down their ideas, thoughts and plans. The reason that this is so effective is simply because you can test a variety of scenarios quickly and easily... and make changes painlessly. Better to crumple up a sheet of paper than to deal with a poorly planned action.

Your Personal Journal is a safe place where you can really get to know yourself and become more comfortable with the person you are. Thoughts tend to be slippery and fleeting, but the written word is by its nature more permanent. I sometimes can't remember the details of last week's thoughts but when I write about them in my journal and review it later I can often see how I have grown ... very often growing right through momentary problems. The emotional trap I was so caught up in is now something to smile about and learn from ... water that has long since passed under the bridge. It will certainly be the same for you on many occasions. You gain perspective, which helps you put each experience into a broader context.

Your journal is the place to record your thoughts, feelings, self-observations and records of daily happenings. You can write down the life questions that you feel are the most important ... and the solutions you discover. Good times, bad times ... everybody has their share. How did you feel during the "good" times? What did you learn by experiencing the "bad" times? As you begin to see your "troubles" as learning experiences you can even turn them into positive, constructive insights.

I would suggest that you slant your journal towards finding your own personal solutions to the dilemmas of your life. I went through one extended phase many years ago that was rampant with self-pity. I felt like I was a sorry mess and that's what I wrote about. It was all very negative and self-defeating in content. When I reviewed that particular journal several years later I found that there really wasn't anything constructive in it at all. I ended up throwing the whole thing away ... all except for the cover which I had painstakingly designed. Was this a horrible waste? No, I realized later that I had grown a great deal in working through that particular period ... I just didn't really see any of the growth at the time. I now know that if I had gone in seeking solutions they would have come to me far sooner. That's the suggestion I make to you ... prepare for your next growth opportunity.

An Objective Perspective

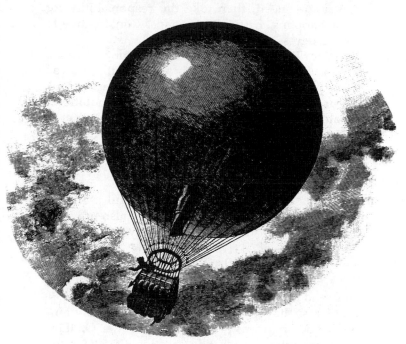

Your Journal can give you a sense of perspective.

Your journal can become a helpful record of your behavior patterns as well. As you write about your life try to occasionally step back and get an objective perspective of yourself and your feelings. Many times patterns will emerge. Do certain types of people always seem to bring out negative emotions in you? See if you can figure out why. And see if you can come up with alternative ways of dealing with these people or with the emotions. For instance, you may become aware of "enablers" in your life ... people who seem to reinforce your negative eating patterns or inactive lifestyle. Like Aunt Minnie who always insists on making your favorite pie every time you visit her. How does it make you feel when she says or implies that if you don't eat her offering it means that you don't love her? Are there any other ways you can deal with this situation? Perhaps you can come up with two or three possible solutions ... once you see the pattern in the first place.

Try "talking it out on paper". You might even try the psycho-drama approach. Try writing a short play with two characters ... you and Aunt Minnie. Attempt to get into the parts emotionally. When you write the parts for Minnie really try walking in her shoes and feeling her feelings. If you can gain insights into her thoughts and actions you may be able to gain insight into yourself as well. See if you can come up with several alternative strategies for dealing with your enablers. Then ask yourself why you allow them to enable you to eat more when you're with them. Give yourself the power you need, then take the responsibility for what happens. Difficult? Perhaps. Constructive to your progress? More than likely.

Your Personal Journal can be anything you want it to be. It's yours to do with as you will. You can write poetry, draw pictures, paste in Dream Book pictures, write down your favorite quotations. Whatever you want. The main purpose is to get to know yourself better ... so really be "yourself".

Pushing Away the Clouds

While I firmly believe that a useful journal is focused on personal growth, you can also use it for things that are just plain fun. I love to save my favorite comic strips from the newspaper. Sometimes they wind up on the refrigerator door, but the best ones, the ones that I really identify with, end up in my journal.

I also have a "joy list". Whenever anything really good happens to me I write it down. On those occasions when I backslide emotionally I have this ready reminder that I have indeed had some good times. This can definitely help snap me out of a snit.

Sometimes I'll write the rough draft of a letter to a friend in my journal before I break out the good stationary. It helps me to clarify my thoughts. Just remember that insights come in some unlikely ways at times ... so you have to be open and receptive to them.

Although having a place to write down my thoughts is immediately stress-reducing and helpful in terms of clarifying my feelings, there are times that I don't really derive certain benefits of the journal until some later time. In fact, this is often the case. I have found that there is definite value in a periodic review. I have used my journal to learn how I think. Sometimes in my day-to-day affairs I tend to be indecisive, and I hesitate on making commitments until I feel that my decision is flawless. Interestingly, in my journal I usually have pretty strong, clear-cut opinions. That's one of the journal's great values. It gives you a chance to reflect on your thoughts, make adjustments to your opinions and observations, and test the waters before making an impulsive decision that you might regret later. I still make mistakes, of course, but I learn the lessons more quickly these days.

Lighting Up Your Mind

It's been said that wisdom is gained by reflecting on our experiences. My journal is helping me to become a wiser individual, who makes fewer costly mistakes. For example, now I know that

buying a dozen brownies is just inviting ... well, you know what. Or mentioning a certain subject to a friend just invites a hostile response. I'm learning to avoid stepping into obvious traps. And I'm sure you will feel the same sense of illumination after you've kept your journal for a time.

Some possible journal "projects" that you might consider include using your writings to help you identify situations and feelings that trigger your urges to eat. Did the cookie aroma at the mall nearly drive you insane with desire for chocolate chips? Now is the time to develop an alternative strategy for dealing with this particular land mine. When are your most vulnerable times to eat "regret foods" ... the ones you later regret having eaten.

Is Friday night your old cue to have pizza, beer and buttered popcorn at the movies? And then wake up on Saturday morning with three or four extra pounds to deal with. How can you change this pattern? You won't be able to do much changing of old patterns until you:

(1) Become aware and recognize it.
(2) Acknowledge it.
(3) Make a list of acceptable alternatives.
(4) Make a commitment to do something about it.

Your journal can help you through all four of these stages, if you choose to act on what you learn about yourself (refer also to the **BAMM** concept in Chapter 14 "Taming Your Stress").

What about that 5 P.M. "grab a burger on the way home" trend? Can you see it for the self-defeating habit that it is when you pick the wrong kind of snack? How does getting on the scale affect your attitude? Are you playing the role of "family failure" ... the poor, overweight, lost soul who just never has been able to get on the "right" side of life? (kind of like the fat, black sheep of the family). Are you satisfied being in that role? Who made the decision that you were the one who needed to play that part? What are your choices now that you can see the issues from a different perspective? There is no right and wrong here. The issues I've mentioned cause problems for lots of people. Your success at losing weight and at life in general really boils down to just making better choices over the long haul, and of being more consciously aware of why you make them. I think you'll find that a Personal Journal is a good start towards self-awareness. It is a very useful tool to help you recognize and heal the areas of your life which presently hold you back. Become aware and change these and you will achieve wonderful new levels of physical and emotional health.

In A Nutshell

1) The journey to weight control can be a great adventure into self-discovery.

2) You are okay right where you are!

3) Awareness leads you closer to your own feelings and reveals possible limiting societal views about being overweight.

4) Don't get caught in denial! You're overweight! And it's compromising your health and every other area of your life as well.

5) Noting the changes that occur in your life can be exceptionally beneficial to your growth process.

6) Your Personal Journal is a safe place to write your ideas, thoughts, feelings, self-observations, daily happenings, plans and solutions.

7) Slant your journal towards finding solutions and learning about yourself.

8) Behavior patterns will emerge over time if you review your journal from an open-minded perspective.

9) A key strategy of successful people is "talking it out on paper".

10) Several projects are listed. Try them and make up your own to get the most out of your Personal Journal.

Troubleshooting Guide

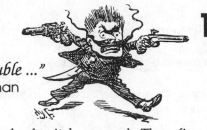

13

"For them to read when they're in trouble ..."
A. E. Housman

Every one of us (yes, me included) runs into temporary glitches once in a while. Life is full of little bumps and surprises that can sidetrack even the most directed and motivated individual. But that's life for you ... just learn to expect it and handle it, and you won't get completely derailed every time something comes along ... which it will, and often, too.

In this chapter you will find what I have identified as some of the most common little buggers and a few suggestions as to what to do to keep them at bay. Read through them now even if you aren't having problems at the moment. That way, when one does come calling, you will be prepared. Reread this Troubleshooting Guide whenever you need extra help, and remember, it was written because I have experienced every one of these situations often enough to know that they can become problems only if you let them. Getting past the mountains time after time will eventually give you the confidence that you can and will climb them successfully ... and presto, they become molehills! A tendency to give up when these things happen just means that either you don't have a clue as to how to combat them, or you have failed in the past and this has eroded your confidence to deal with them successfully. But not this time! With the help of this guide, you are going to get on top of them and each little win will lead to bigger wins. Pretty soon you'll be able to sit in the same room alone with plateful of hot-from-the-oven cookies and not even flinch!

Dealing With Setbacks

First, remember that any setback that you may have is only temporary. The main direction of your weight loss is downward, whether or not there are occasional glitches. Always keep that downward trend foremost in your mind ... never take your eyes off that goal of reduced weight. Remember what Helen Keller said: "It's impossible to see the shadows when you are staring at the sun". You will get there. Now, just get right back on your weight control routine and realize that yesterday is water under the bridge. The longer you wait the harder it will be. There is absolutely nothing you can do about yesterday ... with one exception. You can learn from your mistakes. Remember, there is a seed of equal or greater benefit in any setback. Analyze what

happened and why it happened. Then figure out what you can do next time to avoid the problem. Sometimes this can take many trials and errors before you straighten the problem out. Just keep at it and never, never, never, never give up! Even if it takes longer than you would want, isn't it better to finally get thin than to give up and never get thin? This is not a contest. There is nobody that you are racing to find the food plan and behavior changes that will be unique to you and keep you thin forever. Whatever it takes, you have to go through the actions and complete each step for your own situation before going on. This temporary setback that you have had is one of those steps. This is your golden opportunity to face the challenge, figure it out and get rid of it for good! That way a year from now you won't be stumbling over the same stretch of road ... you'll be miles down the highway.

Be patient with yourself. Forgive yourself for goofing. We all do it, and you're not "bad" because you made a choice you regret now. Be good to yourself. Give yourself a pat on the back right now for looking in this Troubleshooting Guide for assistance. You are doing the right thing since that action shows you are looking for answers instead of just giving up. Be assured, you are eating the best food available and you are following a plan that will get you thin, and keep you thin, the absolutely fastest way you can while maintaining super health. Write in your Personal Journal exactly how you are feeling now. Talk to your support person or group in an unhurried and thorough way about what happened, how you are feeling and what direction you can take now. Write down anything about the incident that caused the setback and keep your Daily Success Planner. This is vitally important. Eat something you really love. If you are on a binge or plateau see the sections below for more specific solutions.

One action I take when I have had a setback may surprise you. I reward myself. Yes, you read it right! I actually buy myself a reward. Why? Because I have taken the time to confront the issue of the setback because I deserve to acknowledge the positive direction I have chosen because I did not give up because it is a positive move to look for and act upon a solution instead of wallowing in the setback and having a little pity party for me, myself and I! You deserve a reward for choosing to do something about the problem this time, too. One of the worst things you can do right now is tell yourself you are bad or you have "blown it again". That attitude is the real culprit! Good attitude ... positive action ... reward!

Congratulations on choosing the right solution and having faith in yourself!   By keeping at it, you will eventually get there.

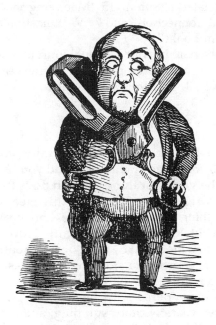

Drastic measures aren't always called for.

Quick Tips - Setbacks
1) Setbacks are only temporary. Keep your eye on your goal and off the setback. What you think about expands. Think control.
2) Let it go, forgive yourself and learn from your mistake by facing and analyzing the incident.
3) Keep your Daily Success Planner.
4) Talk to your support person or group. "Confess" it all.
5) Write in your Personal Journal.
6) Eat something you love.
7) Reward yourself for getting back on track.
8) Keep exercising.

Food Cravings and Urges

Use Chapter 15 "Managing the Food-Mood Connection" to identify exactly what you are craving, if you don't already know. As soon as you know what it is, then plan it into your daily menu as soon as possible. If it's ice cream that you want, see if something else cool and creamy such as yogurt, frozen yogurt or a Cream Fluff will do the trick (see Chapter 30 "Basic Recipes"). If it just has to be ice cream, then decide if you must have a full serving or if just a taste or a smaller serving will do to satisfy you. Sometimes a tempting food in the house can start a craving, and just one bite will stop the craving. (Be careful, though ... sometimes just a bite primes the pump!). I always count each bite of extra food as 25 additional calories for the day. That keeps the number of "little tastes" down to a minimum. If a bite just won't do, then go ahead, figure out what the food will "cost" you in fat grams, calories, etc. and write it down in your Daily Success Planner. Then enjoy! No guilt.

Remember that a craving is not the same as an urge. An urge can be more difficult to handle since it comes on you suddenly and almost demands immediate action. Walking by the cookie shop in a shopping mall where they are unmercifully baking fresh, hot cookies, and getting a heavenly whiff, might trigger an urge. There often isn't time for adequate sensible planning at this point! In this case, get out of the vicinity of the food pronto and get busy with something else. In a mall, I might go into a store and try on that great outfit I've had my eye on, or duck into a book store and browse. Often when the food is out of sight and smell, an urge will leave just as quickly as it appeared.

Whether it's an urge or a craving that strikes, and you want to avoid eating the food altogether then try these techniques. In the case of an urge, get as far away from the food as possible. If you and the food are at home alone together, then either get out of the house or get the food out of the house. Wash the food down the garbage disposal if necessary! Try, at all costs, to avoid taking that first bite. Then keep as busy as possible. Once you give in to the urge or craving it is much harder to stop than if you never get started at all. Boredom is one of the main reasons why people tend to drift towards their old habits of filling up the empty space inside with food. Take a long, hot bath or shower. You'll feel more relaxed and more in control after spending an hour this way. Make yourself a pot of herbal tea, put on a favorite piece of quiet music and snuggle into a big, soft chair for a good hour of fantasy reading. This is a great time to practice meditation (see Chapter 11 "Breathing and Meditation"). Or get out of the house and take a walk, or exercise in some other way such as putting on an exercise video tape and working out. Give yourself a manicure. It will keep your hands busy for quite a while. Call a friend or someone in your support group and tell them what is going on with you. A sympathetic, empathetic ear often helps. Even if you aren't having urges and cravings now, you should think about the times when this may happen to you ... and be prepared. In your Personal Journal, make a list ahead of time, of your favorite activities and diversions that will come to your personal rescue when you need them. Make short-term goals such as getting from breakfast to lunch without overeating. Then reward yourself for doing it and make another goal right away.

Perhaps none of the above suggestions are for you. They are simply things that have gotten me over my own bumps when food seemed like the only thing in the world that would help. It wasn't ... there were plenty of other activities out there just waiting, but I had to work at changing the habit of automatically reaching for food. That was the easy, lazy way out. Make your own list and get it out when you're in need. Ask yourself if you'll still feel good about what you're about to do food-wise if you allow yourself to eat the offending food. Maybe it won't be worth it later. Remember how awful, guilty and hopeless you may feel in an hour or so if you give in. Now, instead, visualize yourself overcoming the craving or the urge and how great you feel by conquering it this time (see Chapter 7 "Visualization and Dream Books"). See yourself, smiling and confident, as you step on the scale the next time.

Above all, don't be hard on yourself. We're all human and there isn't one among us who doesn't have ups and downs when striving for a goal. You are reaching for a big one and deserve a lot of credit for that alone.

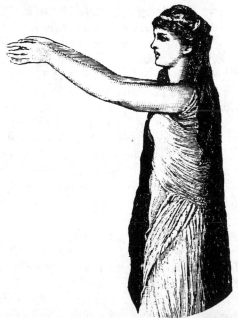

When the cookies at the mall call your name ...

Quick Tips - Food Cravings and Urges
1) Find out what type of food you are craving and how you can safely meet your need. Is it a physiological need such as a vitamin deficiency or a longer term emotional void.
2) Cravings are not urges.

3) To squelch an urge (temporary desire triggered by an external stimulus, like smelling cookies at the mall) remove yourself or the food.
4) Avoid taking that first bite ... it may "prime the pump".
5) Or just take a taste and really enjoy it (if you're in control).
6) Have your alternative activities list ready ahead of time. Be prepared.
7) See related chapters: 15 "Managing the Food-Mood Connection" and 7 "Visualization and Dream Books".
8) Make a note in your Personal Journal of what works - so you'll be ready for the next time.
9) Above all, give yourself credit!

Binge Busting

Okay. Due to temporary insanity you have given in to your urge or craving ... and you can't seem to stop. The very best thing you can do is to put the fork down right now. Not after this meal or after the whole thing is gone not tomorrow not on Monday morning, but RIGHT NOW! Great! Now drink 2 glasses of water, take five deep breaths and congratulate yourself for stopping as soon as you did. Believe me, this is wonderful! As I mentioned earlier, I have personally been on a binge that lasted three years without stopping, and I've heard others say the same thing. So stopping is indeed great. If this cold turkey approach is not working, then taper off ... shovel a little bit slower, and begin adding some planned food into the binge. Eat an apple for every bag of chips you crunch down (hey, it's a start!). Be sure you are fixing your food properly. Start looking at portions again, serving it on a plate and sitting down to eat at the dining table. Do not stand over the kitchen sink and wolf down food. Be good to yourself.

As soon as you slow down ... or better yet, put the fork or food down altogether, get out your Daily Success Planner and write down everything that you ate. Yes, everything. Estimate the serving sizes if you failed to keep weighing and measuring. Most of the time you'll find that it really wasn't as bad as you thought. Two or three sandwiches or a quart of ice cream are really small potatoes when you compare it to all the food you eat in a week. Even if you went whole hog and pigged out on Mexican food supremo for dinner, the fact is you had to eat dinner anyway, so a lot of those calories were needed. Maybe only 1000 extra calories were consumed, and that only averages out to 150 extra a day or so over a week, so all is not lost! Once you have stopped, written everything down and decided not to berate yourself for the episode, then switch to the techniques for avoiding the cravings and urges as discussed in that sections above.

At this time, the best thing to do is just get on with it. Again, there is nothing you can do about the food you've already eaten. So learn what you can from the experience, determine how to avoid what got you started in the first place and don't even bother punishing yourself for the slip-up. There is a reason this happened and you should try to uncover it (see Chapter 15 "Managing The Food-Mood Connection", especially "Anatomy of a Binge"). Only in this way will you be able to face up to the real motivation and deal with it, instead of trying to stuff it down and forget it with food. Drowning yourself in alcohol, drugs or food will never solve your problems. Only facing them and pushing through the problem to the solution that exists on the other side will effectively eliminate the emotion that caused you to eat. If you are angry at someone, tell them, write it down or tell another person. If you eat instead, you will not only stay fat, but you will still be angry. Food will solve nothing.

Most importantly, treat yourself like you are your own best friend. If he or she called you up, distraught and guilty over being on a binge, what would you tell them? "You stupid fool! Eating like a pig again!? When will you ever learn?" No good friend would ever treat you that way. And you shouldn't treat yourself that way either. Be kind, understanding, and tell yourself, "Well, the worst is over. It's great that you were able to stop and get control of yourself. We're all human and slip up once in awhile. Now it's time to get back on the plan". This attitude will allow you to eliminate the guilty and negative feelings that often can happen after a binge. Associate the bad feelings with the binge itself, with being out of control. Pair feeling good with the times you are on your plan, in control and calling your own shots. Whenever you're on your plan you are doing great!

Plateaus

We've all had the disheartening experience of being absolutely virtuous all week and having that #@!*#! scale stubbornly stick at the same weight. This is called a plateau and is a natural part of losing weight. Your body just seems to need a breather after losing a few pounds. This phenomenon is also one of the best reasons for not weighing every day. It's a kind of desperation that's predestined to be painful. Having your day ruled by the scale is giving away control of your emotions... to an inanimate object, no less. A week will usually give your body time to do something positive with all your effort. But not always.

First, make sure you are watching your portions and type of food, drinking all your water every day, getting some form of exercise at least 3-5 times per week. Check your Daily Success Planner for the past week to see if you have eaten anything particularly salty in the last few days. Often a dill pickle, Chinese dinner out or other high sodium foods can cause you to retain water and show a temporary weight gain at the scale. Check Chapter 34 "Sodium" for sources of excess salt, and ways to reduce it in your diet. Women tend to retain a few pounds of water about a week before their periods, so consider that if it is applicable.

If you are doing everything you should and are still not showing a loss after a good honest effort then perhaps you will just have to be patient. Sometimes your body is losing inches and consolidating the losses you already have made. Often, these will be the weeks when you notice that your waistband is actually a bit looser! And certain people will lose very slowly, as I did ... usually only $1/2$ pound or less per week! My metabolism was extremely low because of genetics and so many years of yo-yo dieting. I often experienced extended plateaus for no good apparent reason. Just continue on your plan and eventually the pounds will begin to come off again. Consistency is critical for your success. Concentrate on working other parts of your plan, such as recipe conversions, exercise or keeping your attitude positive. Remember, you are aiming for optimum health and the weight loss is just a by-product of great health.

If you feel you want or need to try and push through the plateau forcibly, instead of waiting it out ... then let's take a look at a few of the more active steps you can take. If you are eating at the high end of your range of food, consider switching to the low end for a week or going on the Accelerated Plan (see Chapter 37). I caution you again not to limit your food too drastically however, since that may trigger the survival mechanism in your body. This is when you limit food too much and your body perceives this as a threat to its survival ... and actually slows down your metabolism in order to conserve calories. That's the last thing you want! Too little food can also trigger cravings as your body tries to get you to eat more to satisfy its nutrient and calorie needs. It's trying to keep from starving. So be sure you are eating a well-balanced diet with enough calories (about 1200 minimum for women, 1500 for men). Watch your fat grams carefully. Consider dropping to 10% of total calories in fat for a few days or a week. Add an extra aerobic session or two a week, or take a ten minute brisk walk after every meal for the next week. Drink quarts of water and limit your sodium intake. Hang on, be strong and you will get there. This plateau is only temporary and it happens to everybody!

Hunger

When I find myself standing in the kitchen in between meal or snack times, I ask myself the question, "Have you been drinking all your water today?" Nine times out of ten the answer will be "No", and that's when I pour myself a tall one ... mineral water with a fresh strawberry, or a steaming, fragrant, soothing pot of herbal tea. Or I might just have a cool, refreshing glass or two of plain water or herbal ice tea. It's really surprising how much that satisfies the need for something in your stomach. Often, when you think you're hungry, you're really thirsty instead. So start there.

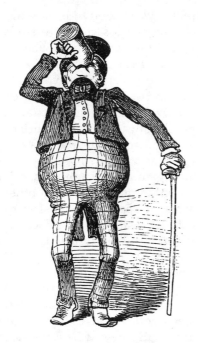

*Reach for the water
when you're hungry between snacks.*

If you haven't eaten in at least two hours consider having a snack. There are many options for healthy snacks depending upon what you have eaten so far that day and what you have planned for the rest of the day. Fiber is the key to alleviating hunger (see Chapter 33 "Fiber is Your Friend"). Vegetables should be first and foremost on your list when considering a snack, especially when you're hungry between meals. Keep your emergency container of raw, crunchy veggies in the front of the refrigerator. Start munching on these first while you are deciding what other veggies you may wish to have. Ask yourself what qualities in particular you are wanting. Something hot and filling? Try a steaming bowl of spaghetti squash with spaghetti sauce or salsa on the top and a sprinkle of parmesan cheese. Craving something sweet and rich? How about an Instant Pumpkin Pudding spiced with

vanilla and cinnamon (see "Basic Recipes"). A big, fresh salad with yogurt and salsa dressing might fill that gap before your next meal. Or a big artichoke with yogurt-mustard dipping sauce. Most of the time when hunger is constant, you are not eating enough vegetables or drinking enough water or both.

Check your Daily Success Planner to see if you have a piece of fruit to use for a snack, or perhaps a dairy serving. I often save my fruit and milk servings for desserts and in-between times. Try a Cream Fluff for instant satisfaction. They are easy and quick and come in practically unlimited varieties. Try to eat bulky, high fiber foods for maximum filling power. A cup of fruited yogurt or a chocolate shake made from reduced-calorie mix goes further to satisfy hunger than a cup of skim milk. A whole apple will give you lots of crunch and munch power while a 6 ounce serving of apple juice goes down quickly and may not be as satisfying.

Certain times of the month a woman's hormonal system may cause undue hunger which can be harder than usual to satisfy. Wild and crazy visions of food pass through my thoughts for about a week out of every month! You've got to learn to recognize this as normal and come up with some options, lest you be thrown off balance every month. I believe that PMS (pre-menstrual syndrome) is not an isolated occurrence that only happens to a few of us women. It happens to all of us! It's just a matter of degree. And, if it happens to all of us, then it's a normal occurrence, right? There are certain foods it is best to avoid at this time, such as caffeine, sugar, salt and alcohol. They tend to exaggerate the symptoms. Pay special attention to eating foods that you absolutely love for maximum fulfillment. Eating especially high bulk foods may help since they physically fill the stomach to the point where you can actually feel the fullness. Sometimes the craving for food continues, but you can at least tell yourself that your stomach is definitely full and the craving is hormonal in nature. Also, be sure you are doing some sort of stress-reducing activity at this time such as stretching, light exercise, hot baths, mental relaxation techniques or meditation. Lighten up a little on yourself.

At any time, exercise can actually decrease your appetite, so consider a long walk or an hour doing your favorite physical activity. Keep busy! Fill up your time with activities that focus on other people, such as volunteer work at a local school, hospital or library. Having other people in your life who depend on you for a daily smile or encouraging word can go a long way to eliminate the need to "fill up the emptiness" with food. By reaching out to others you are also giving yourself a helping hand.

Food Allergies

If you have, or suspect, allergies to certain foods such as milk or wheat, then I suggest that you consult with your physician or a nutritionist. They will be able to help you adjust your food plan to ensure that you still receive the necessary nutrients in your diet. They may possibly suggest that you take certain vitamins, minerals or other supplements to compensate for the missing nutrients.

This should also be your strategy if you are in need of a special diet. This might include a diabetic regime, vegetarian diet, children under the age of 12, pregnant or lactating women, or any type of food intolerance. Don't try to experiment here or guess. A professionals input is best for your health and will give you added confidence in your plan. Make it a point to educate yourself on the foods which can impact your life so greatly.

Too Much Food

Believe it or not, there are actually those lucky souls who feel that there is just too much food on the plan! If you have a hard time fulfilling all of the serving requirements every day without feeling overstuffed, then here are a few suggestions. Rather than skipping meals or required foods, try switching to low bulk foods instead. Drink juice instead of eating the whole fruit, choose to eat salads and soups less and drink just the eight minimum glasses of water a day. Switch to reduced-calorie bread and eat lower bulk cereal such as fat-free granola instead of puffed wheat or rice. Choose also to have few or none of the additional calories or extra servings you are allowed for the week. Eating more often, but smaller amounts may also keep you from feeling too full.

In A Nutshell

1) Everyone has temporary glitches and setbacks.

2) Yesterday is gone! Forgive yourself and get back on the program.

3) Learn from your mistakes. Figure out what went wrong so you can avoid the problem next time.

4) Quick Tips for handling setbacks, cravings and urges were discussed.

5) The best time to end a binge is NOW! Analyze your behavior and take control.

6) Be sure you always treat yourself with love. Out of control behavior does not make you a "bad" person.

7) Plateaus are natural. Consistency is critical for your success. Stay on your program. Drink lots of water and limit sodium.

8) If you're hungry eat extra fiber and drink water.

Part III

Behavior Changes

Taming Your Stress

14

Mac Beth: "Canst thou not ... raze out the ... troubles of the brain?"
Doctor: "Therein the patient must minister to himself."
William Shakespeare

The Alphabet Soup of Stress

Stress, in its typical sense, is negative pressure or tension with which you must deal. Generally, stresses of different kinds are uncomfortable and tend to draw energy away from you as you fight to control it. Stress can cause everything from emotional upset (and a ruined dinner party) to physical diseases like ulcers and high blood pressure. The following A to Z list presents just a few of the possible kinds of stresses and effects of stress that can enter your life. Do you recognize any of these stressors in your life?

Anger, anxiety, "armoring" (overall muscle tension), apathy
Boredom, binges
"Can't do it" thinking, cravings
Depression, dissatisfaction, disgust, drinking too much
Environmental stress (noise, too much going on),
    Eating too much
Fatigue, fear, frustration, fat
Guilt, giving up, grazing (non-stop eating)
Hardened arteries, headaches, high blood pressure,
    high fat-salt-cholesterol diet, hunger, hatred
Illness, irritability, isolation
Jammed lifestyle (feeling pushed into a corner),
    jaded (tired or worn out)
Keeping your feelings bottled up, killjoy
    (destroying other people's fun)
Lack of hope, lack of energy, loneliness
Martyrism (choosing to suffer)
Negative mental attitude, nibbling
Obesity, over-reacting, overly-sensitive to criticism,
    overwhelmed
Pain, pessimism, poor self-esteem, plateaus, paralyzed
Quarrelsome
Resentment
Sedentary lifestyle, self pity, sadness
Too serious, type A personality (never relaxed, hard driving)
Unassertive (people push you around), urges to eat
Vitamin deficient, vague hunger
Worry, weakness
Xenophobic (fear of strangers)
"Yes man" mentality (agreeing with others only to be compliant)
Zodiac dependency (placing responsibility for your life on outside forces or astrology)

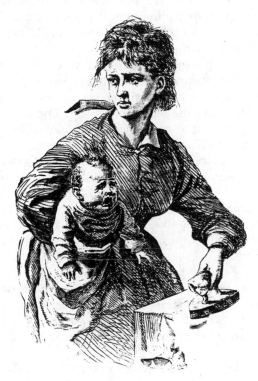

"Stress? What stress?"

If you can't relate to at least one or two of these stressors you're probably either a Zen master or you're dead and just don't know it yet! It's impossible to live a completely stress-free life. There's always going to be something new to cause your stress meter to soar no matter how aware and focused you are on releasing stress (There is even such a thing as positive stress). But there are techniques which you can use to lessen the negative effects of stress that we are all faced with. According to Dr. Norman Shealy, in his book **Ninety Days To Self-Health**, there is only one health-related influence that is completely out of your control: congenital problems with which you were born. Barring that, you can choose to recognize and learn to cope with anything. The health factors that are fully under your control include your personal habits, attitudes, living environment, diet, exercise patterns and faith (personal beliefs). In addition, there are trainable factors you can control such as your body temperature and immune responses which can result in a healthier state of being.

Is This Stress, or What?

We are living in stress-filled times. You can tell from all the antacid commercials they run on TV. More, more, more. Faster, faster, faster. A-a-rg! That must be why they invented remote controls ... so you could turn off the 500 word per minute, non-stop commercials without getting up! They're trying oh-so-hard to control your moods. And you've got lots of them, too. It's not just a simple matter of feeling good or feeling bad. It would be a lot easier to keep your stress levels under control if there were only those two mood states.

Unfortunately, you may have come to rely on food as an all-purpose way to relieve stress. That's counter-productive when it comes to controlling your weight, to say the least. So it's very important to learn to clearly identify your problem stressors and find more effective ways to deal with them then popping a Goo-Goo Pie. Your personal stressors will show themselves in your moods or emotions, but they may initially come disguised as other people or situations that are out of your direct control. What you think about them or how you choose to respond to them is in your control (more on that in a minute).

But first, how do you know when you're under stress? Here are some signs to look for:

1) Eating when you're not hungry, or at irregular times.
2) Drinking too much (more than 2 alcoholic drinks a day).
3) Emotional volatility ("blowing up" over non-critical events).
4) Sickness (colds, headaches, not feeling "well"), especially lingering, resistant symptoms.
5) Feeling overly tired and lacking energy.
6) Sleeping poorly or excessively to avoid people or situations.
7) Avoiding responsibilities, social situations or people.
8) Feeling "flat" or "down in the dumps", unable to enjoy life.
9) Giving up, not caring.
* If you can think of other stress symptoms in your life write them down in your journal.

Handling Intense Stress

You knew from the very beginning that there was going to be more to losing weight and keeping it off than just the issues of food and exercise. You've already dealt with those factors and you're still struggling. Self-awareness is equally critical. One of the most important steps that you can take to get control of your lifestyle is to know yourself well enough to really understand what gets under your skin and causes you to eat. Here is a 4-step strategy for handling problem stress: **BAMM!** (Yes, I know this pushes the limits of cleverness, but BAMM sounds so much better than AAAC.)

1) **B**ecome aware of the stress.
2) **A**cknowledge how you feel.
3) **M**ake a list of acceptable alternative behaviors to substitute for eating.
4) **M**ake a commitment to do something on your list.

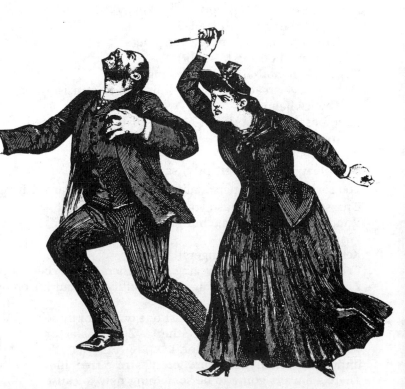

"Moody?! What do mean moody?!"

The following list contains some of my personal emotional states and how I deal with them in terms of eating. Your list will certainly differ somewhat from mine, but this will give you a basic guideline to follow.

Mood	Never Eat	May/May Not Eat	Always Eat
Anger		X	
Boredom		X	
Confusion	X (Only when I'm too confused to find the refrigerator!)		
Defeat			X
Deprivation		X	
Emptiness			X
Fatigue		X	
Fear			X
Frustration		X	
Guilt		X	
Joy		X	
Loneliness		X	
Overwhelmed			X
Regret		X	
Relief		X	
Resentment			X
Sadness		X	
Tension			X
Vengeful			X

As you can see from this list, there are a variety of moods or emotions that I have to be wary of in terms of eating. I know from experience and my own self-analysis that I always ate when I felt defeated, empty, fearful, overwhelmed, resentful, tense or vengeful (!).

These are definitely not pleasant moods to experience, and as you might guess, I avoid them whenever possible. However, during the course of my life I do admit to experiencing them all at one time or another. It is this honesty with myself that has allowed me to acknowledge and cope with my eating in response to stress before it gets too far out of control, and has accordingly allowed me to be able to successfully control my weight. The extra fringe benefit is that by feeling in control of my moods and behaviors I feel good about myself a large portion of the time. And I deserve to. This was hard work!

The same results can happen for you. Make up a similar chart for yourself in your journal or contact THINNER WINNERS for a copy of the workbook for this program. Filling in this chart is a big step towards getting control of your problem eating behaviors. You will be increasing your awareness of the moods that stress causes you to feel.

Once you have become aware of your potential problem moods, the second step is to acknowledge how you feel. Be honest. There's nobody here but you and me so why not take a minute to think and answer truthfully? It's okay to feel what you feel. Most of these feelings are unpleasant enough ... you

don't need to add any extra doses of guilt. Your objective should be to spend as little time as possible stuck in a lousy mood. Be especially wary of the particular vulnerability you may experience if two or more of these moods occur at the same time. This can and does often happen, and takes courage and awareness on your part to stay in charge.

If your mood seems to be caused by another person or some event out of your control, keep in mind that by hanging on to the negative mood you are essentially giving that outside source control over your emotions. You don't have to do that, and nobody can make you. You are in charge of your thoughts and emotions. You can choose your moods! If not you, then who? Why not choose a mood you want right now? What's stopping you? You can be happy or joyful in any situation. That includes working, washing dishes or even paying bills. You can choose happiness any time! Having said that, there will be a number of ways for you to act appropriately for the mood you're choosing to feel. For example, if you've decided to be angry, you could yell (preferably at the sky or some inanimate object). If you're feeling tense you could meditate or take a warm bath to unwind. If you're feeling defeated it's certainly appropriate to cry, call a sympathetic friend or write in your Personal Journal. Remember, whatever the mood is, it will eventually pass.

The third step in effectively handling problem moods is to make a list of acceptable alternative behaviors to substitute for eating. Eating as a way

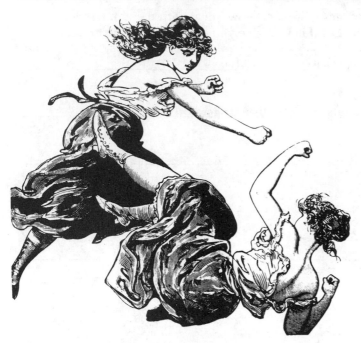

*It's hard to make progress
when you're fighting with yourself.*

of dealing with your moods is perhaps the most costly choice that you can make. Moods will pass. On the other hand, compulsive stress-related eating tends to be of the kind of foods that will stick with you for a long time (see Chapter 15 "Managing the Food-Mood Connection"). You certainly don't want to allow your mood of today to affect your waistline next week. Or even worse, to lead you into a binge cycle.

Instead, imagine that there is no food available. What will you do instead of eating? Here are a few suggestions ... add more of your own.

1) React appropriately to the mood (yell, cry, look for insights).
2) Talk to yourself or your support person about it.
3) Write the issues down in your journal.
4) Exercise, take a walk (this is my favorite mood manager).
5) Go someplace you enjoy (beach, a museum, the movies, shopping).
6) Do something for yourself (take a bath, read, bake bread).

7) Drink water (or eat something appropriate ... veggies are our friends).
8) Tell yourself "I'm only human ... it's okay to feel this".
9) Think positive! Become assertive about your moods (take control - it's your choice how you feel). Substitute positive thoughts for any negative ones. Positive thoughts put you in harmony with solutions and constructive action. Negative thoughts disconnect you from the flow of possible assistance. Pick a positive affirmation such as "I can lighten up and stick my tongue out at this stress!". Then smile and do it. Remember NLP in Chapter 6 "Great Expectations".
10) Laugh it off. Make funny faces in the mirror until you laugh. If that doesn't work turn on the Comedy Channel.

The fourth and final step in the BAMM process is to make a commitment to doing something on your list. This is the critical point. In the past you have probably given in to the urge to eat some kind of "solace food". Now is the time to truly grasp the concept that **"you can't expect anything in your life to change for the better if you keep doing the same old things"**. This is not rocket science. By repeating the coping method that you've used in the past (eating), the same one that has never allowed you to maintain a weight loss for any length of time, you are just setting yourself up for failure. So don't fall for that trap again. Take your list of alternative behaviors and put one of them to use. Now! This may take some concentration and discipline on your part, but by learning to substitute positive behaviors for self-defeating ones you will help yourself achieve your goals.

This 4-step BAMM! strategy will work for you, if you choose not to give in to negative moods and immediate-gratification eating. Become aware of your mood, acknowledge how you're feeling, make a list of solutions and make a commitment to use one of them. You are responsible for your life, and you can take charge of your decisions. It's time for you to make new choices and get new positive results. You can choose to be as creative and individual in this process as you allow yourself to be. Who knows? It could even be fun.

The ABC's of Stress Reduction

The following list is a cornucopia of techniques which you can use to reduce and manage the stresses in your life, and make day to day living a much more enjoyable experience.

Aerobic activity

Your body wasn't designed to sit cramped behind a desk. Activity relieves tension. Take a walk, dance a jig, get moving. Be sure and stretch first.

Breathing

Eastern religions and martial arts emphasize the simple power of breathing correctly. View each refreshing, deep breath as a gift. Close your eyes and take ten deep breaths, relax your muscles and smile. (See Chapter 11 "Breathing and Meditation".)

Count to Ten

Before you make a big decision or jump into the heated fray of an argument take a deep breath and slowly count to ten ... you just might get the insight you need to turn the event into a win-win situation.

Drink plenty of water

Dehydration can cause everything from constipation to headaches. Water lubricates your joints and washes away your bodily waste products. Drink 8 glasses a day. Have a glass now.

Eat right

The American epidemic of heart disease is due primarily to a high fat, high salt diet. A nutritionally well-balanced diet, high in vegetables, fruits and fiber will slim you down and pep you up. Avoid fat, sugar, sodium, caffeine and alcohol. Relax and have a cup of herbal tea.

Exercise

You won't build muscle and burn fat by sitting on your fanny. The endorphins released during exercise will help you feel good mentally. You'll look better, too.

Find your "quiet center"

There's a wonderfully peaceful "quiet center" in your mind that provides your ultimate haven. It's got everything that you need for perfect peace, and it's only one thought away. The next time stress is nipping at your heels, excuse yourself for a moment and head for your own internal paradise. It's there when you need it. Learn how to tap into the energy and power within yourself.

Get enough sleep

One of the classic "brain washing" torture techniques is sleep deprivation. It can cause physical illness and hallucinations. You won't think clearly if you're tired, and you can't really improve your life if you're not thinking clearly. Get a good night's sleep tonight. If you're exhausted now, take a nap.

Have some fun

When was the last time you played with your dog, children or spouse? The happiest, healthiest people always seem to be having a good time. Tickle someone today. Or work on your hobby.

I Can

There is nothing more important that you can say. You'll get more done, feel better about it and relieve more stress when you say "I can".

"Jaywalk"

Perfection is a lofty ideal to shoot for but the rules keep changing. Vincent Van Gogh painted some perfect paintings but he couldn't sell any of them during his lifetime. Relax and bend the rules a little bit ... especially when they're rules of your own making. Take the long way home and wave to a stranger.

Keep a joy journal

Write down the highlights of every single day. After a year you'll have a list of 365 good things that happened to you.

Kick the Kangaroo

Are you driving yourself crazy by jumping around and trying to do eight things at once? One of the identifiable traits of genius is the ability to stick with a single task until it's done. Take a good look at all your tasks, put them in order of priority, and do the number one item until it's done. You'll feel great.

Listen to Music

Put on some peaceful music or a relaxation tape, stretch out on the couch, loosen up those muscles and relax. Or put on some headphones and tune in to a private concert.

Learn to Laugh

NOTE: This is an essential life skill. Without laughter you will not live nearly as long and your life won't be worth much anyway. If you haven't laughed at least once today put on a funny video tape now and laugh your cares away.

Maintain positive health

So many things seem to scramble for your attention, but when your health goes down everything goes down with it. So eat right, exercise and keep your attitude positive.

Nice people finish first

Instead of smashing carts at the grocery store let somebody in ahead of you. Take a long, slow deep breath and browse through the National Irrational Pseudo-News for a few chuckles while waiting in line.

Obsess on positive thoughts

If you don't leave room in your mind for any negativity, it won't be there to trouble you. Plant the images from your Dream Book firmly in your mind. Enjoy a mini mental vacation.

Pray for PMA (Positive Mental Attitude)

Ask your divine power source for help and guidance, know it will come and keep those positive thoughts in your mind. Always focus on the possibilities of a project, never the obstacles. You'll be amazed how quickly help will come your way when you're receptive to it.

Quiet

Shhhhhhh. When your mind is buzzing like a hive of bees and you've got some problem you just can't seem to solve, find a quiet spot, take a dozen deep breaths and give your mind 30 minutes of uninterrupted thought time. Shhhhhhh. Push those distant worries out of your mind. The answer will come to you.

Read something good

No matter what your problem is, chances are good that it has happened to someone else, too. Not only that, they've probably written a book or article about how they solved it. So head down to the library or bookstore and get some help. Worrying won't solve anything, but productive action will.

Stretch

Your muscles are stiff and sore because they're so TIGHT! Take ten minutes and slowly stre-e-etchhhhhhhhhh. Relax and stre-e-etchhhhhhhhh. Ahhhhhhhhhhhh ....

Take one moment at a time

Here and now is where you are. Guilt drags your mind into a long-gone past that you can never change. Worry focuses your mind on the one possible future that you absolutely don't want. So why bother with either of them? Work on the task at hand and give it your best shot. Life is nothing but a series of moments that you get to string together in the theme of your choice. Make a beautiful necklace of gem-like "moments".

Unwind with friends

Sip some tea with your best pals and get it off your chest (whatever it is). Don't carry around the weight of old emotional baggage. Your friends will help you, and you can help them, too. We all need each other.

Visualize

Picture your goal clearly in your mind and visualize yourself with the dream already accomplished. It feels good, doesn't it? And you're on your way to getting there that much quicker.

Volunteer

Help somebody out. If you're able to do this, then things just won't seem so bad for you ... and smiling will come easier, too.

Walk tall

Combine the best of walking (and drawing in that wonderful oxygen) and positive thoughts with their guaranteed energy boost. This is the first moment of the rest of your life, so enter your future with pride. The possibilities for your success are unlimited!

X marks the spot

Here you are! You've had a million adventures along the way and there are a million more to come. Whatever future you plan for, and work towards, can come to pass. Enjoy the trip, it may be the only one you get.

"Yes"

It's the most positive thing that you can say. You've been telling yourself "No" for so long that you've probably forgotten that it's okay to let yourself relax, unwind and enjoy the incredible experience of living on this beautiful planet. Take a deep breath and feel alive! Yes, you can be happy.

Zarf

A small, metal, cup-like stand , usually ornamental, for holding hot coffee cups (no, I'm not making this up!). What! You don't have one? Well, look around at all the wonderful and amazing things you do have. So your cup isn't full yet, is that any reason not to enjoy life? You can get a lot more done by being vigorous, happy and relaxed than by any stressed-out, tension filled manner you could describe. So relax. And if you happen to pick up a zarf, try to stick to decaf.

It's just possible that the solution for your particular form of stress didn't show up on the previous list. If that's the case, here's a few more ideas you might try out: take a long, hot bath; take a shower and sing while you're in there; sex and cuddling in general is a great tension reliever; cook up your favorite treat and share it with a friend; plant a flower or tree; go to a support group meeting; meditate; take a nap, or if it's late, just go to bed early; hug someone today ... a good long one; hug yourself for not giving up; smile at the first ten people you see today; start singing a happy song just because ... "Singin' In The Rain" is my favorite.

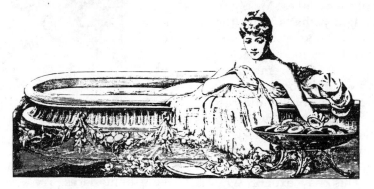

Aaaaaaaaaaaah, a long, hot bubble bath ...

Loosen Up Your Chuckle Buckle

I feel so strongly about humor as a great way to manage stress, and avoid the short-circuiting that stress can cause, that I'd like to cover this wonderful life skill and coping tool in more detail. Surprisingly, embarking on any new project, even a life-enhancing program, can cause you stress. You will be pursuing activities that will, by design, cause you to make changes. And changes almost always cause some degree of stress ... even when you know they're good for you. A weight control program is certainly no exception. It is therefore a good idea to have a handy bag of additional tools to call upon when you're feeling under pressure. The ultimate purpose of this section is to help you stay on the sunny side of the street as you walk towards long-term weight control.

Losing weight can be a complex business and at times you may feel like you're balanced on a high wire while being forced to juggle knives, hum, chew gum and hop at the same time. So it's really important to remember to keep a smile on your face. After all, your final objective is to be thinner, healthier and happier. Admiral Fullgut of the Gravy Navy may disagree, and state loudly that dieting is serious business and must be done in a solemn, sullen manner ... but he's mistaken. The health consequences of being overweight are serious,

but once you start to deal effectively with the issues involved you can take off the undertaker disguise.

One of the greatest mistakes that's been foisted on the American culture in recent years is the concept of "playing hard", as in "work hard, play hard". If everything in your life is hard, you're doing something wrong. Life is a wonderful, experiential, learning process, not an endless race. Laughing out loud with the sheer joy of life will do you far more good than bellowing out that you're this week's King of the Mountain. In fact a recent phenomenon to emerge in the business world is the concept of actually working yourself to death. In Japan, several hundred high-level executives have died during the past few years, and thousands more reported stress related illnesses. It got so bad that the government had to set work-reduction guidelines. All work and no play sets Jack up for a heart attack. So be very wary of taking things too seriously.

If you find yourself pulling out your hair over the horrible state of the world that you see on the evening news, do yourself a big favor and channel-surf your way over to the comedy network or the Travel Channel. Give your poor drained brain a vacation.

For a long time I relied on the expression "No Negs" (no negative thinking) whenever I felt myself getting caught up in the horrors of the headlines. But these days I've got an even better one ... "Positive Only" (you'll note that it's a positive statement ... and it gives new meaning to the phrase "being P.O.'d"). If it's negative news and it's not something that I can do anything about, well, I just let some bureaucrat deal with it ... that's what they're getting paid for. The bottom line: don't waste your time soaking up garbage into your brain. You can always turn off the TV.

Desensitizing Your Fears

You'll pardon the expression, but overweight people are often the butt of many jokes. Mostly of the malicious variety. Certainly that's what the average overweight person thinks. That's one reason why it's important to have a well-developed sense of humor. It's a tremendous defensive tool as well as a powerful coping device. Humor allows us to see the absurdity of difficult situations, and even to laugh at our fears. It also allows us to take ourselves lightly. People who take themselves too seriously and identify too strongly with their difficulties are easy targets for ridicule of various types. This may explain why overweight people often seem so drained of energy ... they're so busy guarding themselves emotionally that it actually drains them physically. After all, we do respond in physical ways to our thoughts.

The greatest fear in the western world seems to be public speaking. It seems as if more people would be willing to store a nuclear warhead in their microwave, than would be willing to speak in public. That's a pretty big fear. After that, the greatest fear most people have is appearing foolish in public (or even in private for that matter). Heaven forbid that you should ever appear foolish. My goodness, what would the neighbors say?

Fortunately, there are cures for both these great fears. Join Toastmasters to take care of the public speaking issue. And practice being silly to take care of your fear of foolishness. What? No, I'm not crazy. There is a tried and true psychological technique called progressive desensitization that can reduce all kinds of fears ... everything from heights to snakes to flying (and perhaps flying snakes?). You can use this method to get over your fear of potentially being ridiculed. How? By gradually allowing yourself to relax, loosen up and get silly, starting in the privacy of your own home. Start practicing the following exercises today. Before each item take 10 long, slow deep breaths.
1)   Spend 5 minutes a day for the next week smiling at yourself in a mirror. Not just any smile, by the way, but a great big Jack-O-Lantern smile that shows every tooth in your mouth.
2)   During week #2, spend 5 minutes a day standing

in front of a full length mirror and make a variety of funny faces at yourself. And keep practicing your smile.

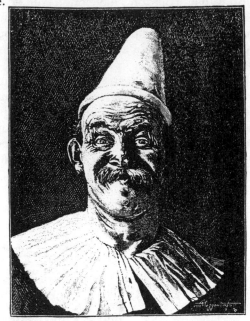

3)   During week #3, practice laughing loudly at your funny faces. Try a range of laughing styles ... from chuckles to guffaws.
4)   During week #4, put on your silliest T-shirt (you know, the really dorky one that you're planning on wearing the next time you paint the garage) and your Goofy underwear and practice #1, #2 and #3.
5)   During week #5, practice #1-4 in front of your spouse or support person. If they don't laugh, tickle them until they do.

Once you've completed steps 1-5 you should have become aware of the fact that you haven't yet died of embarrassment. Yes, you may have been a bit embarrassed, but note carefully that you did not die.

It's a little known fact, but most of the people on this planet are so busy caught up in the doings of their own lives that they rarely see beyond the ends of their own noses. In fact, it's downright difficult to get people to even pay attention to most major news events. So the likelihood of anybody spending a lot of time attending to how you look or what you do is really quite small.

On with the desensitization exercise.

6)   During week #6 (or whenever you're ready) go to the grocery store wearing your silliest T-shirt (and I would recommend wearing pants, too!).
7)   If nobody seems to notice you, make a funny face at a small child.
8)   If you think anybody is ridiculing you, smile at them.

9)   If anybody openly ridicules you, give them your best smile (see #1). Then make a funny face at them (see #2).

I suspect that you will find open ridicule an exceedingly rare occurrence. If it does occur, and you can face it with a smile, you will have won a great victory for yourself. Not only that, you will still be alive and stronger emotionally than ever before. Consider carefully the fact that if a person puts you down for any reason it is defining their personality, not yours. I think we'll save #10, appearing naked on national TV, for another time.

Humor is a tremendous coping skill that has enabled people to survive such extreme ordeals as concentration camps and being held hostage by middle-eastern terrorists. Abraham Lincoln read from joke books during the Civil War to help keep his sense of emotional balance intact. Humor is now used effectively to treat cancer patients, and it is becoming more clearly understood by the healing community that a sense of humor and a positive attitude can truly heal the sick. And that's no joke.

Hugging and Touching

To conclude this chapter on stress reduction, let's look at one of the most important factors in human development: touching. If you don't get enough touching in your life, you're missing out on one of the most critical ingredients in the human recipe.

Periodically, a truly sad situation comes to light that shows us how much we really do need each other. In the 1950's psychologists observed that infants who were placed in impersonal, clinical orphanages literally died from lack of caring physical contact. Additional scrutiny showed that lack of loving touch at an early age can lead to extreme emotional disorders. This led to the knowledge that touch and specifically touching other people in a positive way is essential for our well-being. Think about it. When you bring to mind positive caring relationships, touching is always involved. Mothers carry their babies in their arms, close to their bodies. As children get older they still hold their parents hands ... it's a sign of love and caring and protection. When you're sad you just want to curl up in someone's loving arms.

As people mature the touching evolves into various forms ... almost always affirming and supportive. We shake hands and slap each other on the back. We hold hands and put our arms around people's shoulders. We hug. We caress. It's really a shame that the English language doesn't have more words for the positive feelings that touch can convey. We hold hands to show love and also to express consolation. We shake hands to convey strong friendship and also to express trust, as in business transactions. We touch upon greeting each other and upon parting. It is an integral part of our lives. There is even a form of therapy known as "healing touch".

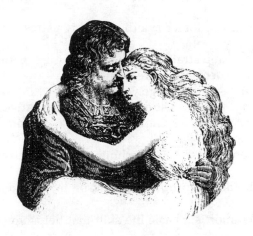

"Thanks, I needed that."

Several years ago I went to see the author and love promoter Leo Buscaglia give a talk. He is definitely an open, honest, caring and sharing person. He's a great believer in the simple power of love. After his wonderful presentation he mentioned that it was something of a long-standing tradition for him to hug the people that he had shared his feelings with. Soon I was standing in line with hundreds of people, virtually everyone in the audience, to get a hug from Leo. He is a very deliberate hugger. He takes his time and puts warmth and feeling into his hugs. It was over an hour before I met him face-to-face. He radiated a pleasant happiness and he asked, with great sincerity, how I was feeling. I told him I needed a hug. We embraced each other for a long moment. I felt accepted. He didn't know me, but he didn't judge me. He accepted me for who I was and shared willingly of himself. I can still feel the power of that hug.

The need to really connect is deeply felt in people at the very core of our being. Beneath all the judgments, past experiences, opinions and anxieties we are all connected in spirit and energy. When you touch that core, you touch our essence. And at that point you can heal pain ... even the pain of being overweight, as well as other addictions, at its very root.

So what does this mean for you? It means that you need to hug somebody today. You'll feel good, and so will they. By the way, have you hugged yourself lately? Go ahead, you're worth a hug!

In A Nutshell

1) Stress is negative pressure or tension that you may typically react to by eating because eating relieves tension for you.

2) See the A-Z list of possible stressors.

3) No one lives a stress-free life, so you must learn to handle stress more constructively.

4) Signs to look for indicating high stress are listed.

5) A 4-step strategy for handling stress: **BAMM!**
   a) **Become** aware of the stress.
   b) **Acknowledge** your feeling.
   c) **Make** a list of acceptable alternatives to substitute for eating.
   d) **Make** a commitment to pick one and do it!

6) See the A-Z list of techniques to reduce and control the stress in your life.

7) Breathing properly should be the first place to start relieving tension.

8) Humor is a basic life skill that helps you stay flexible and see the absurdity of difficult situations.

9) Practicing humor helps you put your life in perspective.

10) Hug someone you love today! Touching heals and connects us to each other in positive, healthy ways.

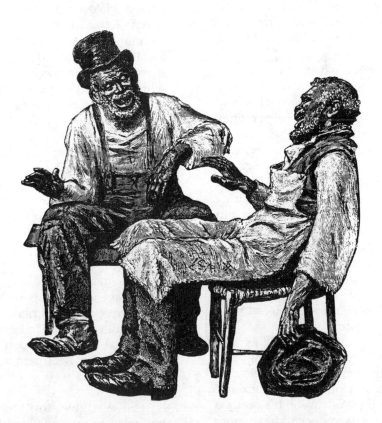

"... and then I tried Dr. Speedy's Two-Hour Wonder Diet!"

Managing the Food-Mood Connection   15

"Let me alone, that I might take comfort a little ... "
The Bible

How the Food-Mood Connection Starts

Chances are good that one of your first official acts as a person was to eat something. When you cried as a baby, more than likely you were picked up, comforted and fed. Food and being fed then became connected with being comforted and loved. Your emotional bond with food thus began. Food and feeling full simply felt good and satisfying. It replaced feeling bad and hungry or distressed.

Later, as a child, this connection was reinforced by getting a goodie to soothe the hurt of a skinned knee or a trip to the doctor or dentist. Again, food made the hurt go away and was a source of comfort, love and caring. At your birthday parties you got to choose your favorite flavor cake and ice-cream as a way for Mom to show she loved you and as a special, fun treat. Nobody stopped you after just one piece either. After all, it was a special day. Tasty food, fun, friends ... and presents to boot! What could be better than this? Not much, really ... and you've been trying to duplicate this feeling ever since. But now that you're all grown up, you may view those magical carefree days as gone forever. Most of your childhood friends have moved away and birthdays just remind you that you're getting older. It may seem harder sometimes to have fun too, with all the responsibilities of adult life. Only the food and the happy memories remain.

However, by simply putting the right food in your mouth it's possible, in a way, to bring it all back any time you want. And it sure is a lot easier to just let yourself go and get swept away by the pleasurable tastes and fleeting happy memories than it is to deal with your life these days. Between housework, shopping and working all day to pay the fifty bills that arrive in the mail every month there isn't much time for kicks and jollies. It seems that there's hardly enough time to talk to Mom on the phone. Thank goodness for food. It's easy, fast, inexpensive, fun and readily available in this 24-hour society in which we live. At least three times a day, whether it's raining, snowing, sleeting or hailing you can legitimately sit down and eat something. And who among us can pass up this lovely opportunity to bring back those warm, pleasant memories ... if only for a short time? And there you have it ... chocolate cake for lunch again.

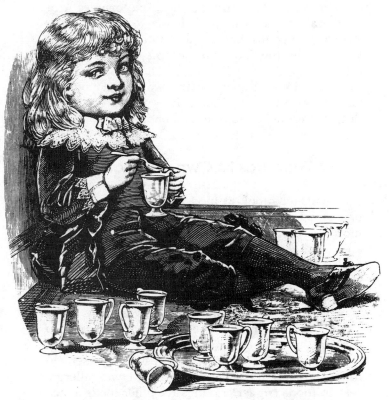

Overeating can start at an early age.

For a brief span of time food can allow you to seemingly be in control of your feelings. Thoughts of drudge-work and unpleasant associates melt with the frosting on the cake. The trouble is that the flavors and the feelings never last very long. The comfort is fleeting. The food has even taken on some adversarial qualities. We have now discovered that some of those yummy goodies we enjoyed as children aren't exactly the healthiest foods for our bodies. But, all too often, the feelings outweigh the facts. Essentially you've been having an affair with food since day one. Admit it! You love food and you can't do without it. Well, food loves you, too. It provides comfort and satisfaction. It is your friend: non-judgmental, totally accepting, always available, entertaining, interesting, fulfilling, attractive, aromatic, colorful, fun and tasty as all get-out. Sometimes it's so good that it can send chills down your spine. Why, in fact, if you're not careful, food can just about take over your life. And that may be exactly the problem. Food has taken over your life.

It often seems like everything good, those happy holidays, family get-togethers and outings, vacations and social events all too often center on food. Cherished family recipes, special holiday meals, favorite restaurants and food at parties and other special events all contribute to the connection of food to social situations involving fun, friends and celebrations. The moods you experience are inseparably intertwined with the foods you love. Rather than controlling the foods in your life to suit your needs, the food has become the controlling factor.

Let's look at some of the ways that you can take back control, and learn how to manage these deeply ingrained emotional bonds that food has formed over the years.

Each Food Has Its Own Characteristics

First, let's look at food itself and the qualities or characteristics that at times make certain foods more appealing. Have you ever eaten something and then immediately wanted something else to eat? I have. I've actually eaten so much that my stomach felt like it would burst and I still wanted something else ... without even being sure of what it was. Rationally, I was not physically hungry.

There are many theories that attempt to explain this phenomenon, including the following: my "appestat" (appetite thermostat) was set too high I craved the foods to which I was allergic certain foods trigger cravings for other foods a lack of certain vitamins or minerals kept me from being satisfied I was eating to fill up the "emptiness" in my life, and on and on. I'm sure some of these theories are valid. But I found that relationships with food are pretty straight-forward most of the time, and by understanding the nature of this relationship, the searching for satisfaction could be met with more success.

There are certain qualities that foods have, such as sweet, salty, cold, smooth, crunchy, rich, etc. If you eat a food that is salty and what you are really craving is something sweet, then you may still want something sweet long after the salty calories have entered your body to do their dirty work. But if you ate a food with the quality that you were actually craving you could perhaps satisfy that need.

Unfortunately, for me this didn't turn out to be quite so simple (is anything ever simple?). I usually craved foods with 3 or 4 different qualities at the same time! Oh, well. This actually turned out to be a blessing in disguise since it started me on the road to concocting dishes with all my desired qualities in them. (As you'll see in Chapter 30 "Basic Recipes"

and Chapter 31 "Converting Your Favorite Recipes" the techniques and strategies you will learn are designed to enable you to have healthier versions of all your favorite foods.)

To be prepared before the urge strikes, check off the food qualities below that you enjoy the most and list several foods that could satisfy those wants. Then design several dishes you can eat whenever the mood strikes you for those qualities. Keep a copy of this food qualities list handy in your Personal Journal: Bready, Bulky, Chewy, Cold, Creamy, Crunchy, Fluffy, Hot, Juicy, Light, Rich, Salty, Savory, Sour, Spicy, Sweet, Tangy, Thick. If you can think of any more food qualities feel free to add them to your personal list.

My favorite qualities turned out to be rich and creamy, sweet and crunchy. All at once! I came up with several recipes that I could eat at the times that I craved these qualities. These dishes acted to stop my cravings and ongoing eating, and satisfied the need for further food. Sweetened peanut butter or ricotta cheese on toast or crackers or rice cakes did the trick. A Cream Fluff with crunchy cereal, such as granola, on top was also a good choice.

The point is that I could now identify what I was really wanted. Then I could give myself the healthiest approximation of that food in order to halt, or at least slow down, the urgent craving for a particular quality. So instead of frantically eating my way through every morsel that drifted into my path during the day, I could slow down enough to be aware of what I was needing, and satisfy that need.

Remember also that your preferences will change according to your moods and circumstances. For example, in high stress situations, I need lots of bulky foods. Lots of crunch and munch. When I'm in a festive mood I like to have some fun food to celebrate! When I'm at home alone, I like warm, comforting foods.

Know your relationship with different foods and plan ahead for maximum satisfaction. This awareness can save you quite a few calories and help stop those searching-for-something forays before they begin. It can give you back a sense of control.

Anatomy of a Binge

There is no single word in the vocabulary of overweight people that strikes as much terror as the word "BINGE". In its way a binge isn't much more comforting than a notice of impending death. A binge signifies a total lack of control when it comes to eating. It also implies a complete loss of emotional control. The strongest physical and emotional needs are involved. Certain stages of a binge often feel about three times as bad as losing an IRS audit, losing your job and being hit by a train ... all on the same day. A binge is bad news.

The basis for this discussion is the "Anatomy of a Binge" diagram later in this chapter. Please refer to the diagram for clarification as you read. If you suspect that you are the victim of an eating disorder, bulimia or anorexia nervosa, you should contact an eating disorder specialist to help you find a solution to these serious problems.

The ultimate objective is to help you avoid future binges by understanding why they happen. If it's too late to stop the binge from beginning then your goal is to shorten its duration and minimize any weight gains and the resulting negative emotional impact. The very concept of weight "control" means just that ... you are in control. Binges are periods of being out of control. They can have a crushing impact on your weight and your attitude. However, there are elements of binges which are surprisingly rewarding. In fact, at the very heart of a binge there is a paradoxical place where it's possible to get a sense of great power because of the intensely reinforcing qualities of the food. Looked at from an objective point of view, every binge has a beginning and an end. It's important to know that they do end. It's also important to know what causes them to occur in the first place. What factors can trigger a binge? How can you possibly head one off before it gets started? And how do you shorten the duration of a binge if you're in the middle of one? The answers to these questions will help you get control.

I'll be the first person to admit that none of this will be easy. I have had many episodes of "out of control" eating during my life ... including a binge that lasted close to three years. Three long, miserable years that I wouldn't wish on my worst enemy. But for some reason I wished it on myself. Which tells me, in retrospect, that I felt more negativity towards myself at that time than I did towards my worst enemy. And I've managed to learn a thing or two in the process.

The "Anatomy of a Binge" diagram has been of tremendous help to me in identifying the destructive cycle of bingeing that I was caught in. In the days when I was still bingeing I had little understanding of the thought processes involved ... and I was perpetually in danger of being controlled by food. The diagram evolved as I analyzed my thoughts and behaviors before, during and after binges. In its present form it's like a map that will help you identify the emotional eating stage you're in and assist you in regaining control of your mood and attitude. (Refer also to Chapter 13 "Trouble-Shooting Guide" for additional binge solutions.)

The binge process begins with a craving. This can be for food or due to an emotional need that isn't being met. This can result in immediate "out of control eating" which is the beginning of the binge. Or you can try to substitute a positive alternative behavior (something other than eating). Any alternative strategy is going to involve taking control of your thoughts and actions and will involve some delay of immediate gratification. While this is sometimes quite difficult it is definitely a trait of a THINNER WINNER ... the ability to "hold off" eating when food is being used for something other than physical hunger.

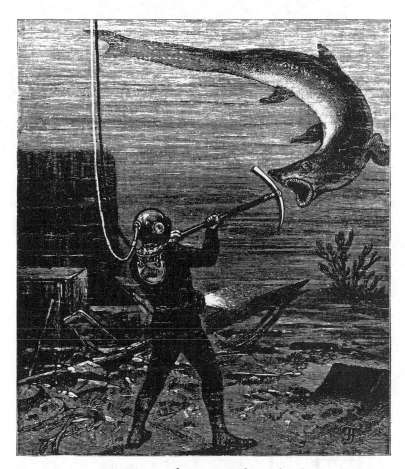

Binges ... the great white shark of your dietary ocean.

If you do begin to binge you will notice that the eating becomes immediately self-reinforcing. The food itself acts as a continuing reinforcement for bingeing. This was the first big surprise that I discovered about bingeing ... it feels good during the initial stages. All thoughts of anything other than food are quickly tossed out the window and for a while you can feel like you've hit the million dollar jackpot ... with the prize being an endless "all you can eat" buffet line. As long as you shovel in the food, and it's satisfying your craving, you can develop a tremendous sense of power where

Anatomy of a Binge

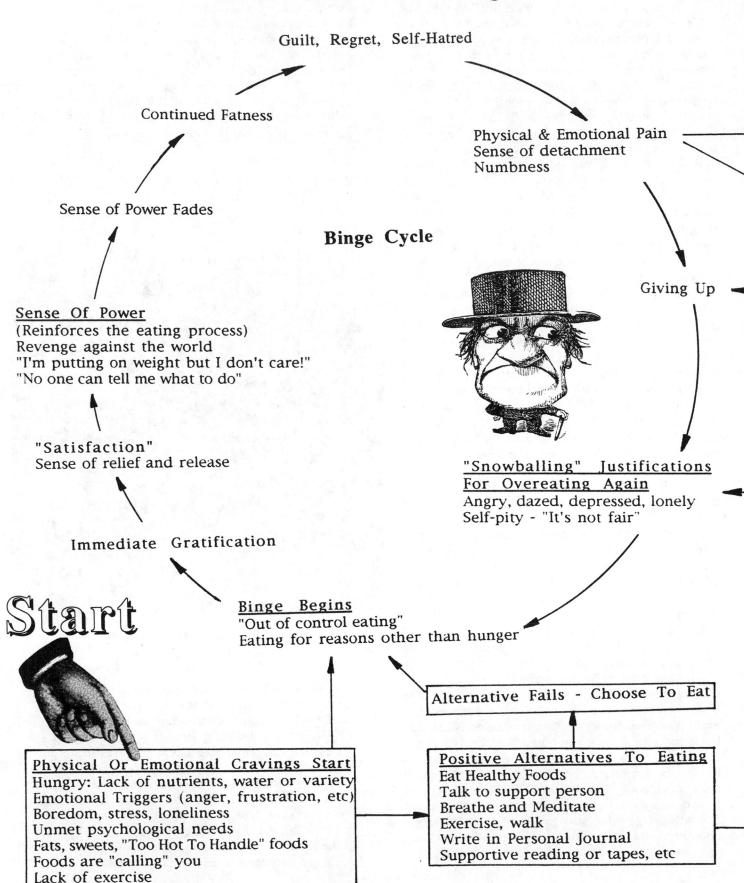

Guilt, Regret, Self-Hatred

Continued Fatness

Physical & Emotional Pain
Sense of detachment
Numbness

Binge Cycle

Sense of Power Fades

Giving Up

<u>Sense Of Power</u>
(Reinforces the eating process)
Revenge against the world
"I'm putting on weight but I don't care!"
"No one can tell me what to do"

"Satisfaction"
Sense of relief and release

<u>"Snowballing" Justifications</u>
<u>For Overeating Again</u>
Angry, dazed, depressed, lonely
Self-pity - "It's not fair"

Immediate Gratification

Start

<u>Binge Begins</u>
"Out of control eating"
Eating for reasons other than hunger

<u>Alternative Fails - Choose To Eat</u>

<u>Physical Or Emotional Cravings Start</u>
Hungry: Lack of nutrients, water or variety
Emotional Triggers (anger, frustration, etc)
Boredom, stress, loneliness
Unmet psychological needs
Fats, sweets, "Too Hot To Handle" foods
Foods are "calling" you
Lack of exercise

<u>Positive Alternatives To Eating</u>
Eat Healthy Foods
Talk to support person
Breathe and Meditate
Exercise, walk
Write in Personal Journal
Supportive reading or tapes, etc

Breaking the Binge Cycle

Transition Zone   **THINNER WINNER**

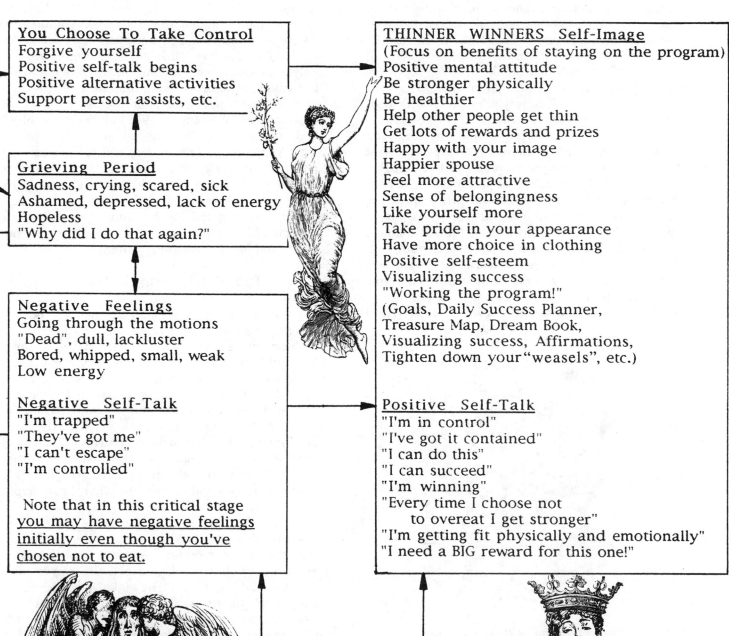

You Choose To Take Control
Forgive yourself
Positive self-talk begins
Positive alternative activities
Support person assists, etc.

Grieving Period
Sadness, crying, scared, sick
Ashamed, depressed, lack of energy
Hopeless
"Why did I do that again?"

Negative Feelings
Going through the motions
"Dead", dull, lackluster
Bored, whipped, small, weak
Low energy

Negative Self-Talk
"I'm trapped"
"They've got me"
"I can't escape"
"I'm controlled"

 Note that in this critical stage
<u>you may have negative feelings
initially even though you've
chosen not to eat.</u>

THINNER WINNERS Self-Image
(Focus on benefits of staying on the program)
Positive mental attitude
Be stronger physically
Be healthier
Help other people get thin
Get lots of rewards and prizes
Happy with your image
Happier spouse
Feel more attractive
Sense of belongingness
Like yourself more
Take pride in your appearance
Have more choice in clothing
Positive self-esteem
Visualizing success
"Working the program!"
(Goals, Daily Success Planner,
Treasure Map, Dream Book,
Visualizing success, Affirmations,
Tighten down your "weasels", etc.)

Positive Self-Talk
"I'm in control"
"I've got it contained"
"I can do this"
"I can succeed"
"I'm winning"
"Every time I choose not
    to overeat I get stronger"
"I'm getting fit physically and emotionally"
"I need a BIG reward for this one!"

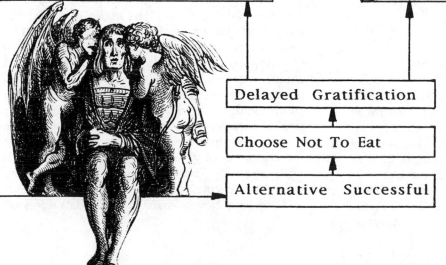

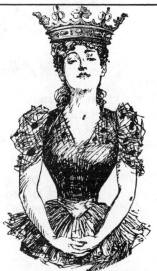

Delayed Gratification

Choose Not To Eat

Alternative Successful

thoughts of obesity and weight control are temporarily nonexistent.

Unfortunately, like all "highs", this will eventually pass. And then it's a quick plummet to the depths of despair. You realize that you blew it again and you're fatter than ever. Now you're filled with tremendous guilt, regret and self-hatred. Eventually you enter a painful, enveloping state of emotional detachment (when you realize that your runaway train has finally crashed). At this crucial point you can "give up" and start the binge cycle all over again. Or you can break the binge cycle by entering the transition zone.

In the transition zone you're faced with both positive and negative alternatives. It's possible to snap out of your "grieving period" by forgiving yourself ... first and foremost. A very important step. Then begin plugging in some positive thoughts of your choice by using techniques that you've been learning about in this book. You can pick yourself up, dust yourself off, and get back in the game ... heading towards your goals of health and thinness with another well-learned lesson under your belt. Remember, mistakes are for learning. Or you can give yourself a "pity party" and spend some time wallowing in misery. If this happens you are in danger of re-entering the binge cycle ... so BEWARE!

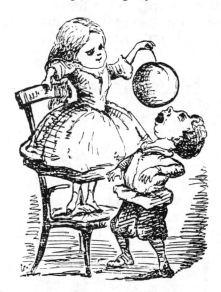

Don't let food pull your strings.

In the lower section of the transition zone you'll notice another mine field. The second surprise is that delaying gratification and not eating can sometimes result in negative feelings. This was the opposite of what I had always thought ... that binges were always "bad" and self-control was always good. In terms of my weight on the scale, this was true, but in terms of my emotions it threw me for a loop. The transition zone is a dangerous

place to be, so stay aware.

That's why this program puts such a strong emphasis on mental self-control. Our actions always follow our thoughts and that's why it's so important to take tight control of your thoughts in terms of your weight and your health. Being a THINNER WINNER requires the extra effort that winning performance always entails. You have to seek out the positive alternatives when you become aware of your cravings and you have to make certain that positive, "in control" thoughts are the only ones you allow into your mind. Sure it's work, but staying in control of your attitude and behaviors also becomes highly self-reinforcing. Look at all the benefits of winning and see how much healthier and rewarding positive self-talk is.

Your binge cycle may very well differ from this one. If it does I suggest that you take a closer look at the great white shark of your dietary ocean. The more you understand about the way you think and act the easier it will be for you to stay on your program. Make your own binge cycle chart. Become aware and break the vicious patterns.

Too-Hot-to-Handle Foods

Sometimes certain foods are just too-hot-to-handle. Of course, these foods will be different for each one of us. How can you tell what yours are? They will be the foods that cause automatic eating, even when you're not really hungry, and you find difficult to stop eating once you've started. Foods that seem to call your name relentlessly in the night. It's very important that you identify them consciously in order to take control and manage them. They should send up a personal red flag that you will immediately recognize. Sometimes I visualize a skull and crossbones when I run across these foods.

First identify the foods that cause you trouble. You probably already know what yours are, but let me list a few common red flag items. Chocolate is on almost everybody's list, and actually has enough caffeine and sugar in it to make it addicting in sufficient quantities. Pizza, chips and crackers, peanuts, peanut butter (my personal nemesis), cookies, ice cream, soda, candy, lasagna, potato salad, alcohol, cheese, etc. Ask yourself this question: the last time you can remember being out of control with food, what were you eating? Bingo, red flag! Whenever your red flag foods are available, you are susceptible to losing control, especially at the beginning of your weight control program. This will gradually change as you get some weight control success under your belt (or out from under it!) and you learn how to manage the foods successfully.

Taking Back Control

Now that you've focused on the offenders, let's take some action to correct the situation. For right now, while you are getting started, don't have them around. This is the easiest way to not eat them. If you have to get in the car and make a special trip to buy a peanut-butter cup then it may just be too much trouble. If it's in the house, it's more available. I've often asked Howard, who is mercifully slender, "Honey, will you please eat this up?". Especially if it's something I love and will probably devour if it hangs around the kitchen long enough. I usually have a small pang of regret for not getting to eat the goodie, but then my mind does a funny thing. Since the food is now gone and unavailable, my mind let's it go. Out of sight, out of mind.

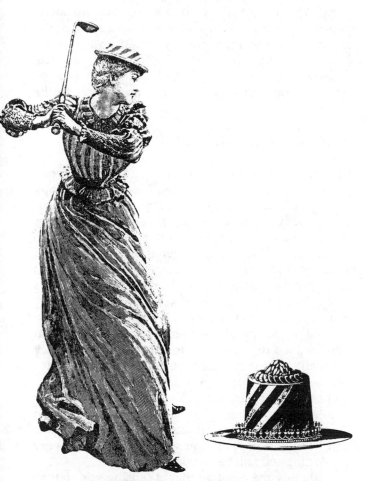

There are some very creative ways
to get troublesome leftovers out of your house.

Another technique is to make use of your garbage disposal and just wash the trouble-maker down the drain. Hold on! People are starving the world over, you say? But, does it make any more sense to be fat while people are starving? Why should you eat an extra piece of cake because a person in a third-world country is starving? If you could hand it to them, you probably would. But you can't, so flush it! Remember, the end destination is Thinland, and you must resolve to do whatever it takes to get there. To win the war, you must also triumph in the battles. Sometimes I will ask my long-suffering and patient husband to take some food that I know I may have trouble with and not to let me see it, actually hide it. The deal is, if I "accidentally" find it while cleaning then it gets thrown away. This insures good hiding places most of the time. (Who says you can't have fun with this?)

Although I'm sure I could sniff out most of the goodies, it does slow me down and give me time to think. I've also given away bags of groceries to charitable groups like soup kitchens and church-run food banks. Then I don't feel guilty about wasting the food. I have actually thrown an entire box of See's chocolates in a trash dumpster! (It had to be a big container where I couldn't go back and retrieve it later.) Although that act haunts me to this day, I do hesitate to buy a whole box again. Oh, I may buy an occasional box as a gift for someone else. That way I can eat a piece or two and still get out alive ... and thin.

The next step is to find an appropriate food that will satisfy you. Remember, substitute, don't eliminate. Don't make the mistake of tossing out all unhealthy foods without replacements and leaving a big empty hungry hole. Plan in advance to fill your cupboard space with healthy foods of your choosing. If it's pizza you crave, buy a healthier version at the grocery store and keep it on hand. Or learn to make one of the quick and easy pizza recipes in this book. If candy is your thing, try the "Babe Rosie Bar" or other healthier sweet in the Recipe section. Substitute Cream Fluffs for ice cream. Identify the qualities of the food you desire and substitute a food with similar qualities. The Food Substitution Chart in Chapter 31 "Converting Your Favorite Recipes" is a good place to find appropriate alternatives for your problem foods.

When you're feeling stronger, you can begin to work the target food back into your program if you wish. Plan an evening out at the local pizza parlor. First, enjoy a big salad, then indulge in your slice or two of pizza. Go through the salad bar again if you're still hungry. If you fail at this attempt, just accept the fact that pizza is too "hot" for you right now and avoid it for a bit longer. Try again when you are feeling more in control. You can buy some foods such as potato chips, peanuts or frozen dinners in individual serving packages. This helps you avoid having a whole package around to tempt you. Buy one fresh cookie or brownie from a bakery. That way a whole bag won't be lying in wait for you in the pantry. If you find yourself slipping back into uncontrolled eating, whether it's one bite or the whole thing, then go back to square one. Avoid the food for a while, find a substitute, plan it into your food program and reintroduce it gradually when the control returns. Realize that there are certain foods that will always be more tempting for you than others, perhaps because of early associations. You can learn to manage them, but you must always maintain your awareness of your relationship to them.

There will definitely be times when you'll find yourself more vulnerable to the call of the wild cherry cobbler. Know and expect this. It happens to everyone and you can be prepared. Hormonal changes occurring in women during their monthly cycle may cause a craving for certain foods or just food in general. Be aware of this, if you aren't already. Before I figured this one out, I would eat the world the week before my period and then hate myself for being so "weak". Now I handle this with flying colors since I plan special, extra-nourishing and satisfying foods to keep me balanced and stable at this time. Whenever I get too busy and forget that this week is coming up, I usually go nuts for a few days before I realize what is happening. And when I realize that it's just my hormones playing their little tricks on me again, I breathe a sigh of relief and begin stepping into my safe and sane mode of nutrition to counteract the craziness. Men also have unique biorhythms and should learn to recognize times when they have especially urgent food cravings.

During the day, observe yourself and identify the time periods when you are most vulnerable. It may be in the mid-afternoon or the middle of the night. Observe other times when food pops into your mind and it is not meal or snack time. Once you know when a stray urge may strike, then you can PLAN a snack to fill that void. Or better yet, plan an activity that will keep you busy through that time if possible. Keep a list of activities in your Personal Journal that you can substitute for food. These can be such things as taking a hot, relaxing bath, meditating, gardening, calling a friend, reading a book, going for a walk or shopping for fun. Sometimes just getting out of the house can break this cycle. Make it something really enjoyable, and preferably relaxing and soothing. If you simply must eat make it something healthy and filling. Fix the food properly, serve it on a nice plate and sit down to eat. You deserve better than to gulp something down over the kitchen sink or in the car on the way home. With a little forethought, planning and practice you will be able to thwart these pitfalls.

Other occasions such as weekends or celebrations, vacations or visits from friends or relatives can also stimulate you to go off track. When you become aware of these times, you can plan ahead for them, intervene and stop the automatic eating habit. Take them one at a time, and reward yourself for every triumph (see Chapter 17 "Rewards—A Feather in Your Cap"). They will all add up to a thin you eventually, no matter how many there are. Keep plugging away at them. They are finite in number, and eventually you'll face them all and succeed at turning them to your advantage. If weekends are your weak points, then realize it ... share that fact with your support person (who may have a suggestion or two) and structure your weekend time more closely to gain control. Substitute foods or activities that will replace the eating binges and cravings. Between the stimulus and your former response you can learn to place a response of your own choosing. You are not an automatic eating machine. You do have a say in the matter! You can reprogram yourself and develop healthier habits. This will take time and practice, so be patient and never give up. If you fall down, get up and keep going. It's the only way to get to the finish line.

Separating Your Moods from Foods

By far, the most common reason for eating when we are not hungry is emotions. These can be happy or sad ones. Relief, joy, boredom, loneliness, fear, stress, being tired or anxious, resentment, anger, frustration, confusion, even being ill ... all of these emotions, and more, can trigger a need for extra food when you're not really hungry. The need to eat when feeling threatened or down in some way is a basic biological response of your body. It naturally tries to strengthen you by stoking up the fire.

Your goal should be to minimize the times that you use food to manage your feelings. If you are sick or lonely, try doing something "warm and fuzzy" for yourself. Brew a cup of your favorite tea, put on your favorite relaxing music and cuddle into a big chair with a juicy mystery or romance book. Be good to yourself. Plan a "comfort food" such as warm cocoa and healthy cookies if you wish. Food can be very comforting and still be on your program.

Identify the emotion that is causing you to turn to food. If it is anger, then figure out who you are angry at and go holler at them! Or imagine the offensive person is sitting in a chair opposite you ... and then tell 'em what for! Or write your way to releasing those feelings. Write a letter to that person. You don't have to mail it, just slug it out with them on paper. Get it off your chest, and you'll feel a lot better (both now and later) than if you sedate yourself with food or hold your negative feelings inside. If you're happy about something then smile and laugh. Share the feelings with your support person or someone else you trust. Even your dog or cat can be very sympathetic at times. But avoid stuffing the emotions down inside yourself with a bag of cookies. It won't do you any good anyway. The emotions will still be there whether you deny it or not, ready to flare up again long after you've eaten the whole thing. Learn to face up to the object of your fear or anger. A fear faced, disappears like smoke. Becoming assertive will often release enough pressure that you can more easily control the pull towards food. Talk to a friend or join a support group of people who are concerned about similar emotions. Sometimes just the fact that you are overweight and feel ugly, inadequate or left out from life will cause a cycle of anger, resentment and eating. If you can't seem to break through your emotions, you might consider seeing a therapist. You can break this cycle. Also see Chapter 14 "Taming Your Stress" for further insight into the connection between emotions and food.

Feel Your Feelings

As you begin changing some of your relationships with food your feelings may become more intense for a while. After all, you aren't obliterating them with chocolate chip cookies any more! They are just out there and you have to deal with them. Let's face it, it's a lot easier just to forget that you're angry or stressed out by going out to dinner and ordering all your favorite goodies. But how many times have you faced the cold light of morning knowing that you "blew it again" last night, even after swearing to never do that again? If you are like I was, a lot. When you really get tired of being fat and feeling bad about it, then you must be willing to experience those feelings. Really stay with them and allow yourself to feel the sensations fully.

I was always so afraid that someone might find out that I wasn't such a "very nice quiet young lady" all the time. That I had thoughts that weren't so sweet. Well, I found that I could learn to (and had a right to) express my own feelings and

thoughts in a non-aggressive way that didn't hurt anyone and that, lo and behold, the world went right on anyway. I had to get past being afraid to put the real me on the line. I had to take a risk, live with my feelings and put them out in the world for this incredible (to me) change to take place. And so do you. Try it. Stay with the fear, anger or other emotion without doing anything. Just let it be there. You might be surprised at what happens. It will be different for everyone, of course, but quite often I found that the feeling just kind of faded away after I had thought about it or talked to someone about it. It loses power. You might not even remember what the dickens you were so upset about. And you won't have to deal with the guilt and "oh-no" feeling of just having eaten next week's groceries while you were stewing about it. I respect and admire your courage beyond measure in doing this because I know, believe me I know, it is not easy at first. But I also know, having been through it and making it to the other side, that it is more worth it than you can imagine. Who knows what incredible potential is being squelched by that bag of French fries today? Only you have the power to find out.

Success as Its Own Reward

As you begin to succeed in your weight control efforts, you'll realize that each success breeds more success. Begin now by concentrating on your accomplishments. Fill your life up with people, plants, animals, books, activities and fun. Crowd your life with the joy of living, and it will bolster you through the rougher spots along the way. You are a great and wonderfully unique person. In all the history of the world there has never, ever been anyone just like you! And there are important contributions to life that only you can make.

Eating is not the only response to unpleasant feelings. More than likely it will just be the aspirin to ease the pain for a short while. Learn to zero-in on the real emotions causing your urge to eat. To heal a destructive emotional wound you must remove the splinter entirely. This will take time, attention and loving care. Choose your responses to emotions with health, energy and love for that special you in mind.

In A Nutshell

1) Match what you eat with the food you are wanting for maximum satisfaction and control.

2) Develop recipes to satisfy each of your most common food desires.

3) Identify your personal too-hot-to-handle foods and take steps to manage them.

4) Identify times and emotions that trigger your urge to eat. Stay aware.

5) Emotions, more than anything, trigger overeating. Learn your personal emotional triggers and plan to deal with the emotions themselves in ways other than with food.

6) Keep an alternate activity list in your Personal Journal.

7) Try feeling your feelings. Stay with them and just notice what happens.

"Reward yourself for successes, and soon success will become its own reward."

Roseanne

Creating a Powerful Support System   16

"May he support us all the day long, til the shades lengthen and the evening comes ... "
Cardinal Newman

Finding Someone to Lean on While You're Getting Lean

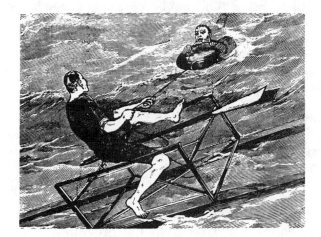

*Your support person
can be a real life saver at times.*

Emotional support. Without it you are a young vine left to struggle along on your own. With it, you can grow tall and straight ... and when you are strong enough, support yourself. For now, in the very beginning, it will help immensely to search for and find an anchor, a source of emotional understanding and support. Of course, the needs and the support will be different for everyone. You may need the entire population of Wisconsin to be on your side before you feel confidant and supported in your efforts. Then again, keeping your weight control plans to yourself for now may be your preferred cup of tea. It may also be difficult to ask for support when you have had unsuccessful results with twenty or thirty different "diets" in the past. Your credibility may be a bit besmirched at this point. Personally, I give the majority of families of "fat folk" a lot of sympathy. I'm sure they really want to help, but sometimes have become just as discouraged as the fat folk themselves, after all of the repeated unsatisfactory efforts.

Still, after evaluating a weight loss plan and making the decision to follow it, you are well advised to enlist the aid of someone close to you for emotional support. The person you select could be your spouse, mother, sister, best friend, or anyone who cares about you and truly wants you to succeed.

Take your time and pick your support person carefully. Make sure they are not competing with you and that they really want you to come to them when the need arises. They must be sympathetic, but firm when you stumble, and able to help get you back on your feet. Preferably they should not be a walking skeleton, but should have some mature relationship with food. You don't want someone who will turn into an accusatory watchdog, jumping down your throat at the first potato chip. Ask them if they would be willing to be in on this with you. If they understand what you're asking for and commit to the cause, then explain your basic weight control plan to them.

Have them read the THINNER WINNERS program. Then discuss it together, clearing away any questions. (Yes, you can have peanut butter sandwiches and dessert every night.) That way there won't be raised eyebrows or questioning looks when you eat. Give them lots of credit for this interest and commitment. Thank them often for their support and belief in you. Let them know they will be your anchor and support, but that the ultimate goal is for you to learn to stand on your own two feet.

This is a lot to ask of any one person or even a family. You may not be able to garner enough support in your immediate surroundings to get going. When even the suggestion of help with another "diet" is greeted with stony stares or rolled up eyes and the statement (implied or spoken), "spare me! Oh please, not again", then you know and it's time to move on to a better resource.

One of the primary premises of this book is that the supportive, non-competitive buddy system is built right in. You're already working with someone who's been there and knows all the twists and turns ... that little ol' fat-burner, me. I'm a real person, living in Oregon with my husband, a dog, 2 cats and a kitchen. Like I said, we're all in this gravy boat together!

Diet Buddies

What about a dieting buddy? This approach can be motivational for some competitive-type individuals ... and if it works for you, fine. Pair up with a fellow employee, friend or family member and work at it together. However, in my experience this can lead to several undesirable consequences (besides the urge to strangle them), especially if they are losing faster than you are. First, you may be doing the "diet thing" for them, not for you. You'll show 'em you can lose that weight! Also, you tend to cut nutritional corners to "win".

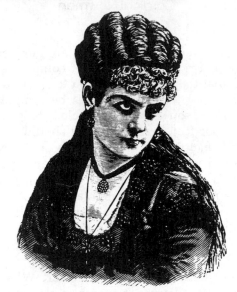

"If he lost more than me again this week I'll just scream!"

If they swagger in on Monday morning and announce boldly to the office that they lost 4 pounds last week, then you just might have the urge to skip lunch to catch up ... or even worse, get discouraged and give up entirely, sending your confidence plummeting. Another problem is that we're all individuals. It's just not a fair or equal fight. It's like comparing lemon meringue pie with chocolate cake. No comparison, right? No matter how closely you feel you are matched, each of you will have different rates of metabolism, different plateau ranges, different body fat ratios, etc. This is especially true between men and women, so watch out gals! Men almost always will lose weight faster because of several factors including higher muscle to fat ratios and consequently higher metabolisms.

So buddy up at your own risk. This is not a race or a contest, but a personal learning process that will help you find the permanent answers to weight control along with a thin, healthy body that is yours and yours alone.

Group Support

Group programs offer another strategy that works well for some people. Or that may be helpful during certain points in your weight control journey. After I lost about 70 pounds I got "stuck". Following a few years of struggling, my new strategy included

joining a group. It did help in this place, and that is one way they can be used effectively ... as a tool when you need them (not as a permanent crutch). There are literally thousands of groups of people out there who get together for the specific purpose of sharing their weight loss and maintenance experiences so that they do not feel so alone in their efforts. People who work at something together have a better chance of finishing the job. It works like a good marriage. When one person is down, the other bolsters him or her up and vice versa.

A group such as Weight Watchers, Overeaters Anonymous or TOPS can be a big help to you if you can't find a good supporter among family or friends. The information in these group programs tends to be geared primarily towards either diet or behavior changes, depending on the program. If one of these areas is your weakest, then it may be a good supplement to the complete THINNER WINNERS program.

THINNER WINNERS now offers groups as well. The difference is that our own groups are member-run. They are personalized support groups with the basic goal of studying the THINNER WINNERS principles. There is no weigh-in or other embarrassing activities, and members take turns presenting materials from the program to each other. If you would like more information about starting up a group, we will be happy to send you start-up information. Oh, yes ... another way THINNER WINNERS groups differ from the others ... they're FREE!

A group that gets to know you little by little (assuming you're an active participant) will be there when you are down, celebrate with you when you are up, and just listen when you need a friendly ear. Your family and thin friends may think you have flipped out if you mention that you actually live in mortal fear of chocolate chip cookie dough (who, me!?), but a group of fellow thinness seekers can instantly relate, nod knowingly and chuckle understandingly without judging you totally insane.

Another wonderful spin-off from being in a group is the fact that you can help others. The first group meeting I went to, I arrived late, after the speaker had begun, crept as silently as possible in the back way, sat in the last row, talked to no one and left immediately after the meeting. I felt like Spy Incognito with a heavy, long black coat and sunglasses. I guess I really thought I could be invisible, but all I really succeeded at was frightening small children on the way to the meeting. Sometimes I didn't even stay for the meetings. I just crept in, paid my dough, tipped the scales and headed off to the nearest eatery to bury my shame in hot chocolate. I was so embarrassed and humiliated I didn't dare to hope that this simple meeting could help end the nightmare. But it was a place to go, a touch point of sorts.

From this minimal beginning, I actually came to believe that my struggle, week to week, would be of some use and encouragement to the next humiliated and embarrassed 272 pounder who came slinking late into class. And guess what? It was. People began to ask questions and since I was succeeding, I had some answers. I was actually helping people even before I had lost all my weight. So can you. That realization can be a high point that affects your whole life beyond measure. The world is good again.

All this work and change that you are doing can be shared with other people who are still in the dark. And the funny thing is, by illuminating their lives, you light up (and lighten up) your own as well. So search for your support now. Think about it. Ask for it … "Ask and you shall receive". Because this support can do more to move you towards healthy, permanent weight control than you can now imagine.

Groups can be great, but they unfortunately have a downside, too. In lecture style groups contact with the leader and the other members tends to be very limited. At the meetings there are only a few brief moments to talk with the leader (usually while you are balanced on a scale) and the meeting itself tends to disrupt any private conversations with other members (at least it should) … and you usually only see them at meetings. Another unfortunate reality about franchise groups is that the qualifications to be a group leader are rather minimal. They may only need to lose as few as 10 pounds. While this may qualify them to deliver a generic lecture, it doesn't provide the insight to relate to members who have considerable amounts of weight to lose. The quality of the group stands or falls on the skills of the lecturer, but you have to pay your membership fees whether or not the lecturer is helping you personally.

Accepting Insight with Love from Your Spouse

If there is any other person in the world who really wants you to succeed in your efforts to lose weight, it is probably your spouse (husband or wife, present or future). Other than yourself there is no one in the world who cares more and knows more about your desire to be healthy and thin. Trust me, he (or she) really wants you to lose weight and look your best. He wants you to succeed and will help you in any way that he can. The trouble is that he may not know all this. It's up to you to inform him of your need for support.

When you are unhappy with yourself because of the way you look, it's a painful time … for both of you. When you hurt, he hurts. He not only wants to help you improve your health and looks, he also wants to end his own discomfort. He would be happy to help you in your efforts if he only knew how. Knowing this, it's possible for you to turn your spouse into a support resource even if he lacks sophisticated skills for the task.

The trick is to find a way to turn this potential supporter into someone who can actually be of some legitimate help to you. The place to start is with honesty. Listening objectively, to both constructive criticism and praise, is a communications skill that you need to develop to be successful in your weight control efforts. When he talks to you in a straightforward, honest manner, try to listen to the messages being given without allowing your emotions to turn them into something else. For example, if your husband mentions that one of your dresses looks tighter than it used to, this does not necessarily mean that he loves you any less, or that you are an unworthy person. It does mean that he is aware of how you look, and that you have probably put on a few pounds … which you already knew. Try not to fly off the handle or revert to automatic pouting. Turn this into a positive learning experience by acknowledging him and ask if he wants to help you or talk about it more.

This will probably be one of the most challenging, yet beneficial things that you can ever do for yourself. In order to be successful with your weight control program, you're going to have to be intensely honest with yourself. Following the plan is your responsibility, and remember, you're doing it for yourself anyway (see Chapter 5 "Motivation and the Success Mindset"). You will have to explore many of the little nooks and crannies of your mind. There may be some pain or complex issues in there, but there will also be tremendous insight. It's the insight that will free you emotionally, and allow you to make the necessary changes in your attitudes and behaviors relating to food, which currently cause you to make the choices that make you fat. This is because your inner search is going to reveal many of the reasons why you are overweight, and the reasons why you want to lose weight. It may be difficult for you to think about the emotional reasons for overeating, but in order to dissolve an obstacle you must first see it for what it is. A carefully prepared support person can help you do this.

Here's how to set yourself up for success: Explain to your husband or wife that you're serious about losing weight in a healthy, realistic way, and ask for their assistance. They will probably offer to help if you are sincere and they feel up to the task. Make sure they understand this is a win-

win venture. You both stand to benefit from your success. Make it clear that you need support and possibly guidance, not someone to take over for you and carry you. And certainly not a judgmental watchdog.

Agree to a set of ground rules that will assist you in gaining insight into your attitudes and behaviors regarding food, exercise, motivation and self-awareness. They will be able to help you most effectively by actively joining your team, reading this book and helping you develop specific solutions to your problem areas. Present this as a challenge that the two of you can work on together. The focus should be on positive solutions and reinforcing statements when you are doing something right.

They can help you:

1) Come up with new affirmation statements.
2) Work on your Dream Book and Treasure Map by finding inspiring pictures.
3) Select possible rewards for your successes.
4) Re-focus on positive self-talk if you should happen to slip into old habits.
5) Plan your daily schedule of eating and activity.
6) Review your Daily Success Planner and make suggestions for improvement, either on a daily or weekly basis.

Tell them you want honest feedback. Allow them to make observations about your behavior ... either positive steps they see you taking or things you are doing which seem counter-productive. It may take a while before you can learn to accept helpful, objective criticism, even from a person who you know loves you. But this attitude is a critical obstacle to face and overcome. Once you get to the point where you can listen to a less-than-totally-complimentary analysis of your behavior and accept it as being helpful, you will have gained the insight necessary to see these things for yourself. Then you can make the necessary changes to really control your weight for the long term.

When your spouse sees that you are gaining self-control and making progress, you'll be amazed at how truly supportive he can become. He'll see you in a whole new light. Then you can start talking to him about some of the big rewards you would like to have for successfully reaching your weight loss goals (see Chapter 17 "Rewards - A Feather In Your Cap"). When your weight control journey starts turning into a positive adventure for the two of you, you'll be surprised at how wonderful your relationship can become. And who knows, maybe you'll even get him to start thinking about improving his own lifestyle.

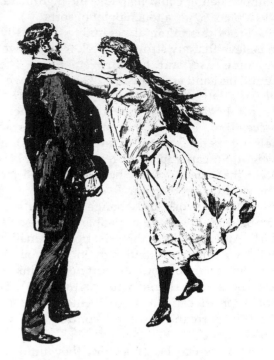

*"... and when I get to goal
I want to go to Hawaii!"*

Support Yourself from the Inside Out

In addition to finding a source for outside support, also begin building up your internal support. One pursuit that must become a priority if you are to truly succeed for the long term, is one that many overweight people do anyway. At least the ones who have not given up hope of being thin. And that is to read, study, listen to and learn everything that you can get your hands on about weight control and diet research, psychology of eating and in fact, anything that relates to behavior, exercise, attitude and nutrition (remember BEAN).

Make sure that you go for quality information. There's a lot of bogus news circulating around on the ever popular subject of weight control. Gossip in the beauty salon, supermarket tabloids and off-the-wall fads are not reliable sources. Be picky ... this is your health at stake. Knowledge is power, and the more you know and understand about your particular situation, the easier it will be for you to change the aspects of your lifestyle that are causing you problems. Subscribe to one or more of the many fine magazines that offer articles and condensed versions of health information that will help keep you aware and informed. Or if that's not in the budget, then go the library and spend a few hours every week or two browsing through the books and magazines. Empower yourself! It will pay great dividends ... and who knows? ... maybe you'll find just the answer to a particular question you've long been wondering about. For example: "Am I the only person in the world who has ever been afraid of being thin or afraid of attentions from the opposite sex when I get thin?" There are tons (no pun intended) of great books in libraries and bookstores that have stories of real people who have fought to understand their problems, and who have won. Information and inspiration are just waiting for your discovery. Develop a passion for learning. In doing this myself, I discovered a sense of belongingness that I sorely needed. Instead of being the only fat person in the world who hid cookies in the bathroom hamper so I could eat in peace, I discovered that I was not alone after all. Plenty of overweight folks, if not a majority of us, had stopped at a fast food joint on the way home from work, devoured enough food to feed a major league football team, and then innocently sauntered in the door asking, "What's for dinner?". I used to think I was so-o-o clever! These and other charming stories are available for your reading pleasure in countless related books and magazines. Become curious and seek out information and answers.

One of the sad but true facts of life is simply that nobody is going to come up to you with a magic elixir on a silver tray that you can swallow in a few gulps and become instantly thin, living happily ever after. If you wish to solve the weight control riddle once and for all, answering how you can be thin for life, then continue the good start you have made by pushing to understand through other peoples' experiences, too. Support your own curiosity and watch it develop into a strong understanding of the real meaning of a healthy lifestyle. The understanding will help lead to actions which will bring results.

Awareness

Unless you know that cheddar cheese has 110 calories per ounce, mozzarella cheese has only 80 calories per ounce, and lo-cal cheese has only 40 calories per ounce (oh, the wonders of modern day science!) then you will continue to eat the higher calorie cheese without being aware of the lower-calorie and fat option. You will pack on pounds needlessly. I am constantly reading the labels in the grocery store and I'm often surprised and sometimes amazed at the ingredients. Some things I thought were "healthy" turn out to be full of fat, salt, preservatives or other junk that I don't want in my body. Another source of information about the foods you are eating is a good paperback reference book listing food contents: calories, sodium, fat grams, sugar , nutrients and anything else you may want to know. The more you know, the better informed choices you can make. The new food labels also make it a lot easier to really know what you're eating.

Until you learn (and everything about this subject is learnable) to tell when a recipe needs readjusting to a more healthful orientation, you will continue to make your macaroni and cheese the old way. Your body and health will reflect this lack of awareness. Take a bit of time to study your particular habits and preferences to become aware of the areas you need to change the most. If sweets are your downfall, then congratulations! You are aware that sweets are your weak point, and now you can do something about that. But if you just keep on the way you have been going, nothing will change.

Are you aware that you can have a "candy bar" (Babe Rosie Bar in Chapter 30 "Basic Recipes") for a snack, or anything you are used to having for dinner and still eat healthy and be slim? Yes, you can! That's what is really so great about the information you are learning in the THINNER WINNERS program. You can eat delicious foods with joy and satisfaction, and still be thin and healthy. You just have to uncover the ways to do it. You do that by becoming aware that there is a better way. This program will help you become aware of these "tricks", and how to apply them. But the ultimate responsibility for knowing what it is you want and need lies with you. You may choke at the thought of 6 muffins for breakfast, but need eggs and hash browns instead. Or maybe you can't even stand the thought of food until noon. You must "know thyself" in order to help thyself!

Become aware of the standard American diet. Listen to the words of the American Heart Association when it says that "the typical American diet may be hazardous to your health". On average, this is a diet that is 42% fat, 24% sugar and 5% alcohol. That's 71% unhealthy junk! Look around at the 64% of American males between the ages of 40-49 who are obese, according to a study done by Dr. Ancel Keys. Many of them will stay that way until they die an early death. What a phenomenal waste! Most of them aren't even aware of what they are missing, because the human body and psyche learns to adjust to the situation in which it finds itself. It endures and adapts. "Things really aren't so bad as long as I can have my chocolate cake and ice cream for a snack while watching TV." Well, I'm aware that I can have this and be healthy, too. And I know that you are also becoming more aware.

Suggested subjects to increase your awareness: (All are found in related chapters of this book.)

* Healthful substitutions for the not-so-healthful foods you crave.

* Your target zones for fiber, fat & cholesterol, sodium and water.
* The most healthful ingredients for recipes.
* What to have on hand to satisfy your particular cravings.
* How to handle your too-hot-to-handle foods.
* How to survive in a restaurant.
* Ways to enjoy holidays and other celebrations while eating healthy.
* The healthiest methods for cooking.
* What exercise does and the best ones for your specific goals and body.
* Your specific needs and how to meet them.
* How to plan ahead for better management of food.
* How to push the right buttons for yourself.

Without AWARENESS of these and other subjects, pertaining to your thoughts and your health, you will not be able to take the weight off, increase your level of health and especially maintain any improvements. You'll be blissfully unaware and not so blissfully fat.

Use your Personal Journal to explore these topics. Concentrate first on the areas that are a problem for you. Do you "blow it" every day at 4:00 o'clock? Then focus on that and study it, and try new approaches until you've got it licked. Then go on to the next problem. Spend a little bit of time every day on problem solving. You don't have to crack this nut all at once, because it may be a tough one. But the kernel of knowledge you gain is going to do a lot to propel you ever faster towards Thinland. Everything that you learn will move you closer to being Thin. It is cumulative. And some great news is that once you realize the power of Awareness, you will find that returning to your old habits is unnecessary. You don't have to go back! It will be like a wonderful game where you are always winning. You can have your cake and eat it, too!

In A Nutshell

1) Choose a support person to act as your anchor who will understand the program, support you emotionally, listen and offer help.

2) Join a group and share your experiences and successes.

3) By helping others you can gain incredible insights and strength.

4) Turn your spouse into your head cheerleader by asking for honest feedback, and then listening to it with an open mind.

5) For internal support - read, study and learn from quality sources. Go for the positive.

6) Develop an attitude of awareness. The more you know, the better choices you can make.

7) Some subjects to begin increasing your awareness are listed. Work in your Personal Journal to explore them for your benefit.

8) Everything you learn moves you closer to being thin and healthy. It all counts and adds up.

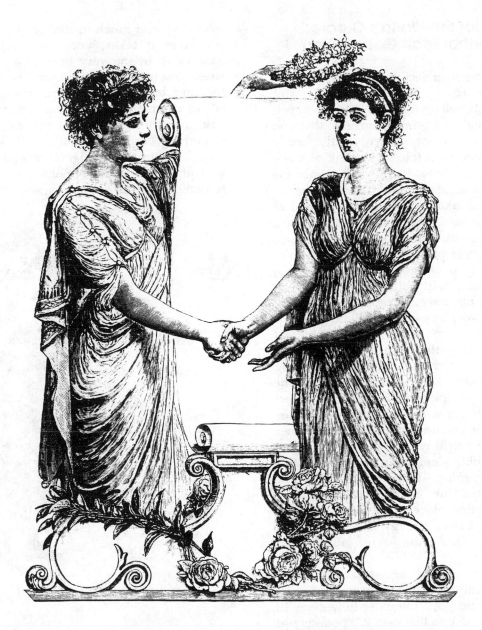

"Congratulations! Another THINNER WINNER gets to goal!"

Rewards - A Feather in Your Cap! 17

"For thou rewardest every man according to his work."
Prayer Book

The Trophy for the World's Greatest Weight Control Effort Goes to You

Let's talk about a subject near and dear to my skinny little heart ... namely rewards and recognition for a job well done. Yes! Now, I want you to imagine with me for a minute. Imagine that you go to work every day, dressed perfectly, apply yourself diligently to your job, even think of a few suggestions or innovations to help your boss increase business. You put a lot of thought into it, really "live" your job and take it seriously. At the end of the week your boss says, "Hey, thanks a lot. Have a nice weekend". Sometimes he or she even forgets to say that. Just a couple of days off and then you're expected to do it all over again. Week after week, month after month, with little recognition, no paycheck, nothing but the expectation that you will either go full tilt every day or you will be labeled a loser or a quitter. "Impossible!", you say? "Not fair!" It most certainly would take a very motivated, self-directed individual to keep up producing at a constant level of excellence if no one even noticed. But isn't this what most people expect of their mighty efforts with weight control? They just try to tough it out until the end, month after month, with little or no recognition of the many smaller but incredibly significant accomplishments and changes happening along the way. It's like doing penance for the horrible sin of being overweight in the first place. Well, folks, it's not a sin , it's just misdirected energy ... which can be channeled into a much more joyful journey and destination.

Some "experts" will disagree here with my viewpoint. "You must be totally inner-directed", they'll pompously purport. I wonder how many of them have stood on a scale that read 272 pounds and thought, "How in the world can I lose 10 pounds, much less 130 or more ? Even if I lost 50 pounds I would still be grossly overweight! Even if I lost 100 pounds!". Well, I have and I know that when something works, use it. Use everything that works. And recognition coupled with rewards works. So start picking out those rewards and acknowledging your efforts.

If you have to give yourself a reward for making it from breakfast to lunch without bingeing, do it. A little success under your belt, recognized and

rewarded, and lunch to dinner will be a bit easier. Whatever it takes, you are worth it and you deserve it. In the very beginning, or in times of stress, you may have to put your rewards very close together or make them something very special. (Well, twist my arm a little. Okay, I'll do it.) If you give it a little thought you can come up with something besides food that will keep you from reaching into that refrigerator again. You'll build up your list of reward options over time, and you'll have more choices as you practice.

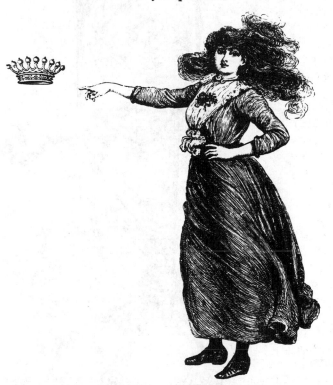

"And then I want one of those!"

Why Rewards Work So Well

Perhaps you are familiar with the story of "Pavlov's dog". Ivan Pavlov was a Russian physiologist who experimented with the use of reinforcements (rewards). He took a dog and designed a device that would measure how much his dog salivated just before being fed. When the hungry dog expected to get some food he would start salivating in anticipation. Then Pavlov would feed the dog. He did this for a while to establish a "baseline" average and then Pavlov started ringing a bell when he prepared the dog's food. The bell had nothing to do with the feeding other than the fact that they occurred at the same time. After "pairing" the bell and the feeding together for a while Pavlov discovered that all he had to do was ring the bell and the dog would begin to salivate just as much as when he was actually being fed.

Much of the way in which modern advertising is used is based on a similar process. Don't you start salivating when you hear those bouncy burger jingles? When you innocently park yourself in front of the tube they lambast you with an image a second of people eating, paired with some snappy little tune, and run the ads every three minutes around mealtimes to entice you up to the drive-thru window. That's the whole idea.

From this simple beginning behavioral psychology made great progressive leaps in the use of observation and reinforcements. Essentially it was determined that positive reinforcements can be used to increase the frequency of behaviors. Just about anything that you do will increase in frequency if it is followed by a reward (the reward can be anything that's meaningful to you). By observing your behavior carefully it's possible to modify your actions very precisely.

One of the most powerful and useful features of behavioral psychology is its quality of accountability. This means that precise records can be kept and by analyzing the data you can get a very clear picture of what happened and why it happened. This is exactly what you want to be doing with your weight control program. Think of all the advantages of taking the guesswork out of your weight loss efforts. If you know that by averaging a certain number of calories each day and exercising a certain number of hours each week you can lose weight at a predictable rate, over time ... and that by receiving periodic rewards you can stay motivated to follow your program in a steady fashion, wouldn't that take some of the mystery and anxiety out of the weight loss process? This is one of the great weight control secrets that you're looking for ... a critical piece that makes the THINNER WINNERS program more than the sum of its parts. (Hint, hint.)

This reinforcement process also shows the importance of keeping written records like Daily Success Planners, your Personal Journal and weight and measurement records. If you know what you're doing, why you're doing it and the results you're getting you'll also know how to duplicate your successful efforts. That's what you want more than almost anything else ... to find out what works for you and be able to repeat the process whenever you choose. By being systematic instead of impulsive you can finally stop feeling like a yo-yo who's riding a roller coaster.

Picking Your Prizes

Your decision to begin this program with positive expectancy and commitment should be applauded, recognized, supported and rewarded heartily! Every step along the way should also hold a predetermined reward. If you feel this is childish, let me tell you that it is not. It works. Some of the finest, most expensive and successful programs for weight loss include gold stars, ribbons, pins, plaques, certificates, applause and other simple, inexpensive forms of recognition. This one technique is a major key to your success. And it just happens to be a fun one, too! So put aside your thoughts of silliness about rewards and put the power to work for you instead.

Here's how: Your participation in this program shows that you're ready to do something about your weight. Great! Reward yourself right now with something you really want that will be appropriate for your accomplishment so far. How about a brand new scrapbook or photo album with an inspiring cover and a stack of magazines to cut up to get you started on your Dream Book? Maybe a blank book with a fancy cover for you to use as your Personal Journal. You need someplace special to write your deepest feelings, wishes, hopes, triumphs and solutions while on the journey to Thinland. Believe me, you will learn so much about yourself, and it is a great opportunity to watch your growth. If you keep a photographic record of your progress you'll be amazed at the changes when you reach goal. These are just suggestions for your first reward.

Next, you can give yourself a predetermined reward for finishing, say, one week of a successful food plan. Here are a few more suggestions for the first successful week: a professional manicure, a health-oriented magazine you don't usually buy, a bouquet of fresh flowers, an afternoon at the movies with a good friend, a juicy paperback novel, a new exercise video or two hours to do whatever you want to do ... no questions asked!

What would you choose? Go ahead, pick it out now and when you succeed, immediately give yourself the reward with a little fanfare and some pat-on-the-back type recognition. Don't wait until next week. Immediate rewards are much more reinforcing. Smile and be proud of your accomplishment.

The emphasis should be on rewards other than food most of the time. However, a special night out at your favorite restaurant can be very motivating and give you a chance to show off your new restaurant survival skills (see Chapter 36 "How To

Survive Eating Away From Home"). Just don't get carried away and promise yourself a total hog-fest for being "good". That defeats the purpose of learning all those new ways of dealing with the "pig-out" mentality. Now, guess what? It's time to pick another reward for your next accomplishment! Who said weight loss can't be FUN?

Using Rewards Effectively

Give yourself a larger reward for one full month of successful effort. Maybe a new hairstyle, a new blouse or shirt. Maybe a special gift that you normally wouldn't buy for yourself is in order. You deserve it! You earned it! Make it even more fun by purchasing your reward ahead of time and wrapping it as a gift in fancy paper and ribbons. A nice decoration for the coffee table is a pile of pretty gift boxes. They're inexpensive and motivating every time you look at them. I happen to love rings, so every time I lost 10 pounds, I picked out a special ring that signified that success. Every time I see those rings on my fingers it reminds me of my accomplishment. And that's just what your rewards will do for you, too. When I finally hit my goal and stabilized for 6 months, my wonderful husband escorted me to Hawaii to celebrate! Complete with a new size 8 wardrobe, including a bathing suit (not black)! Do you think that trip was on my mind a few times during the months it took me to lose the weight? You bet your butterscotch it was! I got pamphlets from travel agencies and dreamed about that trip for months. I could really visualize myself being there. And when we finally went, the trip meant so much more because I had earned it.

Meaningful rewards can certainly be small, too. Every day that went by with a successful effort, reaped a gold star for me at the top of my Success Planner (I bought a whole box at the five and dime). Silly? Who's wearing a size 8 now?

To use rewards most effectively, really think about what you want and has special meaning for you. My motivators may not work for you at all. Start a personal rewards list in your journal to keep track of your current goodie wants (see Chapter 12" Your Personal Journal"). If you find that nothing on the list works any more, then change it to something that will really ring your chimes when you think about it. Be flexible. This is also a great way to get to know yourself and your personal tastes. Then when you find that certain "something", give it to yourself for your efforts. It's the payoff for positive effort! By putting this very powerful technique to work you can watch your goals materialize in your life over and over. And each little step along the way will move you happily along the road to The Big Goal: permanent, healthy weight control.

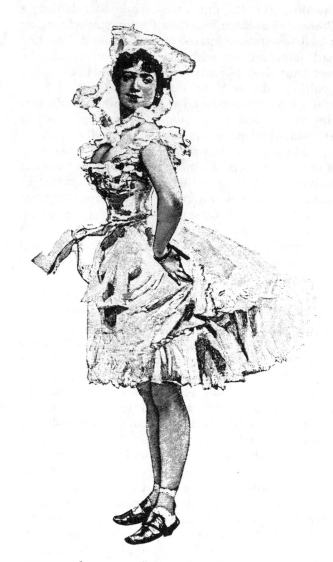

A new dress can do wonders for your attitude!

Look Good, Feel Good

New clothes? While you're still overweight?? Yes! Absolutely! A must! Why wait until you've lost every ounce to buy clothes that you love and that look great on you? Taking care with your grooming as if you were going to dine with the Queen of England is a sure sign of positive self-esteem. You should always have at least one entire outfit that fits you perfectly, makes you feel great and flatters you no matter what your weight or size. You deserve this! You're working hard to change fat-producing habits into healthy, thin ones, so don't walk around in baggy, shapeless tents. It damages your self-image. Think back to the last time you were going out for the evening and you really got dressed to the teeth ... I mean an all-out effort in your Sunday best. When you finally made your entrance what was the reaction from your friends or family? "Wow, you really look great!" or something similar to that happy observation. Well, why not look like that all the time and get that reaction from others regularly? It will do wonders for your self-esteem and motivation to know that you look your very best at all times.

Start Wearing Your Dream Now

Whether you're 300 pounds overweight or ten pounds from your goal there is a store or catalog offering your size, and clothes that both fit and flatter you. Study the catalogs and order clothes that look good on models that are similar to your body type and weight right now. If cost is a concern consider making some of your own clothes, buying at good second hand stores or swapping with other weight losers.

My dream was always to wear a pair of blue jeans. At the time, they didn't come in size 24 $1/2$ plus, even when I got down to that size. But when I finally hit size 20, that was the first thing I did ... bought a pair of blue jeans. I also treated myself to another new pair for every 20 pounds or so that I lost after that. That way they never got too baggy. I topped these with various comfortable, knit shirts and sweaters in pretty colors that flattered my personal coloring. These simple styles tend to look good, even if they become quite large because of lost weight ... so I could wear them even as I shrank in size. I then dressed up the outfits with jewelry, scarves, hair goodies, bright socks and shoes. Although my feet were about $1/2$ size larger (!) when I was at my highest weight, most of my shoes still fit.

Prizes that You Can Wear!

Use items for rewards that will still be wearable when you're thin. That way you can start building a great wardrobe now. Get a color analysis done (men, too!) if you haven't already. Check out a book on fashion styles and decide on a major style that's "You" ... one that you love and feel great wearing.

Here are some reward items you can start with: shoes, slippers, socks, stockings, bracelets, rings, watches, earrings, necklaces, night wear, robes, scarves, hair decorations of all kinds, make-up including nail colors, perfumes, belts, all kinds of accessories such as hats, purses, gloves and neckties.

When I got down to around 180 pounds, I promised myself a colorful, stretchy leotard and exercise tights. This really opened up a whole new category of fun togs! What fantastic colors! I never could have imagined myself in a blue leopard-skin unitard, but now ... wow! These exercise clothes are really comfortable and can be very flattering, as well as uplifting for your spirits. Try them just for fun and you may end up wearing them around the house, too. They make me feel like an athlete. I have lots of head bands, leg warmers, tights, leotards and unitards that I just cinch in with a belt now that I'm thin. The real point here is if you've ever wanted pretty salon nails or a great mustache (guys, not girls) now is the time to give it a try. Don't wait. Get that terrific new hairstyle or hair color. Why not? The better you feel about the way you look, the easier it will be to treat yourself with respect. Remember "Attitude Determines Altitude" and you want to fly high!

My Size 8 Red Bikini

When I was at my very heaviest, I bought myself a size 8 bikini ... a red one. I still have it and it has given me a lot of inspiration along the way. It was just fun to hang it up and dream about where I would wear it and what my life would be like when I could. I don't recommend this too often. Most of your clothes should fit. But if this helps you, go for it. Clothes are so much fun for me now, but I really used to hate putting on that caftan in the morning and having no other choices. I got tired of feeling unattractive, so I began sewing fancy trim on the caftans and making them in prettier colors and fabrics. Just start wherever you are and make the best of that place. If you're a size 3X , then be the sharpest size 3X ever seen on the face of the Earth.

There is no excuse for grumping around in a baggy smock, with no thought to your hair , make-up or colors. Do this right now. Look at your outfit and grooming. Uh-huh. I see. Well, get busy and strive to look your best all the time. There are plenty of gorgeous large size models to use as examples. You may just start to feel like a model, too. Use catalogs to put a few pictures in your Dream Book (see Chapter 7 "Visualization and Dream Books"). You'll feel better about yourself and find it easier to make an appealing meal and sit down to eat it at the dining room table rather than gulping cold leftovers standing at the kitchen sink. You deserve better. You've suffered enough. It's time to give yourself permission to look your best, feel your best and spend a bit of time, energy and money on yourself while you're in the process of losing your weight. "Clothes make the man ... and woman!", so have a little fun, gain some respect for yourself and take a giant step towards being your own inspiration.

In A Nutshell

1) Recognition and rewards for accomplishments and positive changes will keep you motivated and happy with your progress.

2) Behavioral psychology has shown that activities followed by rewards increase in frequency, so reward yourself for your positive behaviors.

3) Keeping records of your program will allow you to duplicate your successes in the future.

4) Rewards are a key concept to your success. Keep a current list of your rewards and wants in your Personal Journal.

5) Tailor your choice of rewards to your accomplishment.

6) Use smaller rewards at first and then more substantial rewards for bigger accomplishments.

7) Give yourself the reward immediately. DON'T WAIT!

8) Respect yourself always - look great for YOU!

9) Buy items that you can still use when you're thinner.

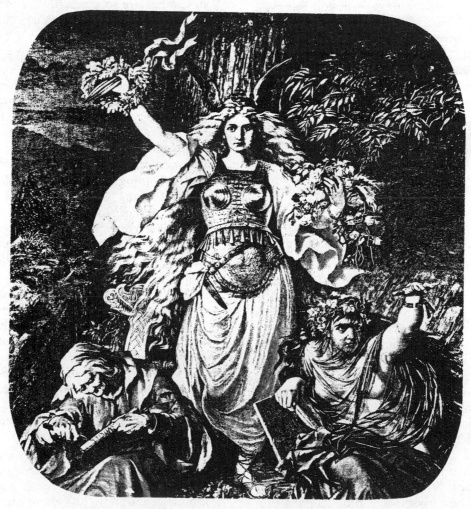

You can even wear all your rewards at once!

Daily Success Planner   18

"When society requires to be rebuilt, there is no use attempting to rebuild it on the old plan."
John Stuart Mill

One Giant Step

The above quotation restates a message that has been given several times in this book ... you will not get new outcomes by following your old methods. The old ways didn't work. By doggedly resisting learning new approaches to controlling your weight you will continue to get the same unsatisfactory outcomes. A big complaint that many dieters have is how much work is required by some programs. At this point in the book you have already learned that you aren't going to get something for nothing. There ain't no free lunch. This leads us on to the issue of record keeping.

Studies have now isolated the #1, most important and effective step that you can take to insure success with any plan to lose weight. Additionally, it has been shown that without this vital step, success is limited and short-term. This powerful technique is simply keeping track of what you eat and do by writing it down daily .

This is so simple that most people tend to dismiss it as hooey. Reasons for not keeping a food and activity journal are as common as fast food commercials ... "There's not enough time", "I did it once and it's a pain", "I don't want to be tied down to a journal", etc. However, the benefits are hard to deny, and personally I have found this technique to be invaluable in keeping myself at goal for over six years. I fill out my Daily Success Planners without spending a lot of time on them. Once you've got the technique down, they go very quickly and prove well worth the effort. I don't keep them all the time now that I'm slim, but I certainly did when I was losing weight and I go right back to them, first thing, whenever I have to "tighten down my weasels" (see Chapter 38 "Secrets of Successful Maintenance"). Daily Success Planners are the very quickest way to get yourself on track right now.

My reluctance to keeping these planning sheets was softened when I discovered that athletes always keep what they call Training Diaries. I liked the sound of that, and it inspired me. So now I just think of myself as an Olympic athlete in training (going for my seventh Gold Medal in the event of Weight Maintenance!) and ... no problemo. With such wonderful Olympic company as Kristy Yamaguchi, Bonnie Blair, Dan Jansen, Jackie Joyner Kirsee and Carl Lewis how can I go wrong? And you certainly want to learn to use the #1 best tool for getting your weight off for good too, don't you? Take heart, it's not so bad after all.

Let's take a look at why these journals are so important, how they can be used effectively and what can be learned from them. Maybe then you can use them to your advantage, like me, without slaving over time-consuming details.

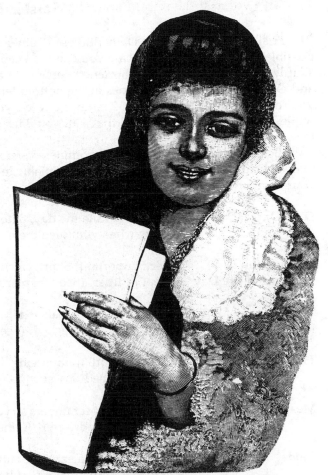

"Daily Success Planners really work!"

But Ma, Do I Hafta?

The main goal in keeping your Daily Success Planner is to keep track of what you are eating and doing. Quick, what did you have for breakfast Monday morning? How about dinner the day before yesterday? I see. Well, how are you going to plan for your big night out this weekend if you aren't sure what went on earlier in the week? Can you afford to skip exercise today? How about a glass of wine? Does it fit in with your goals this week? You can see the first advantage right off the bat. To be able to tell at a glance if you are right on track and how much leeway you've got. Actually, writing it down will save you time! Plus it gives you the assurance that you aren't blowing it.

Also (and this is probably the main reason why these little devils are so effective) you will be much more accurate and honest when you have to write your meals and exercise down in black and white and have someone review and initial your form (your support person). Thinking (or just remembering) that you had a "sandwich" for lunch is a lot different from writing down the truth about the "Super bacon-slathered, double-patty, triple-cheese, quadruple-mayo Monster Burger" that you had with a large side of fries and an extra-large chocolate shake. It keeps you honest (and thin).

I usually keep my planners one week at a time just because it's easy to handle and compare what I've done from week to week. Then I can sign them off as one week down and a job well done. I keep a weekly graph with my weight, number and duration of workouts, calorie average and anything special that happened that week such as a night out, house guests or any down-time such as a cold. Refer to Chapter 19 "Keeping Track of Your Progress" for further suggestions and examples.

Pssst ... Here's the Plan

First, take a peek at the Daily Success Planner at the end of this chapter. Now don't get excited. I put every possible thing on there just in case you want to keep track of everything. There are shortcuts for rushed days or simply if you choose to use a shortened version for any reason. The basics are: what you ate, fat grams, calories and exercise. Also, the little boxes at the bottom left make it easy to assure that you eat a balanced diet. If you're feeling great and losing 1-2 pounds a week, you can just write down what you ate and your exercise. After a while, you'll be in a groove and that's all you'll need. But be careful about those fat grams and calories. They tend to sneak up on you.

Below is an explanation of this complete version. In the beginning I would recommend filling in all the blanks. Daily Success Planner forms are available in our THINNER WINNERS Workbook or you can also design your own form and make copies.

Day/Date	Be sure to note the day, date and year. Your diaries will be more valuable later if you know when you filled them out.
Affirmation or Thought of the Day	Very important! Short, catchy and in the present tense is best. Repeat at every meal at least. (See Chapter 9 "Self-Talk and Affirmations".)
Goals	Choose realistic goals that you can easily meet at first. This will give you confidence when they are reached. (See Chapter 8 "Goal Setting".)
Time of Day	This is important for seeing how long you go between meals and snacks and revealing different schedules, such as work and weekend.
Meal Check-Boxes	These are just reminders so you get a balance of foods at each meal and you don't forget the veggies and water! A line is provided for the total number of fat grams for the meal.
Foods	Write in the type and amount of food that you eat, then follow the line across filling in the fat grams, calories, fiber grams and sodium for that food. You don't have to keep all four of these every time. Maybe you are just concerned with fat this week, or calories.
Totals	Add up the number of fat grams, calories, fiber grams and sodium milligrams you ate during the day. You can do this at the end of day or while planning in the morning to make sure you reach your goals. Sometimes you need to change something during planning if you tend to go over your targets. I usually check after lunch to see what I have left for dinner.
Servings Check-Boxes	These are reminders of the number of servings of each food type that you need to eat to be balanced and get all your nutrients. (See Chapter 25 "What To Eat".)

Exercise   Fill in your goals for how many minutes and the type of exercise you will do. The time of day you will exercise is also very important. Then record your actual time and pulse. I record my average pulse range.

Weekly Weight   Once a week is plenty. Don't be ruled by the scale.

Success Score   Check off all boxes that apply to your day. Then add up your score for the day. The higher the better. These are the habits you want to have every day for the healthiest and fastest weight loss. Be sure to give yourself a gold star for a +25!

Notes/Comments   Anything noteworthy goes here and can be very revealing and helpful in the future. If you have a problem, note it here and make suggestions for improvement next time.

Reviewing Your Success Planner

Now let's take a look at the sample Daily Success Planner that is filled out and see how this person did and what can be learned from her efforts.

She starts off with a great positive and powerful **affirmation**: "I enjoy being healthy today". This will certainly make it easier for her to make strong health-promoting food choices during the day.

Her **goals** are realistic, although fiber might be a bit high if she is just starting out. The typical American consumes just 10 grams of fiber a day. She might try 15 gms for the first week, otherwise she may experience some bloating, gas, etc.

Our Olympian is drinking **water** or herbal teas with every meal and snack! Destined for greatness. This is an easy way to get in your 6 minimum glasses a day. Add another glass both before and after exercise and you're right on target!

Beautiful low fat, sodium and calorie **breakfast** with good balance and ability to keep her fueled up for several hours. If she is going for a total of 30 grams of fiber, then she should aim for about 10 grams at breakfast. She could accomplish this by choosing a bran cereal instead of oatmeal, mixing the two cereals or adding bran on top.

Snacks are well-chosen at about 100-150 calories each and she doesn't eat sweets alone which could affect her blood sugar and cause hunger. She always adds in a grain or dairy to slow absorption (see Chapter 27 "Choosing Healthy Foods"). These snacks can carry you over for a couple of hours and keep you from devouring the refrigerator the minute you get home from work. Water or herbal tea helps her feel full.

Soup and a sandwich is a great **lunch** choice for satisfaction and ease. A salad would also be a good choice, especially if she doesn't have one planned for dinner. She adds yogurt as her dairy item which can often be more filling than milk, since it's thicker and richer. Most of her sodium is eaten at this meal, since bread, eggs and dairy all have high amounts.

Good, high energy and fiber **dinner.** Maybe just a little heavy if she eats much later than 6 P.M., doesn't exercise in the evening or goes to bed early. Wait about 4 hours before retiring after a meal like this with an evening snack of cookies.

How did she do on her **totals**? Only 14 grams of fat! Wow! She should keep in mind that her body needs some fat and so she shouldn't push that figure any lower than 10 grams. Did she feel hungry today or munchy between meals? This may indicate a need for a little more fat at mealtime. The fats she did choose were not saturated though. As matter of fact, since she appears to be a vegetarian, only vegetable fats such as olive oil and those naturally occurring in foods were eaten. Excellent. She tended to "round up" her fat grams and not record every fraction of a gram. For instance, since apples and veggies have some fat in them she probably ate another 3-5 grams.

Calories are just under her goal. Very good as long as she measured accurately. Studies have shown that most people on weight loss plans tend to underestimate the calories of foods they eat by as much as 50%! Always measure highly concentrated foods such as oils, dressings and cheese. Also rolls, bagels and breakfast cereals.

She ate 23.5 grams of **fiber** with a good ratio between soluble and insoluble. That's an excellent amount for just starting out! As you can see, it's just not that easy to get 30 grams of fiber a day. She'll have to work at it, looking up higher fiber foods such as beans, apples, berries, and certain veggies until she knows what to add, and when.

Sodium just about on target. Although she chose low sodium products for dinner and made her own soup, the rest of the foods were of the processed variety without particular attention paid to sodium.

Excellent on the **Servings Boxes**, fulfilling all her requirements and a bit more of the grains and fruit. She's discovered the wonderful world of vegetables and how they can add variety, color, satisfaction, fiber and nutrients with a minimum of fat, sodium and calories! Congratulations!

Her **exercise** goals were realistic and she met them easily. She even notes she might try more time tomorrow.

This is an outstanding **Success Score**, and points out her need-to-watch areas for tomorrow, namely fiber and meditation. She's very close on fiber so her score will go up rapidly with just a little more effort and adjustment. If she loses weight this week, continues with her exercise and excellent nutrition, and keeps feeling energetic, she will move along steadily and swiftly to her goal with this plan. If she gets off track somewhere along the line, she can refer back to this particular planner to see just exactly what she was eating and doing when she was losing weight and feeling great.

Meditation is another critical area of which she needs to be aware. I feel that this is such a critical weight control element that it's worth 5 Success Points. Most people are so used to running around at a mad pace that scheduling in some quiet time seems unimportant to them. Nothing could be further from the truth. Meditation allows you to recharge your mental batteries and get more energy and focus for the rest of your busy day. Our greatest insights and intuitions come during meditation. These are the factors of life that can make you feel wonderfully alive and truly in touch with your world.

Her **notes and comments** indicate she does feel great, with lots of energy and little hunger. Being a little hungry is okay because your body is running at a deficit to lose weight. Use water, veggies and fruit to keep from getting too hungry before your next meal or snack.

If she had noted such tendencies as cravings, hunger, low energy level or headaches, then looking at the Planner could give her important clues as to what might have caused them, and of course, how to avoid them next time. She may learn that chocolate is something she craves the week before her period or that a breakfast of fruit and oatmeal allows her amazing energy for the whole morning.

All kinds of patterns and relationships can reveal themselves over time. You might learn that you do great in the morning sticking to low-fat foods, then start wanting high-fat foods in the afternoon or after dinner. By realizing this, you can make adjustments. You can also pinpoint certain foods that you eat as being high in fat or sodium for example. By using the Food Substitution Chart in Chapter 31 "Converting Your Favorite Recipes" you can replace those troublemakers with healthier versions. You might also choose to reduce the serving size instead. You can check at a glance whether you're eating foods that are high in vitamin C every day or beta carotene or other nutrients and add them if you need to.

Perhaps you notice the tendency to eat the same foods day after day or several times a week. This is a common occurrence. People tend to get stuck on their favorites and most families have about ten dishes that they eat regularly. But variety is extremely important to balanced health. Food sensitivities may develop if you overdo it on one type of food. A wide variety of nutrients provided by a wide range of foods is the healthiest (and least boring!) path. So keep your eyes open and periodically review your Planners. I also check them out occasionally for foods or dishes that I have forgotten about, but used to enjoy. When I "remember" a long-lost dish in this way I transfer it to my Favorite Meals list in my journal so I can enjoy it more often (see Chapter 29 "Sample Meals"). This can work for exercise patterns, time of meals, amount of fat or sodium, etc.

When you eat healthy, use your affirmations with belief, exercise regularly and are committed to record keeping like this THINNER WINNER, you can certainly expect major positive strides towards your goals, too. Doesn't look like she's suffering much in the tasty meal department either.

In A Nutshell

1) The #1 most important step you can take to control your weight for the long term has been isolated: keeping a daily journal of food and activity.

2) Daily Success Planners have been an invaluable tool for keeping me at goal for over 6 years. Try thinking of them as "Training Diaries" such as the Olympic athletes keep.

3) Writing it down will actually save you time in your planning.

4) You are more accurate when you keep a journal since you can't "forget" something that you ate.

5) Keeping Planners one week at a time makes planning easier.

6) How to fill in a Daily Success Planner is explained.

7) A sample Daily Success Planner by a beginning THINNER WINNER is analyzed and discussed to see how she did and what she could do even better.

8) All sorts of patterns and relationships can be revealed when you study your Planners. Then you can make adjustments and improve your personal plan.
    Areas you could look at include:
      * Wanting certain foods, such as fatty ones, at certain times of day
      * Relationships between food and energy levels
      * Pinpointing foods high in fat, cholesterol, sodium or sugar
      * Checking your nutrient intake, such as vitamin C, beta carotene or calcium
      * Avoiding boring or repetitive meals and foods
      * Keeping track of favorite foods and meals
      * Time of meals or exercise and how these effect you

9) Study your planners and get the most out of them! You'll find a wealth of clues to help you target the problems that have been holding you back. Use this very effective tool to move you on to the fast track of weight control success!

DAILY SUCCESS PLANNER

DAY/DATE Mon. 1-1-95

AFFIRMATION/ THOUGHT:_____I enjoy being healthy today!

GOALS:_____20   1200   30   1200

			Fat	Cals	Fiber	Sodium

BREAKFAST   Time of Day _____7 am

			Fat	Cals	Fiber	Sodium
WATER	[x]					
FRUIT/VEG	[x]	1 cup fresh strawberries	0	45	3	0
GRAIN	[x]	oatmeal - 3/4 cup	1.5	105	2	0
DAIRY	[x]	1/2 cup skim milk	0	45	0	60
PROTEIN	[ ]	herb tea, coffee w/milk	0	10	0	10
FAT GRAMS	2.5					
WATER	[x]	1/2 toasted raisin bagel	1	80	1	100
SNACK		1 tsp all fruit jam	0	15	0	0

LUNCH   Time of Day _____noon

			Fat	Cals	Fiber	Sodium
WATER	[x]					
VEG/FRUIT	[x]	veggie soup - homemade	0	50	2	100
GRAIN	[x]	2 slices whole wheat bread	2	160	2	270
DAIRY	[x]	fruit yogurt	0	90	0	85
PROTEIN	[x]	1/2 cup egg substitute omelet	0	50	0	160
FAT GRAMS	2	lettuce, tomato and fat-free	0	20	0	125
		1000 island in sandwich				
WATER	[x]	baked apple and cinnamon	0	80	4	0
SNACK		1/4 cup vanilla yogurt	0	25	0	25

DINNER   Time of Day 6 pm

			Fat	Cals	Fiber	Sodium
WATER	[x]	steamed veggies (in sauce below)				
VEG/FRUIT	[x]	plus large mixed salad	0	100	5	0
GRAIN	[x]	1/2 cup pasta	1	80	1	0
DAIRY	[ ]	chunky spagetti sauce	2	60	1	125
PROTEIN	[x]	1/4 cup garbonzo beans in salad	2	55	2.5	0
FAT GRAMS	9.5	1 tsp olive oil on salad	4.5	40	0	0
		1/4 cup fat-free ricotta cheese	0	40	0	15
WATER	[x]	(blended into sauce)				
SNACK		Chocolate frozen mousse bar	0	30	0	30
		Totals	**14** gms	**1180** cals	**23.5** gms	**1105** mgs

Grains [X] [X] [X] [X] [X]
Veg [X] [X] [X] [X] XXXXX
Fruit [X] [X]
Dairy [X] [X]
Protein [X] [X] [X] [X]
Water [X] [X] [X] [X] [X] [X] [ ] [ ]
Vitamin/Mineral [X]

EXERCISE

GOAL MINUTES___30____
ACTUAL MINUTES___30____
TYPE____walk_____
PULSE___132-136___

WEEKLY WEIGHT

REVIEWED BY ___Roseanne_____   175

NOTES/COMMENTS

Felt great! Lots of energy, not too hungry.
Try 35 minutes walking tomorrow!

SUCCESS points

[X]	AFFIRMATION 3 TIMES	+3
[X]	Met all goals & reviewed	+3
[X]	COMPLETED EXERCISE	+3
[X]	COMPLETED PLANNER	+2
[X]	FAT WITHIN LIMIT	+2
[X]	CALS WITHIN LIMIT	+2
[X]	WATER /6 MINIMUM	+2
[ ]	FIBER/25g MINIMUM	+2
[X]	NO SKIPPED MEALS	+1
[ ]	MEDITATION	+5

SUCCESS SCORE   +18
(+25 possible)

*There is a blank Daily Success Planner in the Appendix for you to copy.

Keeping Track of Your Progress   19

*"Progress, far from consisting in change, depends on retentiveness ...
Those who cannot remember the past are condemned to repeat it."*
George Santayana

When you change your dietary and activity habits on the THINNER WINNERS program you can safely expect your body to respond by losing pounds and inches. What remains to be determined is just how many pounds and inches will come off over a given period of time. It is far too subjective and easy to lose track of how your body is responding to a change in diet and exercise without keeping some kind of records. It's important for you to eliminate as much guesswork as possible. The way to most effectively demonstrate and track your progress is through the use of weight and measurement charts and graphs. That way you'll know you're winning.

Your weight and inches ideally will come down in a gradual and steady manner until you reach your goal. But realistically there will be times when you hit plateaus or even have gains when it seems as though you have been doing all the right things. These can be emotionally trying times to say the least. Through the use of consistent record keeping it is often possible for you to study these slower periods for clues that will keep you on the gradual, safe downward curve. Seeing your pattern of weight loss and related behaviors revealed over a period of months and years helps keep that small loss or slight gain in perspective.

Pretzel Logic

Molly O'Golly is a yo-yo dieter. She's a devoted reader of the National Irrational Pseudo-News and is a self-confessed "diet junkie". She wants to look thin, trim and athletic ... and she wants it now! She fully intends to lose 39 pounds in the next three weeks.

One of the honest-to-goodness, reality-based factors of a truly positive, health-directed, long-term weight control program is that the progress you make often seems quite slow (at least compared to the miracle claims you see at the checkout line). We have become so enamored with the concept of "instant results" that anything we do that takes more than about two days just doesn't seem to be working somehow. This is a dangerous and misleading trap that you would be extremely wise to avoid. Products like "Skinny Minnie's Miracle Instant Weight Loss Pills" advertised on the pages of the Pseudo-News always sound great . It's hard to ignore the promise of being thin by next Tuesday, especially when the product comes with a ten-day money back guarantee and is touted by a size 3 model, who claims to have lost 80 pounds on Minnie's pills. How can you lose? Well, if you really want to know, there are a number of ways to lose at this game.

Molly is a ready buyer of Skinny Minnie's pills. She sends in her coupon and her money and stops eating in excited anticipation of the arrival of this wonderful new super-product that will magically transform her into a size 3 starlet. She loses 5 pounds sitting by her door waiting for the mailman. When the pills finally arrive she follows the directions to the letter. She takes ten pills a day for the next 30 days ... and loses about 15 more pounds. During the first few days she has a bit more pep than usual, and she doesn't feel like eating very often. She also starts talking faster and seems to lose her train of thought every few minutes. After those first few energized days she starts sleeping poorly and feeling rotten, and seems a bit more irritable than usual. For some reason, when the pills run out, she falls into a blue funk even though she has lost some weight. Over the next two months she seems to spend a considerable amount of time sitting in front of the TV, eating like it's going out of style. She's absolutely starving, and nothing seems to satisfy her.

A graph of Molly's weight during this period tends to resemble a "V" , a rapid loss followed by a rapid gain. When she recovers from this particular bout of "dieting" (or forgets about it) a few months down the line, she's going to try it all over again with some new secret formula just developed by the aliens who live high atop the Andes.

Poor Molly has not only failed to learn from similar past experiences, she has jeopardized her health as well. She has also struck a major blow to her already fragile self-esteem.

Engineered Weight Control

When engineers build a road they have to grade the hills along the sides of the roadbed to a "critical angle". If the slope of the hillside is too steep when they're done, rocks will roll down on the road and accidents will occur. The same rule generally holds true for weight loss. In order to be safe and healthy over the long haul you should lose weight gradually. The graph of your weight loss should have a gradual down slope to it ... a critical angle. Try to avoid becoming a "Falling Rock" by losing your weight too rapidly. People who lose weight too quickly tend to bounce out of control and gain it back. The surveys that report a 95% diet failure rate bear this out.

In order for you to get a handle on the way your body loses weight, there are a few essential variables that you need to be aware of. These are measurable factors that will have a direct effect on your weight loss ... and on your ability to maintain your loss.

These are items that you can track with some accuracy. Most of these are kept on your Daily Success Planner. (See Chapter 18.):

1) The number of fat grams you eat in a day.
2) The average percentage of fat in your diet.
3) The number of calories you eat in a day.
4) The average number of calories you eat in a week.
5) The type and amount of activity and exercise you do.
6) The approximate number of calories you burn during your exercise.
7) Your body measurements and body fat percentage.
8) The number of pounds you lose in the average week and average month.

By tracking the interactions between these measurable variables it is possible for you to determine:

1) The approximate average rate at which your body loses weight on your program over time.
2) How long it takes you to stabilize your weight after a day or more of heavier eating or less activity ... and how long it takes to show up on the scale (lag time).
3) The amount of excess weight that shows up on your scale as a result of either (A) overeating (B) under-exercising (C) having your period or other variables unique to your lifestyle.
4) The average daily fat & calorie intake that allows you to lose weight safely and steadily.
5) Your target fat and calorie/activity relationship for optimal results.
6) Your personal pattern of weight loss.

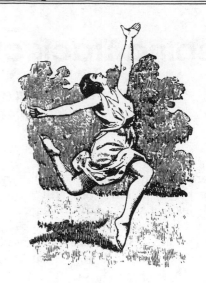

"I lost an inch! YES, YES, YES!"

There is no question that in order for you to gain a high degree of control over your weight it will be necessary for you to pay attention to your body and your behavior. Yes, it is possible to simply eat less and lose weight ... at least for a while. Tens of millions of yo-yo dieters are living proof that this can be done. But the goal of THINNER WINNERS is to help you develop the skills necessary so that you can take control of your weight and health for the long term. This means learning some new skills and changing some old habits. Keeping track and learning your patterns is an important step in increasing your awareness and your skills.

The following lists some important records for monitoring your progress.

1) Your **Body Fat Percentage** (see below).
2) Your **Body Measurement Chart**. Get out your tape measure and record your body measurements once a month (or every 10-20 pounds should be enough). Measure all the critical locations: neck, upper arms, chest, waist, hips, thighs, knees, calves.
3) Your **Weight Chart**. Weigh yourself weekly and keep track by date. Coordinate your weight changes with the information on your Daily Success Planner.
4) Your **Exercise Record** (see Chapter 21 "Get That Body Movin'").

Body Fat Percentage

The question as to how much you should weigh is not a simple one. It used to be. You looked on the standard height-weight chart and found a range of weights within which you should fall to be a normal weight. Well, in case you haven't heard, there's a lot more to ideal weight than that nowadays.

The biggest change is the importance of your body fat percentage and muscle-to-fat ratio which shows the amount of muscle tissue in relation to the amount of fat tissue in your body. This is important because it's possible (and probable if you have dieted frequently) that you can weigh the perfect amount listed on the chart and still be overfat and thus at risk for health problems. Type of weight, fat or muscle, is the real issue. Women should have between 18-22% body fat and men should have a 10-16% range. If you are very muscular or athletic, this could go down, of course.

There are several ways to determine this number. Unfortunately, the accuracy varies widely and is affected by many factors such as what you ate recently, water retention, medications you are taking and the experience of the person administering the test. Health clubs and facilities may offer electrical impedance or infra-red methods at a reasonable cost. One baseline test and another reading six months later may at least give you an idea of your improvement by way of comparing the two figures. That is, assuming that both tests were given under the same conditions.

The underwater immersion test is just as invasive as it sounds. You actually go to a laboratory and don a bathing suit. Then you get dunked underwater in a huge tank. By displacing a certain volume of water and factoring in your weight your body fat percentage can be very accurately determined this way. I don't believe that the majority of us are going to rush right out and do this one. It's not that readily available for one thing. It can be embarrassing, expensive and ruins a perfectly good hairdo.

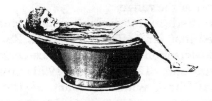

One of the easiest ways to tell if you're too fat is just to take a good, hard look in the mirror sans clothes. If you see lumpy, bunchy deposits that are soft and squoosy and you jiggle a lot, guess what? That's not muscle. True, some may be loose skin on the abdomen after having a baby, or on the inner thighs or under the upper arms. Skin does tend to get loose there as we get older. But I think you can tell the difference if you're honest. Of course, this is just general observation and will not give you the specific information about your percentage of fat.

Skin-fold calipers are another way to determine your percentage of fat. They are inexpensive and have been shown to be fairly accurate when you follow the directions carefully and take readings at several predetermined locations on your body. This is probably the best way to determine fat percentage for most people. It is a more refined version of the old pinch-an-inch test that we all know and love. Remember? Pinch the flesh at the side of your torso just below the ribcage. If you can pinch more than an inch, you're probably too fat. Use this when you get down close to your goal and you want to know if there is still more to lose.

Consider Three Fat Factors: BMI (Body Mass Index), Waist-to-Hip Ratio, Existing Conditions

There are three other factors that you need to consider when you are trying to find an ideal range for your individual set of circumstances. The first is the location of your fat. I know ... everywhere! (Sometimes I felt as if even my toenails were fat.) What I mean is that there are two basic types of bodies. Those that gather fat around the middle (apple shaped) and those that store extra fat around the hips and thighs (pear shaped). The apples may be at higher risk for heart disease, cancer and diabetes. Men are often apples and more women are pears. I'm a pear. But as you can see from my after pictures, you can even this out so you look proportioned and are healthy at the same time. This shape may change somewhat after menopause because of a reduction in the female hormones. I hope. To determine what you are, measure your waist (no sucking it in) and around your hips at the widest part. Now divide your waist measurement by your hip measurement. That figure is your "waist-to-hip ratio". You are too fat if it is 0.95 or above for a man or 0.80 or above if you are a woman.

Many health professionals still use the standard weight-height charts because they just happen to correlate very closely with another measure of how fat you are: the body mass index (BMI). The formula for determining your BMI is a little complicated so hang in there. Measure your height in inches and square it, that is, multiply it by itself. Say you are 5'7" tall. That's 67 inches. 67x67=4489. Now take your weight in pounds and divide it by that number (135/4489). Got it? (It's .03) Now multiply the whole thing by 703. The result is your Body Mass Index (mine is 21.14). For women 20-22 is ideal and for men it's 21-23 although anything under 25, especially if you are over 35 years old is probably acceptable.

The last factor to consider is whether you have any existing conditions or risk factors that would affect or be affected by your weight. Conditions such as high blood pressure, diabetes, heart disease and arthritis among others are examples. Talk it over with your health care professional and follow his or her advice on possible adjustments needed.

So to recap, consider these factors when choosing a healthy weight range:

1) Fat percentage: 10-16% for men, 18-22% for women.
2) Waist-to-hip ratio: 0.95 or above for men, 0.80 or above for women.
3) Body Mass Index: 21-23 for men, 20-22 for women.
4) Existing health conditions or risk factors
5) Age
6) Frame size
7) Sex
8) Height

But How Much Should I Weigh?

The fact remains that most people still determine their success and progress on a weight loss program by weighing themselves on their bathroom scale. If this is the case for you, try to get the most accurate scale that you can. Not the kind where you can lean to one side or the other and instantly eliminate a few pounds.

That reminds me of a story about my wonderful, well-meaning grandmother. She was helping me lose weight as a teenager and I was really trying hard to please her. We weighed in weekly on the bathroom scale that was located next to the sink. As we both leaned forward to get a good look at the scale I ever-so-nonchalantly put my hand gently on the sink. With a little pressure I could magically "lose" a pound or more! She was happy, I was happy. This went on for several weeks with my grandmother so proud of my efforts. But each week I was leaning harder and harder on the sink. Pretty soon I practically had to stand on one arm to make the scale show a loss. Then it happened. You know what. You can't fool grandmothers forever ... they've been around too long. Thus ended another humiliating episode of weight history.

To avoid this type of shenanigans, my advice is to get a balance beam type scale like the one at your doctor's office. The smaller ones are not too expensive and are an investment for lifetime weight accuracy. You could also arrange to weigh in weekly with this type of scale at a weight control group

meeting, your doctor's office, a hospital or public health office or a health club facility. The next best thing is a digital scale if you are under 200 pounds or a high quality spring-gauge scale. If you just have to use your old $6.99 special, then at least try to weigh in the most accurate way. Stand squarely on the scale, wear the same clothes (although most of us weigh in the buff), at the same time of day usually right after getting up in the morning and before breakfast. Weight fluctuates for many reasons during the day and week, so only weigh once a week to avoid getting obsessive about your weight.

I believe that it is important that you have a realistic and definite goal weight to aim for, but not necessarily a single figure. As discussed before, normal weight will fluctuate on a daily, monthly and even seasonal basis. Therefore the chart below is given in terms of range of weights. If you are not muscular or athletic yet (you will be getting more muscle as you exercise regularly!), then you need to weigh closer to the lower end of the range because muscle weighs more than fat. As you earn more muscle, you can safely weigh a bit more and still keep your muscle-to-fat ratio healthy.

To find your weight range, first determine your frame size. Most overweight people say and believe that they are "large-boned". Actually, the majority of people have medium-size frames. So to determine the reality, measure around your wrist. For a woman 5 ¼" - 6"is a medium frame. Anything less and you are small, anything more and you are large. For a man the range is 6 ¼" - 7", again for a medium frame. Check the chart for frame size for adults 25 and older. If you are a woman between age 18 and 25, you can subtract 1 pound for each year you are under age 25. If you are over age 50, you can weigh at the higher end of the range.

I studied many height-weight charts and concluded that for THINNER WINNERS this 1983 standard Metropolitan Life Insurance chart was the best guideline. The newest 1990 government published chart which is part of the Dietary Guidelines for Americans is too broad and easily confused if you don't read the fine print. For instance, at first glance I could weigh 172 pounds at 5' 7" and still be within my range! As long as you have determined your risk factors, primary location of your fat as described above and your correct frame size then the chart below is a good reference. It reflects the latest findings on a healthy weight range for the lowest mortality rate.

Metropolitan Life Height and Weight Chart

	Men				Women		
Height	**Small**	**Medium**	**Large**		**Small**	**Medium**	**Large**
4' 10"	—	—	—		102-111	109-121	118-131
4' 11"	—	—	—		103-113	111-123	120-134
5' 0"					104-115	113-126	122-137
5' 1"	—	—	—		106-118	115-129	125-140
5' 2"	128-134	131-141	138-150		108-121	118-132	128-143
5' 3"	130-136	133-143	140-153		111-124	121-135	131-147
5' 4"	132-138	135-145	142-156		114-127	124-138	134-151
5' 5"	134-140	137-148	144-160		117-130	127-141	137-155
5' 6"	136-142	139-151	146-164		120-133	130-144	140-159
5' 7"	138-145	142-154	149-168		123-136	133-147	143-163
5' 8"	140-148	145-157	152-172		126-139	136-150	146-167
5' 9"	142-151	148-160	155-176		129-142	139-153	149-170
5' 10"	144-154	151-163	158-180		132-145	142-156	152-173
5' 11"	146-157	154-166	161-184		135-148	145-159	155-176
6' 0"	149-160	157-170	164-188		138-151	148-162	158-179
6' 1"	152-164	160-174	168-192		—	—	—
6' 2"	155-168	164-178	172-197		—	—	—
6' 3"	158-172	167-182	176-202		—	—	—
6' 4"	162-176	171-187	181-207		—	—	—

Copyright © 1983, 1993
Metropolitan Life Insurance Company

Men: Height in 1" heels,
weight with indoor clothing
weighing 5 pounds.

Women: Height in 1" heels,
weight with indoor clothing
weighing 3 pounds.

You know you're making progress when your clothes get loose.

Part IV

Activity and Exercise

The Basics About Exercise   20

"Reading is to the mind what exercise is to the body."
Sir Richard Steele

Exercise Excusitis

Okay, you didn't really think you were going to go all the way through a weight control program without facing the dreaded subject of exercise, did you? Think again, oh hopeful one! No real attempt to unravel the mystery of weight control would be worth much if it didn't acknowledge the large part (no pun intended) that exercise plays.

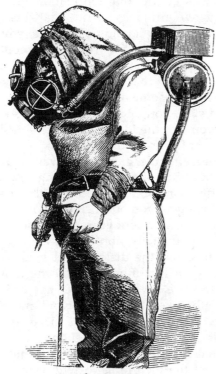

Early attempt to "sweat it off" without exercise.

I tried for years to deny this necessity ... with a wide and well-developed variety of excuses, some of which follow. "If God wants me to sweat my rear off in a contrived classroom full of teeny tight teenagers bouncing and sweating to the loud pounding beat of a rock and roll band then ... I am definitely an atheist!" Then there was "I am a lady, and ladies do not sweat!" I even used "I will not be caught dead being involved in this ridiculous fitness fad. I'll just wait (weight?) it out ... and pretty soon now they'll discover that eating steak and chocolate cheesecake along with being a couch potato is the best way to live a long, healthy life." And so I waited with my excuses, patiently confident that I would soon be vindicated in my choice to not exercise.

The Aging Metabolism

Little did I realize that even as I waited for this miracle of wishful thinking to unfold, time itself was scheming against me. My silly old metabolism was doing what everyone else's does: slowing down as we age. Sorry, but it's a fact of life. We're hummin' beans and that's what our bodies do. Starting at about age 20 (just a few years ago for me, darling) it slows down about 5% by the time you reach age 40. "Not bad, barely noticeable, I can handle it." But you really didn't think it would stop there, did you? Now it's on a roll and knocks off another 5% between ages 40 and 50 accelerates another terrifying 8% between ages 50 and 60, and then caps off the next decade by knocking off an additional full 10% between the ages of 60 and 70! Four times the rate you suffered earlier! If you're keeping track this means that by age 70 you are burning calories at a rate nearly 30% lower than you did at age 20! Whoa, no fair! Stop, stop, stop! I dashed myself angrily against the wall of reality and only got a nasty bump on the noggin for my trouble. My dialogue went something like this: Oh, well, might as well soothe the pain with a banana split and just resign myself to looking like a reflection in a fun-house mirror as I get older. Besides, it's not so bad. My wonderful husband (albeit thin) says he loves me the way I am, and I do have a sense of humor about it all. Being skinny isn't everything. It's what's inside that counts, right? I have a good heart (even though it's about the size better suited to a midget hummingbird). And on and on the rationalizations went, year after year as my metabolism inevitably ground to a halt. I wondered if I lived to be 120 if I'd still be fat even if I gave up eating altogether.

Muscle or Fat?

Then I discovered another nifty trick of aging (besides the wrinkles and sags which I kept plumped up with all that nice fat). One of the reasons that the metabolism does this slow-motion dance is that after age 35, you lose about ½ pound of muscle tissue and simultaneously gain 1½ pounds of fat each year! Each and every year!

It turns out that muscle tissue is active tissue that burns up calories, the actual machinery of the metabolism, whereas fat tissue just sits there clogging up the works, not burning up a blessed thing. So, the more muscle tissue you've got, the higher your metabolism and hence the reason why men (those lucky son-of-a-guns) can generally eat more than women and still lose weight faster than women. They simply have more muscle tissue and therefore more calorie-burning machinery!

After another few chocolate chip cookies to dull this charming news, I rationalized, "Well, these are just statistics after all. I'm an individual, an exception, and a special person to boot! I'm not the average, no sir, not me. But I sure feel for those poor souls who are being poured into their Golden Years like chocolate syrup right out of the freezer ... slo-o-wly". Besides, I figured that nobody would be able to tell if I was one big muscle or a sack of fat, right? That's why they make spandex. So what difference did it make anyway? Well, somebody up there thought of that one too, and they made muscle tissue smaller and denser than fat tissue. That means that even if you weigh the same amount at age 50 that you did at age 30, you'll wear a larger size because fat takes up more volume than muscle. In other words what really matters is not how much you weigh but the percentage of body fat you have. An optimal amount for a woman is between 18-22% and for men 10-16%.

Now one thing I never realized, as I blithely skipped from one fad diet to the next, was that major damage was being done to the actual fat-burning machinery ... the fat-to-muscle ratio. It works like this: Let's say you weigh 200 pounds when you start Dr. Speedy's Lo-Cal Wonder Plan and you are 25% body fat. You actually stick with it long enough to lose 20 pounds. But 20 pounds of what? Hopefully fat, right? Sorry. Weight lost on a low calorie diet is only about ⅔ fat and water, the rest is muscle. So along with your 14 pounds of fat and water you also lose 6 pounds of fat-burning muscle machinery! Less muscle = lower metabolism. Now you don't get to eat as much to maintain your weight because you can't burn it up as fast without that muscle. It becomes easier to regain that 20 pounds. Also, especially if you're not exercising, what kind of tissue do you suppose makes up that 20 pound regain? All fat, no muscle! So now you are actually 28% fat.

Well, you try again since you don't know what else to do, you can't stand yourself this way any more and the high school reunion is just around the corner. You psyche yourself up for another bout with

a new fad diet ... maybe you'll try the Ice-Cream Diet this time. Sounds like you could handle that, and after all, the book was written by a doctor. Off you go paring off that 20 pounds again. What a great feeling. Success! But wait, again you lose only 14 pounds of water and fat and another 6 pounds of that precious active muscle tissue. Then after the reunion, up rockets the weight again. It's all fat, of course, and now you're 31% body fat.

Not one to ever give up, you are again lured into a popular diet by flashy celebrity Sandra Slither and her "guaranteed unretouched" glossy four-color photo advertisements. Where else are you going to turn? Your doctor just looks at you with pity in his eyes, knowing that most overweights are just doomed to stay that way, and then hands you a single sheet of paper explaining the four food groups. So you and Sandra start off again. And again you are rewarded for your deprivation with another 20 pound weight loss. And, (is this getting familiar?) another 6 pounds of muscle, which is in reality your only hope for true weight control and rational eating. When it is revealed in "The Weekly Blabber" that Ms. Slither is actually a bulimic who had some of her ribs removed in order to look so slim, you angrily gobble chips and crab dip until you blot the idyllic vision of your head on her body out of your mind forever.

Of course, you regained the weight as fast as last time and end up with a whopping 36% body fat ratio, all by trying to lose the fat in the first place. Now how many of you out there have been on three low calorie diets in recent years? Four diets? More?

Well, I personally don't have enough fingers and toes to count the diets I tried in the last five years of my fat life, much less all the gimmicks I fell prey to since I was the tender age of 9 when I was officially taken to a "fat doctor" and put on a very strict (and lo-cal) regime of unsweetened grapefruit juice and minced clams in water (try trading that for a cupcake at lunch time!). Now I began to get the picture as to why I jiggled like a bowlful of jello and my metabolism seemed to be going in reverse. I never used to believe those stories of the 900 pound patients put into hospitals on "supervised" (meaning locked in their rooms with 24-hour guards at the doors) low calorie regimes and actually gaining weight, but now I wasn't so sure. The fact is simply this: low-calorie diets (below 1200 calories) increase body fat, especially when used without exercise, and who has the energy to exercise without those needed calories?

The Real Deal that Isn't a Meal

Hold on now, this is really turning into a SITUATION! What is going on? And what in the world can you do about it? Are you going to lie passively on the couch with a bag of chips and watch the march of time and your dieting efforts gleefully plunder your muscle tissue while replacing it with ... MORE FAT!? If you already have enough of that, thank you, then let's get down to the answer. There must be something you can do to hang on to that muscle machinery, to maybe even pump it up a little so you can burn a few more calories (read: be able to eat more). Realization began to dawn. Oh, no! It just can't be! But you finally have to look the monster in it's fiery red eyes and admit that there is only one way to reverse this unfair and relentless trend. Can you guess? Yes, again your archnemesis ... Exercise had reared his vainglorious head.

Now, I don't want you to get the idea that I just logically went through the facts one time and decided that the answer lay in a pair of pink tights and a leotard. No, I'm afraid I'm not that dumb (or smart). First, I had to work my way through a complicated and convoluted morass(!) of rationalizations and excuses and periods of indifference and tete-a-tete's with like-minded friends who were more than willing to be eating buddies. They tolerated my cries of unfairness just as I supported their well-thought-out strategies of denial and justifications. Whew! I was a walking (well, waddling) stronghold of all the "reasons" why the silly notion of exercise was never going to work for such a sophisticated and complex being like myself. So there! Believe me, the wall of resistance I built up around myself to keep out the facts worked wonderfully to shelter my sanity (and fat) for years and years. Impenetrable. They were wrong and I was right. Period. So go away and leave me alone.

Overwhelmed by the Evidence

But ... I just couldn't hold on, and little by little they broke me down with all the studies, articles, books and facts I was reading. "ALL RIGHT, ALREADY!!!", I cried. "You think you're so darn smart, I'll just do it! I'll prove to you once and for all that exercise will never work on me!" And so I took an exercise class. "It didn't work, see? I'm still fat, so there! Now will you leave me alone to eat in peace?"

This is the next phase. Showing the world that you are really "trying" to seriously exercise. I pounded through aerobics classes until I couldn't even breathe. I walked until I actually broke a sweat, and I even tried to jog once or twice just to prove I could do it. I bought an exercise machine and kept it in the living room to show people just how serious I was about all this physical culture stuff. I

bought exercise outfits and expensive shoes and tapes and made lots of loud noise about how much I was working at this thing. Boy, I really had myself convinced that I was giving it my best shot. And I danced along like this for a few years, huffing and puffing for the benefit of the public eye. Nobody could say I wasn't trying! No-Sir-ee, Bob!

To Lose the Weight, Lose the Attitude

So ... why was I still fat? Something must be missing. Well, after a long time spent wondering what in the blazes was wrong with me, I slowly began to put some of the pieces together. And it turns out that dragging myself kicking and screaming, with an I-told-you-it-wouldn't-work-attitude, into exercise was actually holding me back from the benefits. Uh,oh. I can almost hear it now. The newest excuse, right? If I don't really want to do it then it won't do any good anyway ... so why bother? That one worked for a while too, but wore off when I started thinking about square one again. The answer wasn't to give it up, but to lose the "attitude". And this was the part that was harder than giving up peanut butter straight out of the jar with a spoon. I remembered the #1 Rule of all success, the "Strangest Secret" as Earl Nightingale called it: you become what you think about. Here I was, beating myself up again, hammering away at my body and treating it as if it was my worst enemy (other than Dr. Exercise himself, of course). My dominant picture of myself was of a poor, tortured fatty with no hope at all of ever becoming thin and tight and trim like all the other people in the world. I alone must bear this burden. I alone, against the Forces of Nature and the Universe. I alone would struggle and fight like the Man of La Mancha against the evil world. Boy, was I ever a good martyr! One of the best ... Academy Award quality. And so I played around with this role for a while. (If I ever become an actress, just think how much weight I can bring to these roles!)

The Upside of Exercise

Not only was my attitude reigning me in, but I was only working on partial information about exercise. My sources were word-of-mouth, magazine articles and a few talk shows. This is the wrong way to find out about what exercise really can do for you, the best kinds of exercise, etc. And of course, there were also the hundreds of fad diet books I had read, but I already knew that they didn't work. What I really needed was some good, solid "knawledge" as the comedian Jim Varney (also known as Ernest) calls it. Here's what I found out after researching a range of proven sources.

At first, it's hard to believe all the benefits that are claimed for regularly "working out", but believe me (and my photos!) that what you are about to read is all true! First, there are the obvious physical advantages, the ones most of us have at least heard about such as the following: Exercise strengthens and increases muscle tissue including the heart muscle (and now you know what that means ... more muscle = more food). Okay, if I had to work out to be able to eat and still be thin, then ... I'll do it! (More on this exciting phenomenon below.) Ligaments and tendons are strengthened as well. Regular exercisers also have been shown to have a lower incidence of many diseases and ailments such as heart disease, diabetes, osteoporosis, depression, constipation and circulatory problems. In the case of osteoporosis for example, this is done by increasing the density of your bones so they are stronger. Exercise also creates new pathways of circulation in the form of blood vessels throughout the body, because all the extra oxygen that you push through your body needs new pathways (arterioles) upon which to travel. As your new blood vessels are formed you're less susceptible to being cold all the time as I was when I weighed 272 pounds. Of course, when I was hot I also had a harder time cooling off, since there were not enough vessels to circulate my blood fast enough through all that too, too solid flesh. Most of the time I was just plain uncomfortably hot or cold, and now I knew why. Proper exercise also acts as a natural appetite suppressant, just the opposite of what I thought (improper exercise can make you hungrier!). You can actually curb your appetite naturally by working out right before mealtime.

In the physical appearance department (everyone's favorite), the benefits are stellar. Posture improves as all the muscles are strengthened and are more easily able to hold your skeleton in the proper alignment. Aches and pains due to poor posture, such as back, shoulder and leg pain, diminish and disappear. The internal organs are also held in their correct positions more easily, and so can better function in the way they were meant to. No more pot belly. As your posture improves, your body takes on a more balanced and well-proportioned appearance. You begin to look more athletic, lithe and younger (yes!). You enjoy easier, more graceful movement. And as your circulation improves you develop a rosy glow to your complexion and a sparkle to your clear eyes.

Here's a neat fact: a person who exercises and tones up their muscles is smaller, tighter and firmer than another person of the same weight who does not exercise! Let's say that Polly and Dolly both weigh 130 pounds. Since Polly works out regularly and maintains a 20% body fat ratio (20% of her total body weight is fat) she can wear a neat little size 8, but Dolly stays at a 30% ratio and wears a size 12. Really, I'm not making this up! Now, I know that even a size 12 sounds great when you're a size 24 $1/2$ (or larger as I once was), but what if just maybe you could wear a real size 8 (that means the white pants) and look great? Without weighing any less than the person who wears a size 12? Food for thought, eh?

As the disproportionate lumps and bumps begin to even out and diminish you also begin to smile more. And I can think of nothing that makes a person more beautiful and improves their appearance more than a lovely, genuine, easy smile! Are you smiling yet? The best is yet to come!

For relaxation and stress reduction, it seems that mild, consistent exercise just can't be beat. Studies have shown that just 15 minutes of walking releases tension better than a common tranquilizer. How can this be? Well, the answer lies in the fact that muscles, and all your cells, actually build up electrical charges throughout the day. You can chemically release those charges with alcohol or pills, but these don't have any of the other benefits of exercise and can cause other complications that are not desirable. Exercise warms up the muscles, increases the oxygen flow and releases that build-up. That's why you feel so fresh and revitalized after a little spin around the block. Replace the drugs with a walk and make Happy Hour really happy!

Mental Health Benefits

As if all these wonderful physical benefits weren't great enough, the list just keeps on growing! As you become more aware of the connection between the mind and the body, it's just a hop, skip and a little aerobic jump to conclude that your mental health is going to be profoundly affected by exercise, too. Exercisers are more self-confident, emotionally stable and have a more positive outlook in general than their sedentary counterparts. Wow. This sounded like the opposite of my profile when I was fat. Does anybody else out there ever suffer from lack of self-confidence, mood swings, depression and a negative attitude, or was I alone in this? My experience is that just the nature of being fat erodes positive mental health by insinuating the"blame" for fatness on the fat person. The rationale goes: you are responsible for being fat (even though we try to blame it on our parents, society or lard burgers) since you know deep down that it's you that actually places the food in your mouth. Nothing ever fell in there accidentally, right? So there must be something wrong with you. If you can maintain a positive mental outlook with all that in your head, then congratulations. Just think what you could attain if you exercise! Actually, these mental health benefits occur partly because you're increasing the blood circulation to your brain, thus improving brain functioning. You clear away the cobwebs and think better.

These are really amazing claims. But they're true. I really can't say I believed all this stuff before it began happening to me. You had to show me first, like a hard-core Missourian. But I have since become a very excited believer in these benefits. I always keep a pen and pad or a tape recorder in my workout area since I know that I'll get some great insights, ideas and concepts during my workout. And, of course, there are the now-famous endorphins, the chemicals released during exercise that are responsible for mood elevations, the "happiness factor" or the "runner's high". The last mental health benefit I'll mention is the elimination of the nagging guilt that "you should be exercising". A big weight off your mind, as well as your body.

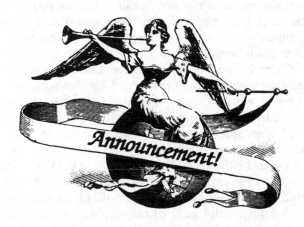

Miraculous Fact: The Kreb's Cycle

And now, for the "piece de resistance", the discovery that tops them all, in the case for being an exerciser. A little phenomenon I ran across called the "Kreb's Cycle" (as in Maynard G.) or what I see as another "miraculous fact".

Just when it seemed that the Laws of Nature were conspiring against my ever being really thin, and being able to eat to my hearts content at the same time, I ran across this little gem of merciful implications. It has a tongue-twisting medical name, which is why some people might miss it the first time around: the tricarboxylic acid cycle (try saying that three times real fast with a mouthful of chips!). This is a chemical process of the metabolic mechanism (yes, your metabolism) that converts all the food you eat into what your body decides is

needed. It can change food into a variety of things such as energy-type molecules, plain old water or carbon dioxide (all pretty good choices for the thin-seeking individual). Or it can produce FAT ... definitely not good. Why does it choose to make more fat? This is the part I really love. It makes fat because it doesn't have enough complex carbohydrates (great stuff like potatoes, rice, whole grain breads, cereals like oatmeal, corn including popcorn ... I could go on and on) to light the fire that burns the fat during exercise. You cannot light the fire to burn the logs of fat without the kindling of carbohydrate. Is this like a dream come true for dieters, or what? All those years of watching and limiting the "starches" was wrong, wrong, wrong. These are really the good guys when it comes to burning up that extra fat.

So the key to burning fat at the greatest possible speed lies in the combination of two things: one, exercise and two, complex carbs. Now, when I first heard this I said, "No way". If I eat extra bread for lunch or a baked potato every night for dinner, I'll blow up like a Steven Spielberg special effect. But then I decided, why not? It couldn't hurt to try since I'd tried eating every other (usually disgusting) food that offered to help, and I could think of lots of things worse than adding extra bread, potatoes and cereal to my daily fare.

The miraculous fact here is that it worked. My body fat ratio came down. Those stubborn, loose globules of fat diminished and finally vanished. I became firmer and more well-defined in places where the fat no longer obscured the muscles that I was busy developing during exercise. I realized that food chemists (that misunderstood group of wonderful folks) had finally come through with a real "scientific breakthrough" that really was worth something to the fat sufferers of the world. Thank you a million times.

Now let me repeat:

Aerobic Exercise
+ <u>Complex Carbohydrates</u>
= Fat Burning

The Afterburner Effect

Besides burning calories while you're exercising, your body gets revved up during your workout and continues burning extra calories even after you've stopped. An afterburner effect is created which has a tendency to reset your metabolism at a higher rate. The rate and the length of time of increased calorie burn varies with the length of time you exercise, the intensity and your general condition. However, the more consistently you work out, the more revved up you can keep your fat-burning engine ... up to 15% faster. This effect can last for hours after you've showered and changed back into street clothes! Stop the presses, hold the phone! I can actually raise my metabolism to burn up all those extra goodies? Maybe this exercise stuff isn't so bad after all.

Skinny Strategy: Eat!

And here's something else you're going to love. If you reduce your calories too much, your body interprets this as an act of "starvation" in progress". So in order to preserve itself, as a survival mechanism, it holds onto the highest food value molecules that it can get hold of, namely fat molecules, because they are a concentrated form of food energy. Fat has 9 calories per gram as opposed to 4 calories per gram for protein and carbohydrate foods. So what's left for the metabolism to convert into energy? Muscle tissue. The very fat-burning machinery that you want to hang on to and create more of. With less muscle tissue the effect is to further lower the metabolism. What was thought of and suffered through (and I do mean suffered) as a heroic effort to stick to a lo-cal diet was actually causing your body to cling to that fat. Your body sends out a message to stop all release of fat (so it doesn't starve), then it diabolically follows up with an order to your brain to crave the highest calorie foods it can think of, like high fat and sugary foods. Double whammy. It's really no wonder that people who have dieted on and off for years have developed a me-against-it separatist attitude toward of all things, their own body. And those lovely sensitive people who actually have a predilection to listening to the world, nature and therefore their own bodies have had to shut that oneness off and force themselves to fight the demon of "overeating". Well, as a former heavyweight champion I'm here to tell you, harmony is on the way and loving your body has just gotten easier. You can now learn to tell it exactly what you want it to burn up, and what you want it to build up. To summarize: eating more carbohydrate calories and less fat and exercising consistently keeps your muscle tissue and metabolism at the highest levels.

So Where's the Downside?

This was starting to get unbelievably good! More calories and more carbs! Well, where's the catch? There's always got to be a catch, right? Right. The catch is exercise. Everything goes better with it. And without it, well, sorry Virginia, there really is no Santa Claus.

Wait a minute now. Maybe I could just dabble in this (choke) exercise thing a little tiny bit. I'd do almost anything to be able to eat more of the goodies I love. Just tell me the facts now. What exactly is it that I have to do? How much exercise and what kind of exercise and how hard does it have to be? I had visions of having to run marathons and live in sweats the rest of my life. I would be harnessed like an ox under the weight of the yoke of Doctor Exercise, methodically plodding joylessly through dull routine calisthenics looking like a refugee from a sheep herd. Grim. I mean you don't get something for nothing, right? And the benefits were certainly not nothing. But as you will soon find out, dear friend, the actual effort is ridiculously easy as long as you follow a few well-chosen guidelines, as I did.

Okay, by now I had to agree that the rewards were overwhelmingly great. And by the way, not exercising wouldn't just keep me neutral either. It had definite negative effects on my health. So there I was, stuck between a rock and a very hard place: either exercise and enjoy the benefits or don't exercise and suffer negative results. Yuck. Who said life was a rose garden? It's more like thorn city. But with the promise of real health, not fad jargon, and let's not forget the goal of being able to eat more (always on my mind) I plunged ahead to find out just exactly what it was I had to do.

And that's what you'll find in Chapter 21 "Get That Body Movin'". Read it next and find out the best exercise to choose for your own use.

In A Nutshell

1) You lose ½ pound of muscle and gain 1 ½ pounds of fat every year after age 35.

2) Muscle is active tissue that burns calories, whereas fat is inactive. Less Muscle = Lower Metabolism

3) Your metabolism slows down as you get older only because of this loss of muscle.

4) How much you weigh is not as important as your percentage of fat tissue.

5) Optimal fat percentage is 18-22% for women, 10-16% for men.

6) Repeatedly losing "weight" on a low calorie diet causes you to lose fat and muscle. You gain weight mostly as fat. Therefore you have a higher percentage of fat after dieting on a low-calorie regime and then regaining weight.

7) The answer is exercise.

8) To lose weight, lose the negative "attitude".

9) Many physical and mental health benefits are discussed.

10) The Kreb's Cycle states: Aerobic Exercise + Complex Carbohydrates = Fat Burning

11) There is an "Afterburner Effect" that keeps you burning calories at an accelerated rate long after you finish your exercise.

12) Low calorie diets cause your body to cling to fat for survival.

13) Eat more carbohydrate calories, less fat and exercise properly and regularly to keep your metabolism at its highest levels and to get, and stay, slim.

14) Not exercising is not neutral! It has cumulative negative effects on your health.

Get That Body Movin'   21

"Our bodies are our gardens, to which our wills are gardeners."
William Shakespeare

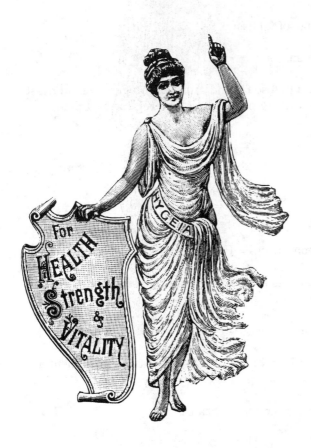

Get Motivated & Stay Committed

We are living in a paradoxical age. The more ingrained that speeding automobiles and zooming airplanes become in our lives, the more we crave a slow ride in a horse-drawn carriage. And the more time we spend lazily parked in a lounge chair in front of our TV's, the more action and excitement we demand in the programs we watch. Life is full of mixed messages. Our heroes and heroines push the limits of physical strength and beauty and all we have to do is sink a little further into the cushions and push the buttons on our remote control. Who needs the ocean when you can go "channel surfing"? It's a dangerous paradox. And your health is at risk because of it. To avoid the trap of a sedentary lifestyle and the health hazards that go along with it you will have to start moving. To develop a truly healthy cardiovascular (heart-lung) system and all the other health benefits I discussed in the last chapter, including fat loss, it is necessary to participate in some type of aerobic activity. At

minimum this means getting your heart rate up to an aerobic level for at least twenty minutes, at least three times a week.

Exercise Rewards

Before I get into all the details of types of exercise, how long to go, how far to go, etc. I'd like first to talk about those twin complaints, the bugaboo and bane of all exercisers, motivation and commitment. It won't do you a bit of good to learn or relearn why you need to exercise, and what horrible things will and are happening to your body if you don't, unless you have a proven plan to ensure you will do the exercise your body needs. So here I offer you such a plan. As Dr. Jon Robison of Michigan State University and head of Michigan Center for Preventive Medicine found in test groups, nearly 97% of former couch potatoes and exercise wannabees are still exercising an average of 3-4 times a week after 6 months by following guidelines similar to those below. 97%! An incredible accomplishment. Especially considering the following sobering facts.

It's a fact that most Americans (about 80%) still don't get enough exercise on a regular basis, even though the benefits have been widely touted. And half of us don't get any exercise at all. It's not that we haven't tried, for goodness sake. I've never talked to anyone who has said they haven't ever started an exercise plan. So the will is there and the need is recognized.

What's missing? One crucial, often overlooked factor ... reinforcement. Nothing works like a good, old-fashioned reward (see Chapter 17 "Rewards — A Feather In Your Cap!"). And not only that, but you've got to get that reward right away. Yes, immediate gratification! You've got to get something besides sore muscles and sweaty hair to want to exercise again tomorrow or even the next day. You need something positive that feels good. Something that will make you want to come back for more. Like having a good time. Like getting thinner, feeling better, healthier, sexier, more in control, sportier or having more energy. If exercise could do that for you, wouldn't it be something that you look forward to instead of trying to avoid? I don't mean dragging through or forcing yourself to endure a workout, but actually looking forward to it.

All these benefits and much more do come to those who exercise regularly. That's why, when a research team wanted to set up a study using people who had formerly exercised regularly for over a year and then quit, they had to ditch their plans because they couldn't find enough participants. And not only that, but the ones who had it suggested to them that they quit just for the study became downright hostile! They wouldn't think of giving up the best thing in their lives even for science!

The period of time between being a non-exerciser to becoming a regular exerciser is crucial. You can count on anywhere from 6 months to one year for the habit to so ingrain itself that you would never think of giving it up. Ever. It sounds unbearably long, but it's for a lifetime of good health. In one year max, you too can be an exercise lover. Use the following strategy, follow the instructions to the letter to get yourself through that 6-month break-in period and you'll never have to say, "Yes, I know. I really should be exercising." You already will be, and enjoying the heck out of the activities and the benefits, too.

1) Find something you like to do.

Later in this chapter, I describe some of the most popular and beneficial aerobic activities. But please, if none of them appeal to you, don't quit there! Go out and find something. (See Chapter 23 "Creating An Active Lifestyle" for some ideas.) Realistically, you don't have to be madly, passionately in love with the activity you choose ... just don't hate it. You can walk on the beach or in a mall, swim in a river, dance, garden, hula hoop or whatever, just keep that body of yours moving according to the F.I.T. guidelines described later. Also, and very important, find several activities that you like and trade off between them periodically to cut down on the boredom factor. For example, I might bike one day, work out with an exercise video the next, walk the mall the third day, run my dog on the beach the next, get on my cross-country ski machine and finish off the week with a planting and hauling session in the garden. Now how could I get bored? You can put the same principle to work. It's called "cross-training" and it's also beneficial because you're working different sets of muscles each day, so you get a more balanced look to your well-toned body. Keep it interesting. You should feel energized when you are finished exercising, not exhausted or dragging.

2) Schedule your exercise sessions.

Each week plan your exercise sessions in advance. Pull out that busy calendar of yours and schedule in at least three exercise sessions ... make an appointment with yourself. Be specific as to

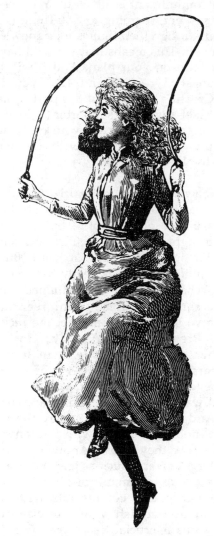

" ...14,226 ... 14,227 ..."

which days, times and activities you'll be doing. Keep in mind that your exercise sessions are more important for you than lunch at the White House. Later in this chapter you'll find specifics about how often, how long and how hard to exercise. In general, a healthy minimum exercise level is 3-4 sessions a week for 20-30 minutes. Be realistic about your exercise goals. You're probably not a professional athlete, so don't trap yourself into a fast burnout. Start with three sessions. Your primary objective is to establish a habit of regular exercise. In six months, exercise will be an established part of your lifestyle ... and you'll miss it if you skip your session (really, I promise). If you're just beginning to exercise, start slowly and build up to the recommended levels gradually.

3) Put it in writing .

Next, turn your plan into a commitment. Write out your personal plan on your Exercise Contract in your Personal Journal. Notice that you must sign it.

That's what a commitment is all about. You need to do what you say you're going to do! There is also space for others to sign their names to acknowledge your commitment. This means that you will have to let other people in on your plan. And it will help keep you honest. I recommend that you read Chapter 16 "Creating a Powerful Support System" and put your chief angel and supporter to good use. Choose a person that you trust and who knows what you are trying to accomplish with the entire THINNER WINNERS program.

4)   Choose a reward and a "booby prize".

Personally, as far as rewards go, my top choices these days are two-hour bubble baths, a new sweater and a night on the town. Pleasant, simple and special. I'm just a romantic at heart. But for some reason similar prizes are really not the most sought after. What is? Good old-fashioned money ... the universal, generalized reinforcer. Most people say "give me the cash and let me pick the prize later". Pretty sensible, really. However, there's another surprise in store ... in terms of exercise, rewards work a lot better when they're tied in to some form of competition. Make a bet with a friend. That way if you fulfill your plan, you get the money. And if you don't, you pay the price. After a while, nobody will bet with you anymore because they know they'll lose. Another approach is to select a large reward, such as jewelry or a trip, and put aside a certain amount of money (say $5-$25, or whatever you're comfortable with) each week that you accomplish your exercise goals. However, and this is crucial, each week you don't meet your goal, you must take out that same amount. I know, negative reinforcement, but here it works. Make sure the reward is for something large and highly motivating to you ... and something that you won't just get anyway. You need to earn it.

5)   Keep track of your progress with a chart.

Get together with your support person or group at least every two weeks and chart your progress. Give yourself a star for every week that you met your exercise goals. That's right! A shiny, bright gold star! It's the very best little reinforcement that I've found. Some very expensive diet groups regularly use stars, ribbons, rounds of applause and other recognition for a job well done. Why do otherwise "mature" adults keep at something to get a paper star? It just feels good to have that little recognition. And to see them all lined up in a row ... well, it's just a wonderful experience. Again, it works. Do it and see.

6)   Get an exercise buddy and form a team.

Find one or more people that you can either exercise with as partners, or people who exercise regularly, though not necessarily at the same time that you do. This is your "exercise team" and it can have anywhere from 2-6 people on it. You can share exercise video tapes with each other and talk about your favorite routines. Research has shown that people who are on a "team" have twice the chance of continuing as those who go it alone! So it's worth it to find someone. Keep looking. If you like doing a solo aerobic activity, that's okay, but choose a buddy who also works out alone and keep yourselves informed by meeting at least once a week and checking each others charts as to whether or not you completed your workout goals. That way you have someone to answer to.

7)   Compete against other teams.

Find another team of exercisers. This could be a mother-daughter against a father-son team, an office-based team or just teams of friends. Use money or stars as rewards for the team accomplishing its goals. If you let your team down, the whole team pays the price. It sounds rather cruel, but that's how competition works. When you see the other members of your team sweating and working, it's a good incentive for getting off the couch and putting your tennies on. Dr. Robison found that when people were asked the most powerful part of this plan, they named not letting down their team members. They knew their friends were depending on them to hold up their end. Use this powerful technique to your advantage.

8)   Don't expect perfection.

I didn't exercise last week. At all. There was a major family event which occurred and my normal routine went out the window. Is all lost? Is that the end of my beautiful new body, my weight loss, THINNER WINNERS? I don't think so. That's just not the way it works. In the world of exercisers, sometimes you miss a workout, sometimes you miss several. It happens. Flexibility is built right in to any good plan.

I know that soon I'll want that good "pumped up" feeling back again and so I'll walk or dance to a tape. No big deal, no guilt, no panic. I'll just do it as I have regularly for the last 8 years. Realize that change is a natural part of the cycle and you'll take a lot of pressure off yourself when you're not "perfect". If your team breaks up, the weather turns bad, you go on a month-long vacation, you get sick or something else comes along to break your stride, don't give up. Just be flexible and find another way to get it done. Or get back to exercising at your very first chance. Believe me, it's worth it. After about 6 months you will "see" yourself as a regular exerciser and if you miss a few workouts, you'll just naturally get back to them as soon as possible. It will become a pleasant habit, like a healthy hobby, that will always be in your life ... a source of happiness and enjoyment that you won't want to give up.

So there you have the ironclad Roseanne Plan for getting motivated and staying committed to exercising. Get started by picking out an activity or two that appeals to you from the list of aerobic exercises later in this chapter. Now I'd like to share with you some more of the reasons why exercise is so good for you. What it really does for your body, your attitude and, of course, your weight.

Burning Fat - Building Muscle

There are two types of exercise. **Aerobic** (with oxygen) and **anaerobic** (without oxygen). You might remember the older terms of isotonic and isometric. The aerobic variety has the ability to burn up the fat, and the anaerobic kind is used to make more muscle, through such activities as lifting weights (don't get excited now, you don't have to become a bodybuilder). This is your goal: get the fat off with aerobics and increase and tone the muscle (fat-burning machinery) by lifting light weights.

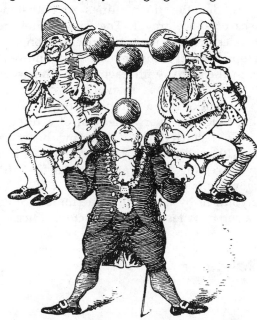

Don't try this at home, kids!
Get expert advice on weight lifting.

To be aerobic, an activity has to elevate your heart rate to an "aerobic training range" and keep it there for about 20-30 minutes continuously. That's optimally, of course. In the beginning for me it might as well have been, "To be physically fit and thin you have to run to the moon and back three times a day". I couldn't even walk one block without

exhausting myself when I started, but hey, I had to start somewhere, right? I mean if I had been in perfect condition I wouldn't have been trying to learn about all this in the first place. So wherever you start, that's the beginning, that's all. You can only get better.

Fat burning itself doesn't really begin until about 10-15 minutes after you reach aerobic levels. Before that, your body is being fueled by glycogen left over from the food you ate yesterday, which is still available in your muscles. But anything after that initial time period is burning mostly fat. That's why the battle cry of fat burners in the know has become "low and slow" or "light and long". This means that exercising at the low end of your heart rate range for longer periods of time is the most efficient way to burn off the fat in and on your body. Exercising for 20-30 minutes will still give your cardiovascular system a good workout and it's great for people not having to burn off a lot of extra fat, but longer is better for fat-burning. An hour of brisk walking (at a rate of 3-4 miles per hour) actually burns more fat than 30 minutes of jogging for this very reason. It's important to know this, so you don't make the common mistake of overdoing your exercise. It's not necessary. You will burn up lots of fat and gain all the benefits of exercise by taking it slower, but doing it longer. This is a major reason for success. The key is consistency. Every day is best, but every other day is fine in the beginning.

Aerobic-type exercises include any activities that get your pulse up to the desired level and primarily use the large muscles of your thighs and buttocks. It really doesn't matter what you choose!

The F.I.T. Formula

Here's a simple formula to help you remember how to exercise at the optimum level. It's called the F.I.T. Formula:

F = Frequency
How often you work out. Your minimum should be three times a week or every other day to start. Work up to a daily routine to maximize your health and weight loss .

I = Intensity
How hard you work (judged by your pulse rate). Below you will find a formula to determine your heart rate range. Keep it low for maximum fat loss.

T= Time
How long you exercise. The longer, the better for fat loss.

Frequency

Back when I was getting started I knew from my research that I had to perform my exercise a minimum of three times a week, about every other day. Five times a week would be even better, not only because it burns more calories, but also because the furnace (metabolism) would be stoked more often and develop a steadier fire to more efficiently burn fat. I started with three sessions weekly. I figured that I might as well leave some room for improvement later. I have found one of the most effective ways to get that body burning fat in a steady flame of metabolic fire is this: exercise more than once a day. Split your time into two sessions daily. As long as you are going at least 20 minutes at a stretch each time you will be getting aerobic benefits. I know this sounds extreme at first, but it's really one of the best kept secrets of all. Try it and you'll see a difference. I now routinely do aerobics during the day for one workout and then do continuous weight sets in the evening that raises my pulse to the low end of my aerobic training range. A walk in the morning and another in the evening is the perfect way to keep that metabolism fired up and humming along.

Intensity

How hard do you need to work to gain aerobic benefits? There is a simple formula to tell exactly how high your pulse rate needs to get before you are exercising aerobically. It's based on your age. First subtract your age from 220. Let's say 220 minus 25 (all right, let's say 35 then. You don't buy that either? OK, the truth is that I'm 46. Sheesh.) 220 - 46 =174, right? That's the maximum recommended exercise heart rate for a person who is age 46. No matter how hard you work out, you shouldn't increase your pulse beyond that point. If you do, you're risking harmful strain on your heart. Don't push your luck, especially if you're out of shape.

Men, especially, have a tendency to try and go beyond their limits, but for this one be careful.

Okay, now I have to bring up my pulse to a level between 60% and 80% of my maximum heart rate (174). So I multiply 174 by .60 and by .80 and I get a heart rate range of between 104 and 139 beats per minute. Anywhere in that range is going to be aerobic for me.

To find your heart rate, take your pulse with your index and middle fingers held together (not your thumb -- it has it's own separate pulse). Place them on either the inside of your wrist below the thumb, or at your carotid artery on your neck (straight down and slightly forward from your ear). Count your heart beat for fifteen seconds. Multiply the number of beats by four. The total equals your heart rate per minute which is the information that you want.

Going back when I began I thought "no problem". My resting pulse at the time was about 100 so I knew that I wouldn't have to push very hard to raise it to 109 (my 60% level at age 38). I also found out that the more fit you are, the lower your resting heart rate will usually be. The astronauts' resting heart rates are somewhere in the 40's and 50's. Can you guess why? They train like crazy to develop the abilities to withstand the stresses of space travel. The reason their resting heart rates are so low is because a stronger, more developed heart muscle can push more blood through the body with each beat. The weak and flabby little heart has to work harder to get the same amount of blood pumped through, sometimes beating twice for every one beat of a fitter, larger heart. So I started with a resting heart rate of around 100 and now, eight years later, it is 56. By the way, resting heart rate is taken first thing in the morning even before you get out of bed. Don't scare yourself by taking it in the middle of the day after a cup of coffee or at your doctor's office.

Aerobic Heart Rate Range

Age

	25	30	35	40	45	50	55	60	65	70
Minimum 60%	117	114	111	108	105	102	99	96	93	90
Maximum 80%	156	152	148	144	140	136	132	128	124	120

This is a general guideline only. The ranges are accurate for about 75% of the population. Before starting your aerobic program check with your doctor (you should have a regular physical exam in any case). If you have any type of health condition that can be affected by aerobic activity, be cautious and increase your workout level very slowly. Listen to your body as you exercise. Slow down if it feels like too much ... even if you're not at the minimum yet. This is not a race. The goal you are seeking is a positive state of health ... safely and gradually.

As mentioned above, for maximum fat burning keep your pulse at the 60-70% level. Remember "low and slow" or "light and long".

Time

How long should you exercise? Start wherever you are able to, 3 minutes or 30, it doesn't matter. The benefit comes from building up slowly and consistently, not by pushing yourself to your limit the first day, then sinking into the couch for a week, a groaning mass of sore muscles. Gradually add 2-5 minutes each week until you are exercising in your aerobic range 20-30 minutes each session (minimum). You can work out for up to one hour if you want. But in the beginning go 20 minutes, then 25, then 30. Up to one hour. It doesn't matter how far you go distance-wise. It's the total amount of time and the intensity that count the most. When you're ready to increase your workout, increase the length of time first, before you increase your speed. Then, after you're at your regular exercise duration comfortably for a while, you can pick up the pace to reach a rate of 3-4 miles per hour. The same principle applies for other aerobic activities as well ... first increase the length of time, then your speed.

Continuous exercise will give you the most benefit. However, recent studies done at Stanford concluded that total time in the aerobic zone is what matters. So if you do 15 minutes 2 times a day, or one 30 minute session, the benefit will be similar. This is great news for the time-pressed.

Start Smart with Walking

If you're not doing any type of exercise now, you will have to build up to the minimum level. A good method is to start wherever you are and build up your aerobic time gradually. If your most strenuous current activity is opening the refrigerator door, you can begin by using it as an end zone. The next time you're hungry and going for the food, walk ten lengths of your house first. And do it quickly. Feel your heart rate pick up and your breathing quicken. This is a clue as to what aerobic exercise feels like.

Your body is essentially a complex machine. What keeps this machine up and moving is a system of pumps. Your lungs pump oxygen to your heart and your heart pumps oxygenated blood through miles of blood vessels to every cell of your body. Like any other type of machine (a car for example), your body is designed for an optimal level of use. Most modern cars are designed to function at their peak at highway speeds. They seem to run the smoothest and get the best mileage at about 55 miles an hour. Likewise, your body has evolved over millions of years into a machine that functions best when it does a certain amount of active physical work.

In reality, the optimum level is probably several hours a day. Our ancestors from the not-so-distant past spent a great deal of their time walking long distances in search of fruits, roots and vegetables, and occasionally running when dinner on the hoof had other plans. It has only been during the last few hundred years, due to the success of modern industrial and farming techniques, that a less active lifestyle has been allowed to exist at all. But that's not enough time for our bodies to evolve into ones needing less activity. We still need exercise for optimum health.

In order to begin your program of aerobic activity, it's recommended that you start with walking. It's an activity that's readily available to you, safe for most people, and it doesn't cost a penny. Take your resting pulse rate before you begin to determine your baseline for the range you reach during your exercise session. Stretch your muscles for at least five minutes after you do your warm-up (see Chapter 22 "Warm-Up, Stretching and Cool-Down").

For your warm-up, walk at a moderate, comfortable pace for about five minutes. Be sure to take a watch with you. Don't try to guess how long you've been moving. In the beginning it may seem like time is standing still.

After your five minute warm-up, stretch out your muscles for several minutes. Take your time and get to know your muscles by concentrating on each one as you are stretching. Then begin your exercise walk, gradually picking up the pace. After about five minutes take your pulse again. Note: continue moving your feet to keep your circulation pumping while checking your pulse or blood may pool in your legs and you could pass out (unlikely, but possible). You need to maintain your pulse above the 60% level to be aerobic. If your pulse is below this level, walk a little faster and swing your arms a bit more.

Your heart rate will vary during the exercise session. Try to find a level where you are working fairly hard but are still able to maintain the pace.

During your initial exercise sessions maintain an aerobic heart rate for at least 12 minutes if possible. This is the absolute minimum time for some benefit to result. Exercise at this level at least three times a week.

After the aerobic section of your walk is completed, gradually slow down your pace for five minutes and then stretch out for five minutes. That's it. A little heavy breathing and a little sweat. No horrible discomfort at all. In fact you might even have some extra energy because of all the oxygen pumping through your body.

Add two minutes of aerobic time each week for the following five weeks. After a month and a half you'll be up to the twenty minute minimum. Once you establish a regular walking schedule you can gradually add more aerobic time and burn more calories. You'll also have a much happier heart.

Walking is easy, safe and inexpensive but it

might not provide you with enough excitement. To add a little spice you could try walking with a friend or taking different routes. You can also "cross-train". That is, choosing several activities you love and rotating your workouts between them.

Getting it Right

It seems, in retrospect, that it took me forever to fall into the correct exercise groove. So, where had I been making my mistakes back when I had been killing myself in aerobic dance class? Well, first of all I would find every excuse in the world to skip a few classes now and then ... like a week or two at a time. This was a big mistake since the first maxim of exercise is consistency. As a matter of fact it really didn't matter if I pounded myself to a pulp once or twice a week because consistency and frequency is much more important than intensity. So, as I began to wise up, I made a solemn pact with myself that without fail, no matter what, I would never miss an exercise session. Never. My commitment was "four times a week forever". This was a giant step in the right direction, even more so than I realized at the time.

Then I discovered strange fact (and mistake) number two. If you exercise too hard and push your heart rate up past the aerobic level, you move into the anaerobic zone and are no longer burning much fat. If you work at up to 70% of your maximum heart rate, you are burning up your fat along with carbohydrates. A rate above that however and your body switches to carbohydrates as its chief fuel because "carbs" are easier and faster for the body to access and break down.

You also will get leaner (use more fat) the longer you work out at a low intensity because you will burn more fat over the longer period. If I needed an excuse to slow down, here was my Golden Opportunity. It's actually better for you if you exercise at a light level for a long time rather than over-exert yourself for a short time. A handy way to tell if you're working too hard is called the "breath test". About 5-10 minutes into your session you should be able to say a few words out loud as a sentence. You should not get out of breath. But you'll know you're not working hard enough if you can sing those same words. If you can sing, pick up the pace. This test will keep you in the all-important aerobic fat-burning range. Of course, use your pulse as an indicator also well, but you should learn to listen to your body and feel when you are in the correct zone. With time this awareness will become easier.

Up and Moving

Armed with this knowledge and a new determination, here's what I did: I got up out of my chair (no easy task in those days), walked over to my front door, opened it and put one foot in front of the other, in whatever direction suited my fancy, for the next ten minutes. Then I hastily spun around and retraced my steps back to the comfort of my chair. I didn't worry about my heart rate at that point because I was definitely huffing and puffing and I instinctively knew that I had performed a great workout. Now all I had to do was wait 48 hours and do it again. I'm serious now. That's it. Even I could handle that. And that was the beginning of my weight control success.

The only hard part was believing that what I was doing four times a week, without fail, was doing a darn bit of good. But to my pleasant surprise I soon started to feel better, and the walks got a little bit easier each day as I kept my promise to myself to be consistent. I actually began to enjoy the fresh air, seeing the neighborhood, being outdoors and my own body moving under its own power. I didn't do much more than that for a long time. That was plenty. After a while, though, I could walk a little bit longer, and I found myself going a full 21 minutes instead of 20 minutes. I even got up to 22 minutes after a month, and it didn't feel any worse! Wow, I was cooking now!

I began taking my pulse with a wristwatch second hand at the height of my workout and, lo and behold, I was pumping away at 109 beats per minute or even a bit more. Right on target. My heart was getting stronger and I was raising my metabolism all at the same time ... without over-straining myself. And I was burning real fat. My measurements started to decrease, my clothes were getting looser on me and I lost a few pounds. And I wasn't even "dieting" yet.

No doubt you're asking yourself, "That's it? That's what all the brouhaha is about? That's the fitness revolution?". Back then I personally was thinking, "This can't be right", so I went over it again. And the conclusion was the same: do any activity you choose that pushes your heart rate up to at least the 60% aerobic level for a minimum of 20 minutes every other day consistently. Yep, that's it! To start basking in all the benefits so eloquently spouted by all the exercise buffs, that's all there is to it. And you can do that just like I did.

Overcoming Excuses

I did have one problem that bothered me a lot and I'll tell you this story because you might find the solution useful. It was embarrassing for me to be seen in public with my caftan billowing in the breeze (I wasn't yet ready to wear sweats in public). I felt uncomfortable about being "watched". So I got my dog into the act. I have a big, black dog named Maxi the Maximum Dog, who is actually the sweetest puppy who ever lived. But if anyone even looked sideways at me, I pretended that she would rip their skinny little hearts out, so I felt more at ease. And the neighbors wouldn't get the idea that I was one of those "exercise nuts". I was just out to do my humanitarian duty with Maxi. Besides, then I had someone to talk to. But even Maxi's evil eye couldn't keep the occasional nitwits in cars from making, well ... rude noises and shouting comments from the windows of their speeding vehicles. So I began driving to a spacious park where there were fewer people, and there I participated in the aerobic craze in peace. Whatever works, right?

This was actually great because I began to see that there is a solution for every problem (excuse?) that can be contrived to stop exercising. Feet hurt? Get better shoes, pads for the shoes, foot-soaker! Bad weather? Raincoat, long underwear, hot tea! Sunburn? Sunscreen! Rotten attitude? Concentrate on the results and just do it anyway! No time? Even I could find 20 minutes every other day! Etc., etc.

I did get a little sore after my vigorous routine for about the first three weeks. I found out that a little soreness is normal in the beginning. After all, these muscles have been under-used for a long time. Pretty soon the soreness fades as long as you are consistent. Proper warm-up, stretching and cool-down along with mild exercise will actually increase circulation and ease the muscular soreness. Besides, it gave me a great excuse to let a lovely long, hot bubble bath take me away from my cares. A little pampering never hurts.

Building the Fat-Burning Machinery

Once I started feeling better about the concept of exercise, I wanted to start building up the amount of muscle tissue I had. So I bought two one-pound weights and started doing easy lifting exercises that I learned from instructors on exercise video tapes. There are many such tapes available at levels ranging from absolute beginner to highly advanced. I recommend them for learning basic weight techniques and terms. Or you can get instructions at a local gym or YMCA. Later, I increased the amount of weight and number of times (repetitions) that I lifted the weights. Pretty soon I could combine my weights and aerobics at the same time, a winning combination for maximum fat-burning and increased muscle tissue in the least amount of time. I walked while holding light hand weights.

Now, if you are a woman, don't worry about building big, bulky muscles from all this weight lifting. That's just not possible for 99% of us because the reason muscles get big is due to testosterone, a male hormone, and we don't have much of it. Even professional female bodybuilders who might want massive, bulging muscles have a very hard time developing them unless they take steroids. So scratch that excuse.

What you are after is increasing the percentage of fat-burning machinery ... the muscle tissue in your body. The principle for building muscle is called "progressive overload". This simply means that if the work is too easy, then nothing is getting done, so you must use a little heavier weight to stimulate muscle growth. In the beginning, use light weights ($\frac{1}{2}$ to 1 pound) and then build up slowly ... very slowly. The tendency is to overdo it with weights, "prove you can", and this inevitably leads to overworked, sore muscles and possibly strain or injury . So, if you start to tremble or quiver, go to a lighter weight. Pick two or three simple exercises such as biceps curls, flies or presses. Follow your instructors explanations and guidelines, making safety and form a priority. And, of course, as always, if anything hurts, stop immediately and get professional advice. You know that!

Technique is very important with weights, so strive for good form and proper alignment. Always use smooth, even movements. Never jerk or tug the weights when you lift them. Concentrate and focus your awareness on the muscle you are working. Try not to lean into the lift with your body. Use the muscle. Go for a full extension.

The Impossible Happened

That's how I began, and that's how you can, too. I asked myself if the benefits were worth the effort ... and I'm still exercising after 8 years. And you know what? The "impossible" happened. I love to exercise. I really do. When I don't do my regular routine, I miss it. I actually look forward to my workouts. I can just let go and feel the joy of my body working and flying along. I really feel a great joy about this part of my life. But I will never forget what it was like standing on the other side of the door marked "exercise" ... not really believing that I could make it through to the other side. But I did, and so can you.

I still amaze myself with the amount of exercise I do now. Is this really me? I do aerobic dance tapes or get on an exercise machine 6 days a week. My favorite one right now is the cross-country ski machine or treadmill. I stay on for about an hour at a time! I also walk or hike, ride a bike (either my 10-speed, a nice recumbent stationary-type or my Mountain Bike Supremo) and I'm generally much more energetic and active all day long. I have even been known to jog at times because it feels so wonderful, but my joints do complain somewhat, so I save this activity for an occasional treat like running on the beach. I also tone with weights every other day.

Actually, I now look for excuses to do something active just because I have this wonderful athletic machine (my body!) and it needs to be put through its paces nearly every day. I really love it when the Olympics are on television. I see myself as an athlete in training, a real dynamo of physical prowess, a force with which to reckon. I'm having fun! With exercise! And if I can, coming from where I came from, then why not YOU? I can genuinely say that the physical fitness part of my life is near the top of my list of favorites, right up there with Mama's Veggie Pizza , and that's saying a lot. It's not something that I would give up lightly. Either pizza or exercise.

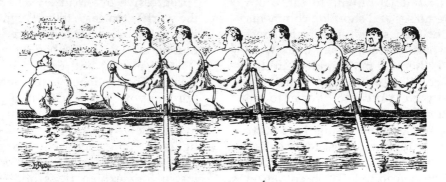

Some activities just naturally build muscle.

Smart Moves for Exercise Success

Let's say that you're ready to change your life for the better ... you're going to start exercising. Seriously do it, not just "try" ... commit! So how can you get started?

1) Get your doctor's blessing. Very important and worth the visit for a complete physical check-up before starting out. Do this for yourself.

2) Follow the 8-step "Roseanne Plan" of action outlined in the beginning of this chapter to get motivated and stay committed.

3) Pick one or more aerobic-type exercises that you like doing. Refer to the list below to help find one that's just right for you. Walking is often the easiest to start with, and is accessible to even oldsters and seriously-out-of-shapers.

4) Calculate your heart rate range and stay within that range while exercising.

5) Always warm up and cool down for at least 5 minutes before and after a session. Walk slowly and do a few easy stretches. (See Chapter 22 "Warm-Up, Stretching and Cool-Down".)

6) Consistency is the key. Three to five sessions a week minimum, 20-30 minutes at a time to start (12 minute minimum). Without fail.

7) Remember the F.I.T. formula: Frequency, Intensity and Time
   a) How often? - Three times a week minimum. Five times is better for fat loss.
   b) How hard? - Stay within your 60-80% heart rate range. Lower is better for fat-burning.
   c) How long? - For at least 12 minutes in the beginning. Then work up to 20-30 minutes. You can go for as long as an hour if you like. Increase your levels as your body shapes up. Find out what exercise levels your body needs to respond with weight loss and then work at that level consistently. If you want to lose fat faster, exercise for a longer time.

Choose Something You Like

Enjoyment is vitally important when starting out. If you don't like the activity, you probably won't stick with it for very long. Look around for something fun. Walking should be your first choice as described above. Many other possible aerobic activities include:

Aerobic dancing - I highly recommend exercise video tapes since there is one for just about everyone: beginner to advanced, oldsters, youngsters, overweight and disabled. They are easy to do in any weather and at any time of the day or night regardless of your schedule. Also, I have found them to be great teaching tools. Sometimes they include mini-lectures about health, nutrition, and exercise. The instructors can be inspiring and entertaining, too. I found a very useful catalog that rates many of the available tapes, hundreds of them, and makes it easy to pick out one just right for you without making costly errors (yes, there are some duds out there). Call Collage Video at (800) 433-6769 and request their free catalog. Choose a low-impact version with an instructor who has a certification or at least a reputation for safe technique. Don't fling, stomp, jump, bounce or otherwise be violent with your body during the workout. Use proper form and listen to your body. A new addition to this category is step-bench classes. Working out with a piece of equipment that looks like a portable step can be very low impact with as little risk to the joints as walking but with a similar aerobic workout to running. It is a very quick way to get into your aerobic zone and the variations in the routine keep the workout interesting. Follow the safety guidelines of your instructor carefully when you are learning to "step".

Aqua-aerobics - Water aerobics in a swimming pool can be very easy on your joints and muscles. Even very obese people can participate safely and get a good amount of muscle-building and fat-burning. The resistance that the water provides strengthens without straining. It's also lots of fun. Check with your local Y or community pool for classes in your area. Lap swimming can also be a good aerobic workout if you are already in good shape. However, swimming for some reason doesn't burn up much fat like the other activities listed. It possibly has to do with the body preserving its temperature core by insulating with extra fat.

Cross country skiing (indoors or outdoors)- There are many cross-country ski machines now available commercially. It takes some coordination and strength to work most of them though, so go to a sporting goods store and try out several before you plunk down a chunk of money. This activity exercises both upper and lower body and so is a very efficient calorie burner. There is a low risk of injury, since your feet never leave the ground, but glide along tracks instead. Outdoor cross-country skiing can be great fun and very aerobic if you live in an area that has snow .

Cycling (indoors or outdoors)- Having a stationary bike in your family room can be a great way to get in your 30 minutes while watching your favorite show. Or it can be a daily reminder that you need to get going on your program. Exercise equipment is designed to be used.

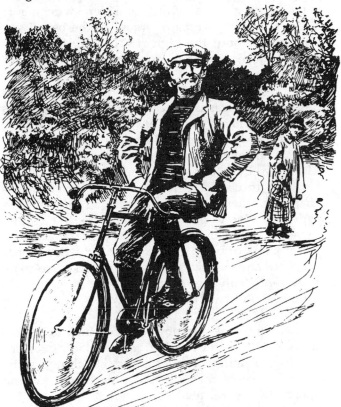

"Look Ma, no hands!"

Cycles are especially good for beginning exercisers who are very out of shape. There is a low incidence of injury and you can even get a recumbent type (with a seat like a chair and your legs out in front of you) that protects your back from strain. Get one with a pulse monitor to make sure you're in your aerobic zone.

Outdoor bikes are really a blast, one of my favorites. They can be expensive, but a reasonably priced one is well worth it. You can also bike for recreation on your off days of course. Wear a helmet and take a class in bike safety and repair. People tend to fall in love with their bikes and the lifestyle it promotes ... freedom and three-dimensional enjoyment of the passing scenery. It's very popular and lends itself well to family and group outings. Did you know that more people world-wide bicycle to work now than drive cars?

Jogging or running - This is for experienced exercisers only because of the high risk of injury or strain to knees, shins, ankles, hip joints and the lower back. People who are very overweight are just asking for trouble if they start right off with a running program. If you do take up running, all you really need to start is a very good pair of running shoes and possibly a hat. Take a class or read a book on running to make sure you're using the proper techniques. If you begin to ache or experience pain after jogging for a while, consider switching to walking briskly which offers all of the benefits of running without the high risk of injury. You just have to walk longer to burn the same amount of calories, that's all.

Treadmills - This is a great piece of equipment that fits the bill nicely when looking for a low impact, easy and safe exercise. Just like walking. Many gyms have them or you can purchase a home model, although they can be expensive. More people continue to use their treadmills after several years than any other piece of equipment. The motorized type is easier to get used to and doesn't require extreme starting motions that may put strain on your lower joints or back. You can adjust the better ones for speed and inclination so you can work up to going faster and with a greater slope. Get at least a 1½ hp motor and handrails for safety.

A few other aerobic choices include: mini-trampoline, roller-skating, roller-blading or ice skating, rowing, canoeing or kayaking, stair-climbing and other specialty machines, racquet sports (tennis, racquetball), handball.

Anything you like to do is fine. This is your workout. Just make sure you stay in your aerobic range continuously for at least 12 minutes in the beginning (especially with racquet sports). I have jogged around the house while cleaning, twirled a hula hoop, roller skated, climbed flights of stairs, jumped rope and used exercise courses in local parks. Someday I'll roller blade!

I'd like to comment briefly on gyms and health clubs. They're great ... but only if you use them. A good gym has high quality, well-maintained, clean equipment, convenient hours, knowledgeable and helpful staff and reasonable rates. Beware of health clubs that ask for a lot of money up front. They know from experience that the dropout rate of members is quite high. Some people move away,

some get lazy. I joined several over the years and what I found was that I personally didn't often get my money's worth. Yes, I admit it, I found excuses not to go ... even after I had paid my money. Today I have a well-equipped, well-used home gym that cost less than a one-year membership in many clubs. Think it through before you spend your money. On the plus side, if you do go to the gym regularly you'll be surrounded by a lot of like-minded people. And when you see a body-builder who's really pumped up it's a great reminder of what the human body is capable of. If you get intimidated or embarrassed maybe it's not for you ... but don't give up without a fight. A good, conscientious gym can be a perfect partner in your health quest and a solid source of information and inspiration. Look for a gym where you can talk to the staff and get a sense of caring and respect for even the most basic questions.

There are some popular activities that you may be surprised to find out are not aerobic. These include bowling, softball, golf, ping-pong, toning tables, intermittent swimming (although lap swimming can be aerobic) and recreational horseback riding. All these activities can be part of a healthy, active lifestyle, however. Remember, if your heart rate doesn't stay in your aerobic range continuously for at least 12 minutes, try something else for the aerobic portion of your exercise.

Try to make your exercise surroundings as pleasant and fun as possible without a lot of clutter. A full-length mirror is helpful if you are doing video tapes (and you're brave!). Don't focus on your "fat roll" the whole time though. Use the mirror to watch your body position so you can check your technique and form against the instructor's. One sit-up done properly is worth ten done with the wrong form, so always strive for good form to get the most out of your workout and every movement.

Wear good, supportive shoes, thick, cushiony socks and loose or stretchy comfortable clothes. Wait about two hours after a big meal or at least an hour after a light one before working out, and always drink plenty of water. You should be drinking at least 8 glasses each day. In addition, drink a glass before beginning to exercise and another glass every ½ hour that you exercise rigorously. Then drink another glass after you finish. Some of the lack of energy or tiredness you may feel while exercising may be brought on by dehydration. The more water you can drink, the better, since you will be losing fluids as you sweat (see Chapter 35 "Water — The Magic Potion").

And, most important, remember to have some fun! Buy an outrageous, but gorgeous, outfit as a reward for deciding to work at becoming active. Or try dressing for your exercise sessions like an

Olympian. Just the act of getting ready to workout will become fun and special. Soon all the excuses will drop away, and you'll see yourself as increasingly athletic, fit and healthy. It will come perfectly naturally into your daily life. You'll soon feel a sense of increased joy and belief in your body as a beautiful part of the world. Harmony is just around the corner, so smile! Your exercise adventure is just beginning!

Your goal is to become active, vibrant and healthy with good prospects for a long, healthy, productive life. Your future will be brighter if you begin today.

In A Nutshell

1)   Use the 8-point Roseanne Plan for ironclad motivation and commitment to exercise.

2)   There are two types of exercise: aerobic (with oxygen) and anaerobic (without oxygen).

3)   Only aerobic exercise burns fat. Anaerobic builds muscle.

4)   To exercise at an aerobic level, keep your heart beating in your Target Heart Rate Zone for 20-30 minutes continuously.

5)   Do your aerobic routine at least three times a week. Consistency is the key! Splitting your time into two sessions a day will increase your fat-burning metabolism even more.

6)   Always warm-up, stretch out and cool-down properly.

7)   Use the Breath Test to stay in your range ... if you can sing, pick up the pace. Or you can monitor your pulse.

8)   Lifting light weights builds strength progressively and increases muscle tissue for more calorie burning. Use video tapes, books or a gym for professional instruction.

9)   Cross-training (varying the type of exercise) helps keep you from becoming bored with your routine and exercises different muscles for a more balanced body.

10)   Strive for excellent form.

11)   Drink extra water.

12)   Wear supportive shoes.

13)   Have fun! Enjoy your workout as your own special time to strengthen and renew your body.

THINNER WINNERS Exercise Contract

By agreeing to complete the terms of this contract you are taking a giant step on the road to positive health and true long-term weight control. You are making a commitment to yourself to get the job done. Make a copy of this contract for your Personal Journal or use the copy in the THINNER WINNERS Workbook, then sign it and get moving!

Commitment To Exercise and Good Health

I, <u>Your Name</u>, commit to change my life for the better. I now understand that a sedentary lifestyle puts my health at risk, and I am worth far too much to allow that to happen. For the next twelve weeks I will exercise aerobically a minimum of three times per week, for a minimum duration of 20 minutes per session in my aerobic heart rate range. I hold myself accountable for getting the job done. No excuses are acceptable to me. My health and weight control are my responsibilities and I will do everything in my power to maintain the highest levels of good health possible.

<u>   Your Name, Date   </u>

Drop us a letter describing your experience during your first 12 weeks of exercise and we'll send you a personalized certificate suitable for framing to honor your accomplishment!

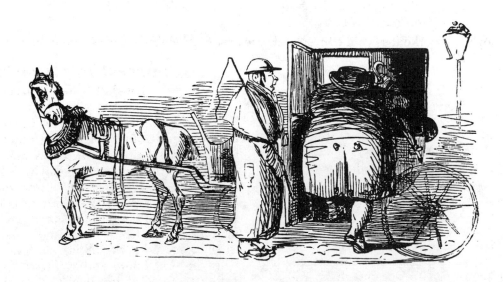

"The gym, Sir? Very good."

Warm-up, Stretching and Cool-down   22

"There was things that he stretched, but mainly he told the truth."
Mark Twain

Slow and Steady Will Get You Ready

Your entire body needs to be warmed up gradually to prepare for activity. Plunging right into a vigorous workout can be dangerous because cold muscles, being stiff and inelastic, can be injured more easily. In contrast, properly warmed up muscles allow you to lengthen and stretch safely, increasing circulation and flexibility so you can get more from the movements during exercise. Also, cooling down the right way allows your body to return gradually to the pre-exercise state. This helps release lactic acid build-up in the muscles which can cause stiffness and soreness the next day and may tempt you to miss a workout (Heaven forbid!). In this chapter you'll learn the proper and safe way to warm up, stretch out and cool down. Aim for a pleasant and relaxing style ... a slow, lingering cat-stretch. This really helps set the tone beforehand for a gratifying exercise session, both mentally and physically, and allows you to appreciate how great your body feels after exercising. Enjoy!

Tips for Safe Stretching

Rule #1: Never do anything that hurts!! If it hurts, it's wrong, so stop. Stretch only to the point of GENTLE tension, then pull back slightly and hold, without bouncing, for 20-45 seconds. Generally, the longer stretch is more beneficial during the cool-down because your muscles are already warm and pliable. Strive to make all movements slow and gentle, smooth and fluid. No jerking and no bouncing. However, a gentle, very slight pulsing motion may be used during the final stretch only, to increase your range of motion. Be sure not to hold your breath! You could turn blue, and besides your muscles need lots of oxygen right now. So breathe normally and evenly. Concentrate on the muscle group you are working and visualize it lengthening and relaxing. Relax into the stretch.

Remember, especially if you are working in a class or with a video tape at home, that you are not competing with anyone. Expand your limits slowly. Never try to force yourself to do something that hurts just because someone else makes the move look easy. Be gradual and moderate and eventually, by working daily, you will increase your flexibility

and range of motion. Be patient. During each movement, listen to your body. Find your own comfort range and progress from there.

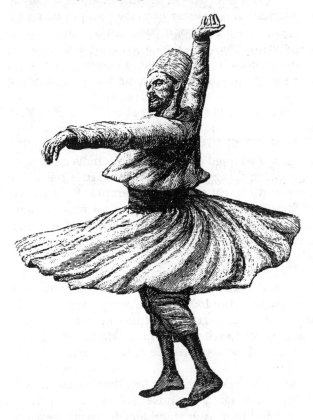

"Warm-up? I thought you said "wind-up."

Warming Up is Essential for Avoiding Injury

You may be so strapped for time or anxious to get right into your workout that you're tempted to skip the warm-up. Don't! It's as essential to your routine as frosting is to cake! The 5-10 minutes it takes to properly warm-up will be well worth the benefits you receive. Like an engine that runs smoother when it's warm, so does your entire body, including your heart, lungs and muscles. It needs time to increase circulation and flexibility. This helps prevent injury and stiffness. You need to be "loose as a goose" to safely gain all the benefits of your workouts! A progressive stretching routine will assure that every part of your body is properly worked and no part is neglected. This will give you a sense of balance and completeness, helping you become aware of all the parts of your body while exercising. Mentally getting ready is important to gear up for the energy to be used and to focus on your movements. Concentrate on the part of the body you are working.

How to Warm-up and Stretch

All a warm-up needs to be is at least 5 minutes of slow movement. The ideal movement is simply a slow version of whatever exercise you are going to do for your workout. So, if you are about to go for a walk, then simply walk at a gradually increasing pace for 5 minutes first. Make a smooth transition into the aerobic portion of your workout. On an exercise machine, simply get on and pedal, walk, row, ski or whatever slowly for about 5 minutes. You can also walk or run in place and do a few calisthenics if that is your style. Just get your body moving and warmed up by continuous movement.

The stretching portion of your warm-up is often done standing up, as in this example. Progressive stretching means to stretch one set of muscles and then to move on progressively to the next set until the entire body has been worked and is ready to safely exercise.

To learn these stretches, you might enlist the help of a friend or exercise partner. Have them read the instructions out loud and correct your form while you perform the stretches. A full-length mirror may make it easier to see what you are doing. Hold each stretch for 15-30 seconds. Be sure to breathe while holding.

Begin by taking 5 deep breaths. Inhale slowly and fully through your nose. Allow your belly to push out and keep your shoulders down and relaxed. This is diaphragmatic breathing. Raise your arms overhead as you inhale. Briefly hold at the top, then slowly exhale through your mouth as you lower your arms.

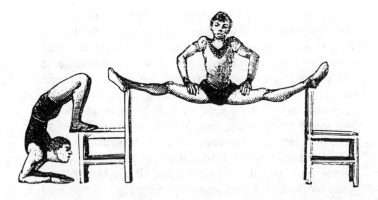

1) **Back of the leg.** Use a wall or upright support if necessary (trees are handy when you're outdoors). With your right foot several feet in front of the left foot, bend your right knee and lean forward, lengthening the back of your left leg by pushing the heel to the ground. Hold.

2) **Hip flexor.** Now bring your back foot in slightly, bend your knee and bring your heel off the floor, tuck your pelvis under and feel the stretch in the front of your thigh and the hip flexor. Hold.

3) **Front of the thigh.** While standing, steady yourself with a support. Take your right ankle in your right hand behind you. Press your right hip forward and your foot into your hand slightly. Point your knee straight down to the floor. Don't lock your left leg. Hold.

4) **Lower back.** Release your ankle. Now hold behind your lifted right knee and gently bring your right thigh towards your chest. Stay lifted in the chest. Hold.

Now repeat the entire sequence for the other leg.

5) **Inner thighs.** Place your feet slightly wider than hip distance apart. Bend your right knee and lunge gently to the right, feeling a slight stretch in the left inner thigh. Hold. Repeat and lunge gently to the left. Keep your knee in line with your toe. Never let your knee jut out beyond your toe. It can cause knee strain.

Breath normally!
Great! Your lower body is ready to go! Let's move on to the upper body next.

6) **Spine.** Stand with your feet pointing straight ahead, about hip distance apart. Slowly roll your head and spine down until you are leaning slightly forward. You'll feel the stretch in your neck and lower back. Place your hands on your thighs and bend your knees. Alternately arch and flatten your back while in this position. Do not bow or sway your back. Use your abdominal muscles to arch. Keep your head in line with your spine or slightly dropped in the arched position. Do not look up. Do this 4-5 times and roll up. No need to hold this one.

7) **Shoulder rolls.** Stand with your arms loosely by your sides. Lift and roll your shoulders in a slow circular motion - forward 5 times , then back 5 times. Way up, way back, way down.

8) **Shoulder Stretch.** Hold your right elbow in your left hand while keeping your right arm straight.

Gently pull your right arm across your chest and feel the right shoulder stretch. Keep your shoulders relaxed and even. Hold, then repeat on your other arm.

9) **Side Stretch.** With your legs slightly more than hip distance apart, lift your right arm straight overhead. Place your left hand on the outside of your left upper thigh for support. Bend from your hip slightly to the left. You'll feel this stretch along the right side of your rib cage. Hold and repeat on the other side. Keep your hips centered when you bend, not pushing to the side.

10) **Neck.** Be careful, move gently! While looking straight ahead, slowly tip your head towards your right shoulder. Move your right ear toward your right shoulder, leaving the shoulder down and relaxed. Hold. Feel the stretch along the left side of the neck. Repeat on the other side. Do each side 2-3 times.

Next, drop your chin gently towards your chest. Don't force. Feel this stretch along the back of your neck and upper shoulders. Hold and repeat 2-3 times.

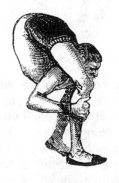

Congratulations! You have first warmed up, then stretched out and now you're ready for a great workout!

Now take your pick of several effective aerobic exercises: walking, aerobic class or video, ski machine, bicycle, one of the new machines ... or the aerobic sport of your choice. All are designed to get your body moving smoothly and continuously to burn fat and improve your cardiovascular capacity. See Chapter 21 "Get That Body Movin" for a complete discussion of choosing an aerobic exercise that's just right for you.

Cooling Down: An Essential Transition

The cool-down is as essential as the warm-up to a complete workout because it allows you to gradually return to normal breathing and body temperature and readies you for the final stretch. The final stretch is really like the cherry on top. Always take your time and enjoy the warm, powerful feeling of a body well-worked. Mentally unwinding helps you prepare for the activities ahead. In a practical sense, stretching at this time helps to release toxins such as the lactic acid that have built up in your muscles during your workout. This, in turn, will prevent muscle soreness and stiffness the following day.

Stiffness can be a cause of those chronic aches and pains that generally make life miserable, and cause you not to want to work out at all! What a terrible cycle to get trapped into! Stiff ... sore ... no positive energy ... no workout ... more pain, stiffness and soreness ... etc.

The final stretch is the ideal time to work on increasing flexibility since your muscles will be at their peak of warmth and pliability. A few extra minutes spent here will go a long way to lengthen and limber you up, and move you toward lithe, willowy limbs. I love to throw in a few ballet or dance moves here and pretend I'm a graceful, expressive prima ballerina or figure skater. Do whatever works for you.

Cool-down and Stretch

The cool-down is exactly like the warm-up! Just continue the same movement you were doing for your workout. Gradually decrease the pace for about 5 minutes. This allows your heart rate and breathing to return to normal.

Following the cool down and right before the final stretch is a good time to do any floor exercises that you would like, such as abdominal work (yes ... sit-ups!). They can and should be done daily to keep your tummy flat and firm. They also help strengthen your back which relieves back pain.

Now you're ready for the best part, the final stretch. This is usually done sitting down, as it is described in this example. If you have to stand, just do a longer version of the warm-up stretch, holding each position for a full 45 seconds.

Always strive for good form. It will protect you from muscle strain and injury. You should look and feel symmetrical and in proper alignment. Keep your knees in line with your toes, shoulders and hips squared and even, head in line with your spine. Your knees should never jut out over your toes in the standing position (this may strain your knees). Keep your pelvis tucked under and your abdominal/stomach muscles and buttocks firm. This helps protect your back. It's a good idea to use a large towel or exercise mat. This provides some extra padding for you.

1) **Back of legs.** While sitting on the floor with your legs straight out in front of you, bend forward from the hips, placing your hands wherever they are comfortable on your legs. Stretch forward with your chest toward your knees, keeping your back flat. Flex your feet towards your head to stretch the calves. Eventually you will be able to have your hands holding your feet and your chest resting on thighs. Hold at least 15 seconds.

2) **Spinal Twist.** Keep your left leg straight in front of you. Place your right foot over your left leg near the outside of your knee. Keep your back straight. Twist your upper body to the right by placing your left elbow on the outside of the right leg, keeping your left arm straight. Turn your head gently and look behind you. Place your right hand on the floor behind you for balance. Don't strain or hold your breath. Hold, relaxing into the stretch, and repeat on the other side.

3) **Inner Thigh.** Keeping your back straight, bend your knees and place the soles of your feet together. Bend forward and place your hands on your ankles and press your knees very gently towards the floor . Hold. Now curve your spine slowly forward and straighten again. Repeat 2-3 times. Now place your hands on the floor behind you. Lengthen your spine. Your knees will automatically move toward the floor.

4) **Front of Thigh.** Extend your legs and roll onto your right side. Bend your right leg to support you and stay up on your right elbow. Grasp your left ankle behind you with your left hand. Press your left hip forward and press your left foot into your hand. Keep your left knee and leg down close to your right thigh. To keep from bowing or swaying your back hold your buttocks and abs firm. Hold. Repeat on the other side.

5) **Straddle.** Sit up straight with your legs out in a straddle position (extended in a "V" shape in front of you as wide as you can). Sit forward on your "sit" bones and don't allow your back to curve. (If this is hard for you, try a modified straddle with the sole of one foot against inner thigh of opposite leg and work one leg at a time.) First, lift your right arm straight up, left hand on left thigh for balance and bend slowly to the left. Reach up and towards your left foot with your right hand. Feel the stretch along the right side of your body. Relax and hold. No bouncing. Repeat on the other side.

Next, reach towards your right foot with both hands. Reach your chest towards your right knee

and don't look up. Hold. Repeat on your other side.

Next, move both your hands into the center of the "V", either on the floor or stretching forward off the floor. Hold. Repeat series 2-3 times in all three positions.

6) **Back and Chest Stretch.** While still in the straddle position, lift your arms up to chest height, with your elbows bent. Pull your elbows back slightly behind you several times to stretch your chest muscles. Then pull your elbows forward and together several times to help stretch your back. Bring your legs together gently. Roll to one side, on your knees then roll up to a standing position.

7) **Spine.** Repeat the Spine stretch (#6) in the warm-up section above. Roll up.

8) **Shoulders.** Repeat the warm-up Shoulder stretch (#7).

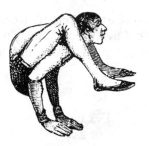

9) **Triceps.** With your legs slightly apart for balance, place your right elbow near your left ear (Only kidding! Just wanted to see if you were paying attention. You're doing great ... almost done). Actually, place your right elbow near your right ear with your right hand reaching down your back. Now gently press your right elbow back with your left hand, stretching the triceps muscle (the back of your upper arm). Hold and repeat on other arm.

10) **Neck.** Repeat Neck stretch (#10) in the warm-up section above.

That's it! You should feel terrific. Warm and loose. Soon these stretches will become automatic for you and you'll move smoothly and easily from one position to the next. Just keep practicing daily and reap the benefits of a graceful, strong and well-aligned body, with increased circulation, balance and flexibility.

Yoga is another effective way to stay stretched out and limber. It increases flexibility, strength and energy. Be sure to consult a qualified instructor.

In A Nutshell

1) Rule #1: Never do anything that hurts!

2) Be gentle, go slowly and comfortably.

3) Wear comfortable, loose or stretchy clothing and keep the room warm.

4) Never force, push, jerk or bounce.

5) Breathe normally, without holding your breath. Relax into your stretches.

6) Learn to listen to your body and work with it.

7) Be gradual and moderate. In time, your flexibility will increase. Be patient and persistent. Little by little wins this game every time!

8) Stretching helps remove toxins from the muscles and prevents stiffness and soreness.

9) Proper warm-up and stretching decreases risk of injury, increases flexibility and circulation.

10) Proper cool-down and stretching allows you to return to normal breathing and body temperature gradually.

11) Consult a qualified yoga instructor to learn gentle stretches and increase your flexibility.

Creating an Active Lifestyle   23

" ... a walk moving freely, without goal. A walk for walk's sake".
Paul Klee

Burning up fat with low-intensity and continuous aerobic exercise while toning up, and whittling down those extra inches with weights is all well and good. In fact, it's great! But what about the other 15 hours that you spend awake and moving around every day? There are plenty of opportunities for using that newly energized body of yours, and moving it closer to your goal (and its purpose) of permanent health, power and vitality. In this chapter, I'd like to offer more possibilities for you to begin building a dynamic, active lifestyle for yourself by rethinking your daily activities.

Why Choose to Move?

By learning to incorporate more movement into your daily activities, and by choosing activity instead of passivity, you will be opening up a whole new world of interaction with your body, as well as with other people. For yourself, you can expect to sleep better, have a clearer, sharper mind, increased energy level and a happier attitude. For every muscle you get into motion, you are also burning extra calories. That never hurts when you've got extra to burn!

Often, being outside in the fresh air and sunshine can give you a boost mentally. Just the fact that you're active and loosened up can be a great "attitude upper", dispelling the blues and leveling out those pesky mood swings that can grab you when your body feels stiff and stuck. I find that the more I move, the better I feel ... and the more I want to move! It's a wonderful cycle to experience, in contrast to those nasty "feel awful ... can't exercise ... feel even worse" vicious cycles I used to have.

There's an interesting correlation between general activity and weight. Thin people tend to fidget and move around a lot. They're almost always moving. Their arms and legs are always shifting position. They get up and walk around. Overweight people, on the other hand, tend to remain firmly parked in place. They don't move their arms very much, or even their heads. The lesson to be learned from this is very much to the point. If you want to become thin you must learn to do what thin people do. Thin people keep their bodies moving. Learn to fidget!

The first thing to remember when you decide to choose a more active lifestyle is to do just that.

Choose it. It will be easier to change your activity level for good if it is something you choose to do, not something you feel you must do. Spend a little time talking to yourself about this. Ask yourself why you want to get active. Write down or just say a few reasons out loud. Listen to yourself, and when you start getting answers like, "I think it would feel good to move and be more active and I'd like to give it a try" or "I just might like it ... sounds like fun", then you know you're on the right track. Answers like, "I just have to ... I must ... I should, etc." are self-defeating. In the beginning you may literally have to drag yourself off the sofa. Unless you find some activity you really like, it will be hard for you to get moving each and every time. So do only what you like ... especially at first.

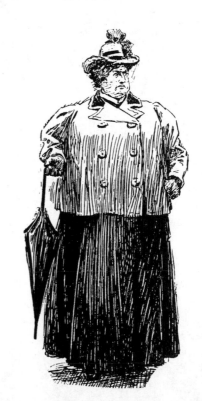

"I'm going for a walk. I need some endorphins."

How to get motivated? Start by spending a little time thinking about the benefits mentioned above and what you really want for yourself. When you get to the point where you feel you deserve all those good feelings that come with moving and using your wonderful body, then you will just easily choose to do that. It will just feel right and good.

Guidelines for Picking Up the Pace

Attitude comes first. Give yourself permission to choose vitality. Don't worry about what anybody else might think. They're too busy thinking about themselves to pay much attention to you anyway.

Next, make sure you do something you enjoy. This is the part where you get to have fun! If you like to pick up seashells or hike in the mountains or play ping-pong, then do it. There are no set rules for becoming more active. Just make sure your choices keep you moving. Anything you can imagine is great. Activities that allow flexibility and variety are important, too. Try to branch out and become more open to the myriad of activities that are available to you. Try something new once in awhile to stay interested.

Now, a word of caution. When I first started out increasing my activity, I ached all over. I remember being sore everywhere. My joints, my muscles, my eyeballs, everything. So I understand the reluctance to even try. But, I quickly learned to increase my activity level gradually (remember the principle of "ease"). And I would recommend that you do the same. Start off slowly ... very light and easy to avoid any muscle strain. Armchair athletes only end up ... well, you know. Those Monday night football jocks who coach their teams from the couch usually end up moaning and groaning after their once-a-month games down at the park. There is a balance point between becoming a full-tilt, all-out, I'm-gonna-show-the-world speed demon and letting dust gather on your hair.

You'll probably have to push-start yourself just a tiny bit in the beginning until you get a taste for the change in activity level. But if you just get started, the effort will be well worth it a few months down the line. Just be sure to take it easy at first. And build up slowly.

Daily Movement Choices

Your everyday situations are the place to begin. Start with some simple changes. You've certainly heard of the "park farther away and walk to the store" trick. It's one of the old standards. That's because it works, and is available to almost everyone. Try it. Once you decide that it's okay to walk a few hundred extra feet you'll really appreciate the benefit of never having to worry about getting a "good" parking place. From the point of view of an active person, you'll begin to realize that there aren't very many benefits to remaining inactive in daily life.

Then there's the old "take the stairs instead of the elevator" ploy. Another good habit you can get into. You could also get rid of that remote control. Or maybe the garage door opener. Try getting off the bus one or two stops ahead of your regular corner and walking the rest of the way. Or just try walking to the store, gym, school or the beach for a picnic lunch. A ten minute stroll can really energize you for the afternoon. Try walking on your lunch hour. It doesn't have to make you sweat up your nice clothes. Just move, breathe and limber up a bit. At home, get your own whatever and refrain from asking a loving family member to "hand it to you". I'm sure you're starting to get the idea, but here are a few more possibilities to get your activity glands jump-started:

* Skip rope, play hopscotch or just play with the kids.
* Help out on the playground ... push the kids on the swingset, throw a ball.
* Take up the hula-hoop or some other active adult toy ... classes abound!
* Adventurous? Try roller-skating, ice-skating or roller-blading.
* Bikes are great fun ... be a kid again or an Olympic athlete.
* Dance at the drop of a hat ... hear a song that makes you want to move while cleaning house? Dance away those dusting chores!
* Western dancing is all the rage and tons of fun ... couples possibilities, too. Or you can try funk, hip hop or ballet.
* Waltz around the kitchen with your mate while preparing your plate.
* Help put away equipment, chairs and charts at your next meeting. Everyone will be grateful and you'll get to talk and move.
* Volunteer to ... take out the trash, get the mail, walk the dog!
* If you must watch TV, at least watch some active shows such as sports events, and get inspired to move yourself.
* Put on a video tape and act out the movie or dances ... when nobody is watching you can really let go!

Healthy Family Fun

There are oodles of fun things you can choose to do with kids, dogs, mates and friends. Everything from flying a kite to swimming by the seashore. From throwing a Frisbee to dancing. All of these activities are guaranteed to produce many more lasting memories than an afternoon in front of "the tube". Why? Well, it actually has to do with the number of senses that you're using to feel the experience. An activity that gets you moving (touch) in the brisk air (smell) with the sounds of nature (hearing) in a beautiful setting (sight) has a much better chance of being remembered in a special way than a couch potato's night at home.

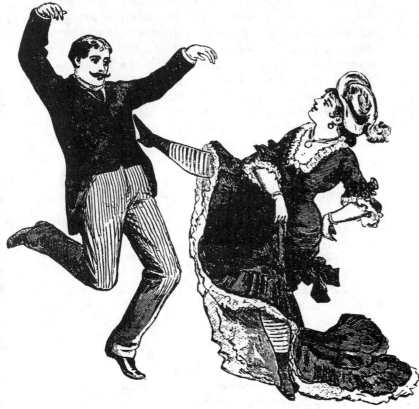

"What did you say this dance was called?"

Back when I was overweight my idea of the ideal night out used to start with a huge dinner ... lots of fatty, salty, heavy food. We would share a bottle of wine and, of course, there would be the richest, chocolatiest dessert on the menu. Then we would head off to the movies. And the very first stop was the candy counter for a large buttered popcorn, a chocolate bar and a soda. Once inside the theater we'd sit in the dark and munch in a womblike reverie of butter, caffeine and sugar. While the munchies slowly settled into (and on to) my stomach, I'd watch the beautiful Hollywood stars live out my dreams on the silver screen of my imagination. Those kind of eating habits are unthinkable these days, but that was heaven way back when. An unhealthy heaven.

If I can change that sad, dead-end, oh-so-fattening scenario one tiny step at a time, then you can move toward healthier activities, too. Social interaction, not centered exclusively on food, can help strengthen relationships and show that you care enough to want to share time and activities with your loved ones.

For recurring leisure periods, such as your days off, when your family has time to be together, choose something active as an essential part of your recreation time. Ride a roller coaster at a theme park, go fishing, garden up a storm, or take a leisurely walk or bike ride on a country road. Everyone loves bikes, and you can start out really slowly for kids and out-of-shapers. It's definitely one of my favorites. Sometimes I zoom ahead of the others, and then circle back. I feel so-o-o athletic, dahling!

By sharing activities with your family you're also teaching your children, by example, that active outings are fun, healthy and normal. The finest gift that you can possibly give to your children is a healthy lifestyle. You are a crucial role model for your kids. I feel so sad when I see overweight children lining up at fast food counters. And it's becoming more and more prevalent. It's a national disgrace as far as I'm concerned. So take your family on the healthy, active route to good health. Your children will copy the lifestyle they learn from you. They'll tend to do it with their kids, too. Those are your grandchildren I'm talking about. The legacy of health you begin will continue far into future generations.

Active vacations are all the rage, too, in case you've been too busy planning your ten-meal-a-day cruise to notice. Hiking through the mountains or biking up the coast are available options for the fit family. They make great memories, too! Simply choosing to go to the lake or river for swimming, boating or any other action-oriented vacation can add zest and fun to your life. Planning some active days during a longer, traditional vacation is a good start. Ski vacations are always a big hit and almost everyone can cross country ski or slide down a hill on a sled. Just tromping through the snow can burn up those calories like crazy while you're having a blast. Think about it the next time you plan a vacation. Even Disney World has gotten into the act and now offers fitness vacations at the Magic Kingdom!

Share your activity-oriented thoughts with your family and watch them light up with the possibilities. And watch yourself lighten up in the process. Both in attitude and body. Enjoy!

Social Outings

The next time visitors are coming, instead of the usual dinner out, sit-around-the-living-room-trying-to-digest-until-the-dessert-arrives-and-talk-about-how-fat-we're-all-getting, why not try something different? How about taking a walk around the neighborhood to talk about old times. If you live in the country take a hike in the woods. If you live by the ocean take a walk on the beach or a light climb to share the sunset from a favorite spot.

I'd sure like to see the old fashioned practice of taking a stroll after dinner come back. People used to put the baby in the carriage or hook arms with a loved one and slowly parade about the neighborhood, greeting the neighbors on their porches and enjoying the evening air. I'm told it was a lovely tradition and it sure sounds great to me. I guess I'm just a healthy romantic. To conclude, it doesn't really matter what you do ... just get moving and enjoy!

In A Nutshell

1) Attitude first! Choose more activity because you want to, not because you have to.

2) Do something, anything you enjoy. This is fun time! Daily active life choices abound. Open up to them.

3) Movement-oriented daily choices can loosen up your joints and muscles, burn calories and be energizing, too!

4) Take it very easy in the beginning until your body loosens up.

5) Active choices bring energy to families and friendships, and social interaction helps strengthen relationships. Choose active visits, outings and vacations.

6) You'll be setting a healthy example for generations to come.

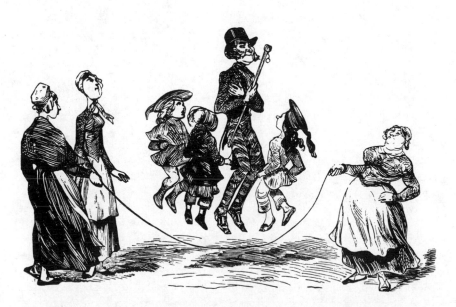

Don't just watch life go by. Participate in it together!

Part V

Nutrition and Food

Real Nutrition — Beyond the Food Pyramid

24

"The Eternal Triangle"
Daily Chronicle

In this chapter you'll learn how your body uses different types of nutrients, including vitamins and minerals, to function at its optimum level. Then you'll discover which amounts and combinations of food create your healthiest ever diet while losing weight (fat weight, not muscle, of course).

The Big Three

The Big Three of nutrition: protein, fats and carbohydrates. You've heard about them your whole life. All foods are in one or more of these categories and they work together to form a balanced diet for a well-functioning body. A healthy, unfat, fit body that is ... the kind that you want. Let's review these food categories and find out how they work together to form the synergy of your perfect body.

A "balanced diet" is something of a cliché. But now you will learn why any diet that asks you to eat only one type of food or a large amount of one type (typically protein on a reducing diet) is out of balance and ultimately will not work, because that's not the way your body was meant to work. These nutritional "tricks" often result in injuries to body systems that can take many years to correct, if they are even correctable at all. Knowledge and understanding about how your body works is the answer to avoiding these pitfalls purveyed by the diet industry of the past. So that you will no longer believe this hooey, and put yourself at risk, let's get the real story.

Protein Redefined

Protein foods have held a venerable position in the American diet for a long time. We've traditionally equated that big steak with strength and affluence ... our dinners as being centered around meat, poultry or fish. Even that plate of cottage cheese was labeled as "fuel food" for burning off excess fat . We've been told and sold in a thousand different ways that protein is what Americans need to eat! That big body builder needs lots of eggs and steak to bulk up those muscles, right? Wrong! You don't need a slab of fatty meat or cholesterol-laden

eggs at every meal (unless you have a secret wish to look like Humpty Dumpty).

Nutritionally, your body needs protein for doing some of the most important work it performs. Namely, building new tissue and repairing everything from blood vessels and bones to hormones and hair. Perhaps that's why the attitude of "more is better" developed. But let's see if this is really true. Maybe overdoing it with protein isn't such a good idea after all, and could even create problems health wise ... just what you're trying to avoid.

Visualize protein molecules as looking similar to a string of beads, with each bead being a substance called an amino acid. Each different protein has a different amount of beads. There are 22 amino acids altogether and your body can make 13 of them by itself. However, 9 amino acids must be supplied by your food. These nine are called the essential amino acids.

Recent research reveals that a combination of animal and plant protein is the most useful for your body, whereas previously it was believed that animal protein alone was the best source of useful protein. Although no single plant food supplies all 9 essential amino acids, a combination of plant foods, such as rice and beans, does the job perfectly.

The real breakthrough news in this area is that you don't have to eat rice and beans (or other typical food combinations) together at the same meal to create a complete protein! This was the message of the "food combiners", and was in vogue for several years. Why? Since digestion takes time, your body uses the food you ingest during one day to make up the complete set of amino acids. You don't even need to eat protein at every meal any more.

Americans, with our tradition of meat-centered meals, eat more protein than they need. Up to twice the amount that is recommended as healthy in the government's Recommended Dietary Allowances (RDA). The amounts of protein needed will vary with your age and weight. However, you should aim to consume 15-20% of your total calories from protein. Your 2 servings daily described in Chapter 25 "What to Eat", fulfills your protein requirements perfectly. It will supply you with 45-60 grams of protein a day for women and 60-80 grams for men.

Protein is Not Pro-Teen

You might ask what the problem is with eating more protein than your body really needs. After all, if a little is good, isn't more better? Actually no. For one thing, excess protein, especially the sort from animals, can cause your kidneys to overwork. This can lead to kidney disease, which is prevalent in American society. In addition, excess protein affects the way your body processes minerals. For example, calcium, which is one of the minerals that a majority of American women are lacking already, can be blocked from being absorbed when excess protein is eaten. Research has shown that excess animal protein can also cause certain other minerals to be excreted in the urine before being utilized by your body. And of course, protein, especially animal-type, has an abundance of calories, fat (especially the saturated kind) and cholesterol ... and we certainly don't need any more of those, now do we?

Now it's time for a bit of an exposé . If you aren't already aware of how food industry lobbies can affect your health, let me clue you in. The meat and dairy industries have extremely powerful lobbies in Washington D.C. (where they decide on the dietary recommendations for all Americans, among other things). Meat and dairy promoters also have well-established places in our schools, where they provide free programs, teaching aids and materials (biased towards heavy meat and dairy consumption, of course). Our kids are being sold on the so-called "healthy benefits" of eating meat and dairy products through these big-budget, one-sided programs. And this has been going on for over forty years. No wonder you're so familiar with the "four food groups" (two of which just happen to be meat and dairy). Few school districts turn down free materials, especially when they're struggling to purchase teaching aids with sagging budgets and overworked teachers. This promotional power has certainly influenced national dietary recommendations, and eventually the nation's health, in the name of profit.

This makes me hopping mad sometimes. But I also see it as another opportunity to pursue self-education and make my own informed choices. You can do the same. Instead of criticizing and being "against" their self-serving efforts, we can focus on being "for" the ability to choose informed, positive health for ourselves. We can work from an intelligent perspective, and base our decisions on good research and realistic conclusions.

Speaking of conclusions ... if you follow the THINNER WINNERS guidelines for protein you will be in the forefront of positive health as determined by the latest nutritional research.

According to these findings, you would be wise to consider the alternatives to having the "traditional" meat every night. You'll improve your health in many ways by adding more vegetarian choices into your diet, such as beans and grains. If you want to be healthy and slim you should lower your consumption of total protein and focus on the true high energy, fat-burning fuel foods, carbohydrates.

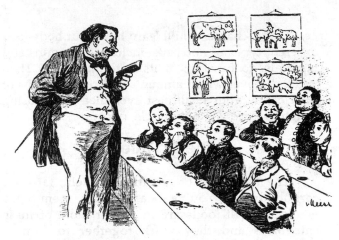

"No Jimmy, a well-balanced meal is not a burger, fries and a shake."

More Carbs Please!
(Sugars and Starches)

By now, most of us have heard the new cry of the nutrition industry. More carbohydrates, such as pasta, rice, bread , and potatoes (yes!) are actually desirable for good health, and especially for fat loss and weight stabilization. Well, hooray! It's about time, eh? Let's look closer at carbohydrates and find out why.

Starches (complex carbs) and sugars (simple carbs) are used along with proteins and fats in a variety of processes. These include breaking down dietary fats, bolstering your immune system, fueling your nervous system and red blood cell functioning. You may have heard that we need more of the "complex" type and less of the "simple" type of carbohydrates. You can see why when you look at what foods are in each of these categories.

Carbohydrates are readily used as fuel by your body. The simple carbohydrates are called "simple" because they are made up of one or two molecules of sugar. They are easily absorbed directly into the blood and can cause dramatic swings in blood sugar with accompanying increase in hunger in a very short time. Simple carbs include glucose, fructose and lactose found in refined sugars, fruit and milk respectively. Fruits can be thought of as the most complex of the simple sugars because they contain fiber which helps slow down absorption. See Chapter 27 "Choosing Healthy Foods" for a complete discussion on simple sugars and the best ones to choose for good health.

Now let's look at those wonderful complex carbohydrates, the dieter's friend. These are commonly referred to as starches and have traditionally been shunned as fattening. Nothing could be further from the truth! They're called "complex" because they are made up of much longer molecular chains than the simple sugars. Because of this they take longer for your body to break down and absorb into the bloodstream. Thus, they don't give you the immediate burst of energy like the simple sugars, but the energy supply lasts longer. Starches are also more filling. With complex carbs your blood sugar doesn't endure the unhealthy cycle of shooting to the sky, then plummeting to the basement (which can cause dramatic mood and hunger swings). Complex carbs keep you on a more even keel, and therefore more in rational control of your food intake. You can avoid the sugar addiction feeling of being prodded from behind with the sharp stick of urgent need for raising your blood sugar NOW. A sugary lifestyle can also lead to hypoglycemia and diabetes.

Another reason that complex carbs are more slowly absorbed is because they contain fiber, another area lacking in the average American diet. Complex carbohydrates are mostly plant foods such as grains, vegetables, beans and fruit. These all contain healthy amounts of fiber, in addition to lots of vitamins and minerals. Refer to Chapter 33 "Fiber is Your Friend".

The THINNER WINNERS daily recommendations call for 65-75% of your calories to come from carbohydrates (with as little as possible from simple carbs ... no more than 10%) and the majority from the "super foods", complex carbs. That's 4-6 servings daily of breads or grains, at least 4 servings of vegetables and 2 or more servings of fruit. See Chapter 25 "What to Eat" for more details. You want to concentrate on starches such as grains and cereals, potatoes and rice, beans, vegetables and whole fruits. I hope you enjoy those carbs as much as I do! Now you know one of the reasons that I'm always smiling!

Let's Take Another Look at Fat

Fats are the third basic type of food that is needed for good, well-balanced nutrition and a healthy body. What? You say you didn't think there was anything good about fats? Unfortunately, fat has really gotten a bad rap lately. I can't say that it doesn't deserve it, though. Saturated fat , found mostly in meats and dairy products (that aren't non-fat), has contributed greatly to heart

disease and obesity among other epidemic health problems in America.

This has caused an all-out assault on fats in general. Many beginning slim-seekers have a tendency to go to extremes with cutting fat. If there is even a smidgen of fat in a food, they won't touch it. That's okay for starting out because the awareness about fat is essential, but keep in mind the important principles of balance and moderation. Cutting fat is not a magic solution, it is part of a healthful, overall dietary change.

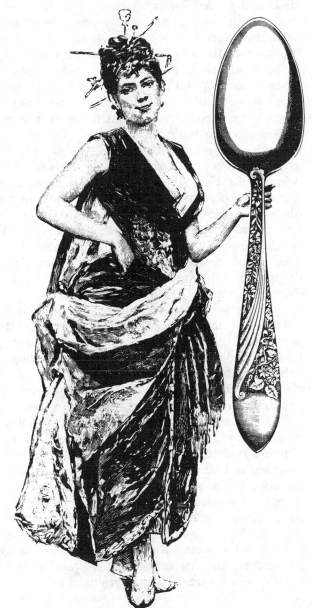

"I'll have another spoonful of carbs, please."

A certain amount of fat is necessary for optimal functioning of a variety of your body's systems. You need it for healthy skin and hair, proper functioning of certain organs such as your gall bladder, cushioning other organs such as your heart and kidneys, temperature regulation and nerve insulation. Your body manufactures some fats, but not certain polyunsaturated fats known as essential fatty acids (such as linoleic acid). These must come from your food, and without them your heart and liver, among other systems, would not be able to function at healthy levels. Fats are also needed to help process certain fat-soluble vitamins such as A, D, E, and K. Certain fats in the unsaturated group, such as monounsaturates and omega-3 fatty acids, have actually been shown to help lower blood cholesterol levels, boost HDL cholesterol (the good kind) and prevent heart attacks.

It's extremely important for you to be aware of both the type and the amount of fat you eat. Researchers have been puzzled by the seemingly paradoxical societies around the world which seem to thrive on high fat diets while not falling prey to heart disease. Eskimos, Japanese and countries around the Mediterranean basin are examples of societies which have been studied. These people eat more than the 30% fat daily while enjoying lower rates of coronary artery disease. Why? Because the fat they eat is mostly derived either from fish (containing omega-3 fatty acids) or from olive oil (primarily monounsaturated fat). This appears to protect these people from disease. The conclusion of this research is that the type of fat is even a more critical factor than the amount. Further discussion of the types of fats and cholesterol can be found in Chapter 32 "Fat and Cholesterol".

Thinner Winner recommendations include a balance of the three types of fats: saturated, polyunsaturated and monounsaturated (with no more than $\frac{1}{3}$ of your total intake of fat being the saturated type). The remaining $\frac{2}{3}$ should be weighted in favor of the monounsaturated, polyunsaturated and/or omega-3 fats. The saturated fat is optional (it's your life). Later in this chapter, I will outline the improved Food Guide Pyramid and this recommendation will be reflected in that new model. The recommendations include 15-20% of your total daily calories coming from fat if you have 20 pounds or less to lose. If you need to lose over 20 pounds, keep the total amount of fat to 10-15%. For example, if you eat 1200 calories per day while losing weight (and need to lose over 20 pounds), then no more than 180 calories or 15% should be from fats (that's 20 grams of fat).

Vitamins and Minerals

Vitamins are "vital amines". "Vita" is Latin for life. An amine is an ammonia based chemical compound composed in combination with carbon and nitrogen. Amino acids are organic, nitrogen bearing compounds that serve as units of protein structure and are essential to human metabolism. (Just thought you'd like to know ... think how handy this will be the next time you're on a quiz show!) Vitamins are organic substances and they are absolutely essential for you to keep on living. They don't supply energy directly but work in synergy with other substances in many different roles. These include: manufacture of DNA coding; metabolic functioning; converting food to energy; chemical actions and reactions of all kinds; absorption of other vitamins; cardio-vascular, nervous and immune system functioning; assisting in maintaining blood cells, bones, teeth and skin.

A new era of nutrition was born when the first vitamin, the B vitamin thiamin, was isolated in a lab in 1911. Since then, 13 vitamins have been identified and 13 minerals have either established Recommended Dietary Allowances or suggested intakes. There are two types of vitamins: fat-soluble (A, D, E, and K) which are stored in your body for relatively long periods (months), and water-soluble (C and the B's with the exception of B-12) which are only stored for weeks at the most. Some vitamins, such as C, need to be supplied daily.

Minerals come from inorganic (non-living), naturally-occurring elements and assist in maintaining healthy nerves, muscles and bones. There are two types of minerals: bulk (such as calcium, potassium and magnesium), of which we need a relatively large amount, and trace, which we only need in very small amounts.

Your body cannot manufacture vitamins and minerals by itself, so the only way it can get what it needs is through the food that you eat or through supplements that you take.

Recommended Dietary Allowances (RDA's)

To help you keep all this straight and to make sure that you are getting all the vitamins and minerals you need every day for good health, government scientists began providing us with Recommended Dietary Allowances (RDA's) beginning in 1941. This was during World War II and the original intention was to insure that our soldiers would be provided with all the nutrients needed for optimum health. They certainly didn't want to risk deficiency diseases like scurvy (characterized by weakness, anemia, spongy gums and bleeding from the mucus membranes). This was the bane of British sailors of the previous century who were getting scurvy simply because they didn't receive their daily requirement of vitamin C on long sea journeys. As soon as they began eating a lime a day, this debilitating tendency stopped (and thus was born the name "Limey" for British seamen). The RDA's are revised periodically to reflect updated research (about every 5-10 years) by the Food and Nutrition Board of the National Research Council.

That's why the RDA's came into being. But just how do they affect your life today? Something you may not have thought about, but is extremely important when learning about the RDA's, is their purpose for the general population. Who are RDA's (present on nearly every food label) really intended for, and what exactly are they supposed to do for you? There seems to be two schools of thought on this subject and the first school prevails at present. This opinion says that the RDA's should provide only the amount of a vitamin or mineral that will keep you from getting sick. That's it. No prevention or cure, just enough so you can function at the minimum health level.

The second opinion, which is gaining in acceptance, is that the RDA's should more adequately reflect the mounting research that these powerful substances can and should be used to help prevent chronic diseases (such as heart disease and cancer) and even cure specific ailments. I believe, as many nutritionists now do, that the way to deal with this dilemma is to provide a safe range of consumption for each vitamin and mineral. The minimum needed to stay healthy and the maximum that you can safely take (some vitamins are toxic when taken in large dosages). In this way, each individual can determine their specific needs and adjust their foods and supplements as needed. This would neatly address the problem of varying needs for each individual.

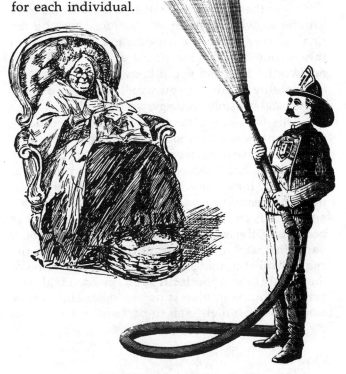

Same vitamin needs? Don't bet on it.

Just think about it for a moment. How can a 6'2" 35 year old male fireman who regularly drinks beer have the same nutritional needs as a 4'11" 62 year old woman who smokes, but doesn't drink, and is a semi-sedentary seamstress? It really doesn't make sense that they might each pop down a once-a-day, one-size-fits-all tablet and be getting their differing needs met, does it? And they aren't!

There are as many different sets of nutritional needs as there are people and lifestyles, but even major categories of factors determining those needs abound here, such as: age (kids and the elderly in particular), general activity level, eating and drinking patterns, general fitness level, general health, medications (for any of 1001 conditions), gender, and disease conditions (with different risks and treatments involved). All these factors come into play, as well as others, when it comes to determining the healthiest amounts of the essential vitamins and minerals you need.

RDA's and Obesity

The RDA's are defined as providing adequate needs for 95% of "healthy adults". This means that with any health compromising condition, the RDA's are not adequate. This includes the noteworthy conditions of reducing food intake while losing weight, increasing activity levels, and being overweight in the first place. Additionally, overweight people often have a myriad of health problems or they develop them over time by remaining overweight (like I did). Note that the RDA's were devised for the mythical, "average" person who, it was somehow determined, eats a minimum of 2000-2400 calories a day! This leaves out an awful lot of people ... notably weight controllers, kids, women and the elderly.

The Recommended Daily Allowances found on food labels are percentages figured for the highest need group in the population ... teen-aged boys. The main value these labels can provide is comparing one processed food with another.

It follows that when you have a reduction in the number of calories or food that you eat (as when reducing), you will have a corresponding reduction in the amount of nutrients that you are providing your body! A diet of 1800 calories would have to be drastically cut in the fat, sugar and alcohol amounts to continue providing the RDA's. When the intake is cut to 1200 calories, like many reducing diets, even the conservative American Dietetic Association agrees that there is virtually no chance that you can get adequate nutrition even from the most carefully chosen and prepared foods. This means you need to take supplements while reducing your weight. But which ones and how much?

The vitamins that are most notably lacking in the reducing diet are B-1, B-6, B-12, calcium, iron, zinc, potassium and magnesium. In a study done of the 11 most popular diets in America, it was concluded that none of them provided even the minimal RDA's needed for minimum health. Many of these programs recommend supplementing your diet with vitamins and minerals while losing weight to fill the gap left by the reduction in food nutrients. After all, you don't want to be a skinny wreck, do you? You want to be slender and glowing with health, right?

Another factor which must be addressed is the quality of the foods you eat. In the past, most foods were grown at home, or at least closer to home, and eaten fresh from the garden or with minimal storage time. Nowadays, produce may have traveled halfway around the world and have been out of the field for a very long time before it reaches your kitchen. The condition of the soil and the types of fertilizer used also have a strong influence on the vitamins and minerals in foods. Unfortunately, soils have become depleted in the last 50-100 years because of the huge yields needed to feed the growing world population. Storing the food properly when it reaches the store, and finally your kitchen, is also a nutritional factor. Also, many nutrients are lost in cooking.

Put this whole picture together and it just makes sense, at the very least, to evaluate the needs for your current lifestyle and take supplements to make sure you're staying healthy. When I began doing this, it was as if my body had been chugging along on 3 cylinders (out of 8!). No wonder I began to break down after years of dieting and the stress related to being overweight in a skinny world. I was treating myself like a run-down old jalopy. It got me there, but it seemed to be getting me there slower and slower. When I realized this and began treating my body like the Ferrari that it is, with good food and supplements, I noticed the difference right away. The engine responded to the quality overhaul, the cylinders really began humming along, and all the wonderful processes my body is capable of were able to come forth in much greater abundance. This propelled me along towards improved health and optimum life force every single day! My energy level of course shot up, and I was able to really do all the things I had formerly just dreamed of, but couldn't do. So don't be a jalopy dreaming of being a sports car, be the Ferrari! It's what you were meant to be.

Thermogenics and Other Anti-Fat Nutrients

"Oh, wouldn't it be lov-er-ly!" goes the song.

And it certainly would be nice if we could just figure out the right combination of magic pills to take so the fat wouldn't accumulate on our bodies at all and what little that did sneak on would be burned off automatically. A biochemical method of ridding us of all this darned fat! Don't hold your breath, darling. I waited and experimented and tried out all the newest and latest "researched and proven" substances for many years and wasted a ton of time and money chasing miracles. It's such a drain on your energy levels. Put your energy into eating healthy, low-fat, high-nutrient foods and getting moderate, low-intensity and regular exercise and replacing all the health-robbing habits (especially mental attitude ones) with strong, productive thoughts and activities. Then the dreams of magic chemical rescues will be just a sad joke to you. You're looking in all the wrong places if you're focused on those pale hopes.

Real health comes from real change that you engineer from a deep understanding of your body's needs and its synergistic functioning within both your physical and mental realms. By looking only outside of yourself, you encourage a schism or split that can only take you further from the union you must form to discover the real "secret" that I discovered. It takes a lot of time and effort to build something substantial. A house of brick will be solid and protect you for years, as opposed to a house of straw which will blow over in a breeze. (I'll bet you never expected to find one of the "three little pigs" coming out a hero in this program!)

Nonetheless, many substances continue to proliferate whose advertisers promise will be the final answer to health, wealth and happiness. In this section you'll learn about a few of the most noteworthy items so you'll know which ones have any validity ... and so you won't waste your time, money and possibly endanger your health.

This first group contains the more reputable and scientifically verifiable substances. Note that many of these will work only in very precisely controlled conditions. But under non-ideal conditions, they cease to be of any value. It's like putting a beautiful new carburetor on a filthy, rusty engine. Even though the carburetor works beautifully, the engine needs to be rebuilt. The more parts that are in good condition, the better the engine will run, that's all. So even though some of these substances perform well in an ideal lab, perhaps your condition is not so ideal. This is why many "magic bullets" fail to perform or backfire in the long run.

Zinc

This is a powerful mineral and is vital for many body functions that affect fat loss including stabilizing energy levels , forming insulin, burning carbohydrates, making protein and helping to digest foods indirectly through enzyme production. You should be getting your RDA of 15 mg of this mineral in your daily vitamin-mineral supplement. Without it, sugars may only be partially metabolized and turned into and stored as fat more easily. Once the fat is stored it's much harder to free up to use for energy. Fatigue is a symptom of this energy conservation effort. Take your zinc.

Magnesium-Potassium Aspartate

Two more absolutely vital minerals for healthy functioning. The addition of the aspartate (an enzyme) works to increase endurance and energy production. This is especially important for the increased amount of exercise that you will be doing to lose weight. In studies, up to 50% of muscle function is lost if there is a deficiency of magnesium and as a two-edged sword, exercise depletes your magnesium stores! This combo supplement helps you burn more fat because you can exercise longer without fatigue. You still have to work for it, but you won't get wiped out either. I wouldn't be without my 500 mg daily.

Chromium Picolinate

Chromium is another mineral that is depleted by exercise and that most Americans probably don't get enough of. Studies have shown it increases sensitivity to insulin which helps metabolize sugars. It tends to stimulate fat loss and encourages the burning of carbohydrates. It also helps you build muscle tissue if you are in good shape and exercising regularly. Muscle is the engine that burns the fat as fuel so you want as big an engine as possible. Picolinate is a niacin derivative that chelates (grabs like a crab) the chromium, making it more readily available to your cells. It was developed by the U.S. Dept. of Agriculture. Keep in mind this won't do you a bit of good until you begin exercising regularly. Otherwise you are wasting your money. 400 mcg daily is what I take. This is not a magic fat-burning pill, just essential nutrition.

Iodine

Another mineral that is essential for health and especially the functioning of your thyroid gland. Warning: This is an example of how unscrupulous supplement sellers try to get you. Yes, you do need it. No, you don't need extra supplements except in very special cases. The 150 mcg that is the RDA should be provided in your vit-min tablets and iodine is also readily available in your diet through iodized salt, fish and kelp. All the salt used in processed foods is iodized, so don't worry ... you're getting plenty!

L- Carnitine

An amino acid-like substance, once thought to be a vitamin, that is responsible for getting the fat to the fat-burning sites within your cells. If it's not there it can't be burned. Our bodies do make some L-Carnitine ... if we have given it the proper building blocks such as B vitamins and vitamin C and iron and we can absorb it. But overweight people, among others, may not be able to absorb what they need. Being physically active also increases your need for it ... it has long been used by athletes since it has been proven to improve heart function and increase aerobic ability. In a well-nourished, active person it can help lower total body fat and weight. It does zip for the junk food junkie sofa spud. Being of the athletic variety, I am privileged to include 250 mg daily in my supplements. Note that D-Carnitine is another supplement that does just the opposite, and can be unsafe, so be sure to get the right one. Remember L for lighten up, not D for danger.

Coenzyme Q10 (CoQ10)

This enzyme may act as an antioxidant along with vitamins E and C which help to protect against free-radical cell damage. The body needs it to utilize all the energy released from foods. Although your body makes some of its own, this ability appears to diminish with age. It helps boost endurance and energy levels during physical activity and so is used by athletes who want to exercise longer and harder while remaining comfortable with their workouts. 10 mg daily is a standard amount, but as with all supplements, check with a qualified and informed health care provider first, especially if you have heart problems or are taking medications which may interact with this substance.

Medium Chain Triglycerides (MCTs)

MCT's are fat molecules that range from 6-12 carbon chains in length, as opposed to Long Chain Triglycerides (regular fats like butter, oils and those in cheese) that range from 18-24 carbons long. MCTs are thus more easily absorbed and not so easily stored as fat ... acting more like carbohydrates to your body. And like carbs, they provide quick energy and increase metabolic burn rate. However MCTs come in the form of oil, and it still has calories similar in quantity to other oils (120 cal per TBL). Diabetics shouldn't use them because of the ketones this quick burning produces. There is great promise for this substance, but more research is needed to fully understand the potential for weight reduction before adding it to your diet.

Thermogenic Herbs and Spices

Here's a fun group that I really enjoy.

Thermogenic means hot and that's just what these herbs and spices are ... HOT! Cayenne (red) pepper, mustards of all kinds and mustard powder, chili powder and chilies of all kinds, hot salsa, Tabasco-type sauces and hot dishes from Southern, Mexican, Indian, Korean and Thai cuisine's, horseradish and spices such as curry and ginger. Some studies have shown that metabolism is boosted significantly after a meal containing these substances. Sometimes you might even sweat or feel hot indicating increased temperature and thus metabolic rate. Spicy foods may also decrease your appetite. Don't go overboard, but a splash or sprinkle could help turn up the furnace. I use them liberally. There is a definite growing underground movement of spicy condiment lovers. Some mail-order catalogs specialize in collections of the hot stuff from around the world.

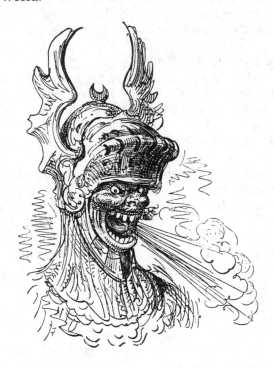

*With some thermogenics
a fire-proof suit is in order.*

Ma Huang

A Chinese herb also known as the ephedra plant. Used improperly, this herb can be extremely dangerous, triggering strokes and even causing death. It is a potent stimulant and should be avoided by people with high blood pressure, heart disease, diabetes or thyroid conditions. Don't give it to children! Don't play around with this one. You could also easily overdose if you took it along with other over-the-counter medications that interacted with it in a negative way, such as decongestants. Although commonly used in "weight loss" formulas, I'd be extremely cautious.

Magic Bullets?

Crossing your fingers and hanging chains of garlic around your neck may or may not keep the vampires away ... and there are many substances that claim to help with weight loss, most of them unsubstantiated or potentially dangerous. A single research study may sound absolutely convincing, but on closer inspection reveal poor technique, very small sample populations and vague or over-optimistic conclusions about the use of the substance. Until more solid research verifies their effectiveness and safety I would avoid such things as ephedra sinica, camellia sinsensis, apple cider vinegar, kelp, lecithin and B6 combinations, grapefruit concoctions, growth hormone releasers, gamma linoleic acid (GLA), lipotropics, DHEA, weight loss coffee and teas, "fat burners", thigh creams and anything else that smacks of popular opportunism.

Such things may "work" for your next door neighbor who swears by her ingenious and sometimes elaborate combinations (and quite often turns out to be a sales rep for those same products), but in the long run you know the real answer for effective, healthy weight control and legitimate mind/body health is not in a pill.

As shown in the "Thermogenic" section above, there are certain substances that can safely encourage your body to cooperate during your fat-loss period. It's like using certain substances during pregnancy or after an operation. Your body has increased needs and it's smart to be aware of them and help your system to function at its highest possible levels. However, don't cross over the line into fantasy land by thinking that you can lose weight and get healthy by simply finding a combination of pills and substances that will automatically lift you from inert fatness to athletic trimness. It just ain't so. Use your intuition to know that this is true and your common sense to choose what is encouraging to your system during this time of additional nutritional need. Make wise and safe choices for your sensitive and beautiful body. There is only one you ... don't risk abusing your health. Maximize it instead.

Your Nutritional Overhaul

First talk with your health care provider about any concerns you may have about altering your nutritional patterns. You should be realistic about the goals that you have right now. Your main objective is to lose extra fat and increase your health by reducing the amount of calories, fat grams, sugar and alcohol you will be eating. You'll also be increasing the amount of activity that you will be doing, reducing stress through meditation and modifying your counter-productive behaviors and thought patterns. Consider specific influences on your life: your age, weight and gender, any medications you are taking, special needs for any diseases, chronic conditions or circumstances such as pregnancy that you may have, your fitness and activity level, the amount of stress that you have in your job, relationships, environmental factors such as living in a crowded smoggy city and driving freeways all day, etc.

Getting as specific as you can regarding your needs will help you get the most out of the supplements that you select. Ask your advisor to help you devise an optimal level of the essential vitamins and minerals for you right now. Be aware that these needs will change as you become healthier and conditions change in your life, so periodically review these conclusions and make adjustments where they're needed.

I believe that you should, at minimum, be taking a vitamin and mineral supplement that supplies the RDA's and in addition take extra vitamin C, E, beta carotene, folate and zinc. Women should also consider additional supplements of calcium and iron.

Be aware that certain vitamins are toxic and should never be taken in doses higher than the recommended minimum daily amount. These include vitamins A, D, B-6, niacin and iron. Certain others can be dangerous if you have an existing condition such as high blood pressure or kidney disease. Discuss these concerns with your health advisor.

Taking a generic supplement each day , or any supplements for that matter, can never make up for a basically unhealthy diet. Watch your food intake carefully. Limit saturated or hydrogenated fats, sugars, alcohol and caffeine (actually known as "anti-nutrients"). They are nutritionally lacking in vitamins and minerals and indeed will drain your somewhat limited supply right now. Also, do your best to limit other negative activities, such as smoking and allowing stress to escalate without taking steps to manage it effectively (see Chapter 14 "Taming Your Stress"). These "drainers" will rob you of essential nutrients right when you need them the most to lose that weight!

Choose your food wisely! Either grow your own, buy organic or at least buy locally grown foods whenever possible. By buying organic foods, you will not only be eating the highest quality food, you will also be supporting the farmers and processors who are valiantly trying to raise our food supply in a more responsible and conscientious way. You'll also avoid consuming any questionable hormonal additives or poisons used by factory farms. Store your food properly and eat it as soon as possible,

using cooking methods that conserve the most nutrients.

Your ability to absorb each vitamin and mineral can be enhanced by following these health-promoting habits. Absorption is a key factor in making sure that you're getting the most from your foods and supplements. That's why certain vitamins should be taken with food or in combination with other supplements. Eating a wide variety of foods will also help ensure that you are giving your system the best assortment of nutrients with which to work.

If you cannot afford, do not have available, or choose not to consult a dietary specialist at this time, I urge you to, at the very least, read up on the issue of vitamins and minerals. Become more aware of this vital subject. I feel it was of immeasurable help in getting me from a 272 pound walking death state to the healthy, productive and very much alive condition I happily find myself in today. These are not miracle pills or magic boosters as so many unscrupulous ads proclaim, but simply the vital components of a well-functioning body. You need these substances to operate your body and mind at maximum levels.

Use a moderate approach and give your body time to adjust to the new regime. Some of the nutrients you will now provide will be soaked up and used immediately because you have been deficient in them. But others will take time for your body to assimilate. Like putting ultra supreme gas in a jalopy, you need to give it time to get used to the change. There is no doubt in my mind that nutritional enhancement can help you in reaching your goals of slenderness and glowing health quicker and with greater vitality than you can now imagine. So go for it!

Four Food Groups - Move Over!

I know it's hard to find out that the world isn't really the way you've been led to believe it was for so long. But now it's time to really tip the cart up on end! Way back in the 1930's, the Home Economics Research Division of the U.S. Department of Agriculture first categorized foods into "groups" in order to give Americans a way to ensure balanced diets. These groups went through several changes until, in 1956, the Basic Four Food Groups were born (with a good bit of help from various food lobbies, as you learned earlier). This standard remained in effect for 35 years, even while much research and debate was taking place regarding the merits of certain foods over others. There were many inadequacies in this model, yet in its defense, it did give us some concepts for healthy eating based on a variety of foods and moderation in servings. That was a good start. But as research became more convincing (especially on the negative effects of certain foods such as cholesterol, saturated and hydrogenated fats, sugar and refined carbohydrates), it was evident that this model was too simplistic and unbalanced to realistically point the way to optimum nutrition.

And as a result, in April 1992, The United States Department of Agriculture (USDA) unveiled an updated guide for recommended healthy eating, the Food Guide Pyramid. This new system replaced the traditional Four Food Groups that we all learned about in school. New category breakdowns reflected the latest findings in nutrition and in promoting the adequacy of America's diet. Additionally, it focused on the role of food in the prevention of common major diseases, such as heart disease and cancer. The consumption of meats and dairy products, and their accompanying saturated fats and cholesterol was de-emphasized. The healthiest foods: grains, vegetables and fruits were once delegated to a minor role, but no longer!

In the government's food pyramid this imbalance has been partially corrected. The pyramid is still divided into four layers or groups. However, the proportionate area of each food group fits the nutritional value of the foods in question. The broad base, which is the first and largest layer, consists of breads, cereals, rice and pasta. The government advises an "average person" (consuming 2000-2400 calories per day) to eat most of their meals from these foods (6-11 servings per day). The second and somewhat smaller layer is made up of Vegetables and Fruits. The combination of the first two layers makes up the majority of your healthful food choices. Choose 3-5 servings of vegetables and 2-4 servings of fruit daily. On the third layer they placed the Dairy group and the Meat group which contribute less nutritional benefit and more fat and cholesterol. Notice that these two groups combined now warrant less than a third of the total area of the pyramid. Quite a change from the combined 50% that they used to command. Uncle Sam says to choose 2-3 servings a day from each group. Fats and Sweets are lumped together in the smallest layer at the very top of the Pyramid and are to be used only sparingly. When you think about it, it might not be a bad idea to turn the whole thing upside-down.

Again, good try guys. I'm sure it was an absolute nightmare to try to get all the scientists, politicians, bureaucrats and food lobbyists together to create this model and I thank them all for their great efforts. But my opinion is that the government's model does not go quite far enough to define the best foods to choose in accordance with the latest research on cutting the risk of heart disease, obesity, cancer and high blood pressure.

Many conclusions of studies are nearly unanimously agreed upon by nutritionists and other health experts, such as the need for less saturated fat, cholesterol and meat, and more grains, vegetables and fruits. Now that we have the research, let's get to work on it and really get it straight.

The New and Truly Improved Food Pyramid

I will continue to use the basic pyramid shape because I think it is a good model that's commonly available and it will be easy to make fairly minor, yet extremely important, improvements while still maintaining the basic structure. So take a look at the THINNER WINNERS Pyramid. This time the pyramid is divided into just three main sections. Each section represents the frequency that the foods in that section should be eaten: Daily, a few times a week (optional) or a few times a month (optional).

Daily

The first and largest section is divided into four layers and all foods in this main section can be eaten on a daily basis (although there are some optional items here also). The very bottom layer, which is the largest, is made up of Breads, Pasta, Grains and Potatoes. There's no need to improve on this foundation for good health. It's just perfect. The next layer is Vegetables and Fruits, but with the important addition of Beans, Legumes and Nuts. I feel that these should not be grouped together with the meat, poultry, fish and eggs for some important reasons. Mainly, they are plant foods and therefore have no cholesterol and saturated fat in them and also have good amounts of fiber. In the case of nuts, some beneficial polyunsaturated and monounsaturated fats are present. They really don't deserve to be grouped with the less pro-health meat protein just because they also offer protein. It reflects their contribution to health far better to place them with the Fruits and Vegetables. These first two layers are the largest portion of the "Daily" section. The third layer of this section is Low or Non-Fat Dairy Products and Egg Whites. These are optional items, but they can still be good sources of protein and calcium without all the cholesterol and fat. The smallest top layer of the Daily section is Mono and Poly Oils. These include canola and olive oil. I don't believe these deserve to be grouped with all oils. They have been proven to be beneficial in lowering cholesterol and risk of heart disease. In other words, research has shown that not all fats are the same when it comes to health.

Be forewarned that when it comes to disease conditions, such as existing heart disease and

The New and Truly Improved Food Pyramid

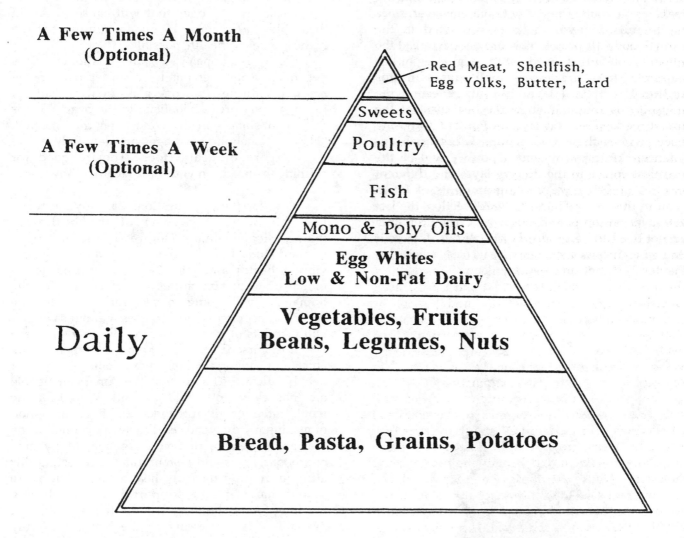

A Few Times A Month
(Optional)

Red Meat, Shellfish,
Egg Yolks, Butter, Lard

Sweets

A Few Times A Week
(Optional)

Poultry

Fish

Mono & Poly Oils

Egg Whites
Low & Non-Fat Dairy

Daily

Vegetables, Fruits
Beans, Legumes, Nuts

Bread, Pasta, Grains, Potatoes

obesity, any fats may make the problem worse. So be sure to follow the guidelines for fat grams in Chapter 32 "Fat and Cholesterol". Make sure your fats are of the healthiest variety (mono's and poly's). That's it for your daily fare. Most of what you eat should come from the foods just outlined.

A few times a week (optional)

The next section, which is much smaller, represents foods that can be eaten a few times a week, if you want. They're optional, however, since all the nutrition you need is contained in the "Daily" foods. (If protein is your concern reread the section "Protein Redefined" at the beginning of this chapter). There are three small layers in this section. The bottom layer is Fish, reflecting the omega-3 oils found in it as the healthiest of the animal foods. The next layer is Poultry. Choosing wisely within these two groups is essential. For instance, skinless white meat poultry will be the healthiest choice in the Poultry layer and different varieties of fish have varying amounts of fat in them. In this "Few Times A Week" section, the last little layer on top is Refined Sweets. They certainly did not need to be grouped with all fats. Use your head when it comes to sugary treats (see "sweets" in Chapter 27 "Choosing Healthy Foods").

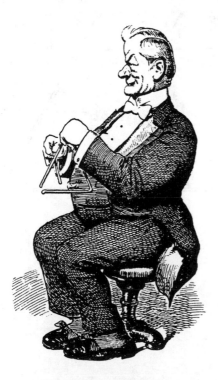

"The new and truly improved food pyramid makes sense to me."

A few times a month (optional)

The last little teeny tiny section on the top is occupied by a group of foods that should only be eaten a "Few Times A Month", if at all, because of their known contributions to high cholesterol, saturated fats and lack of fiber ... to say nothing of their direct ties to obesity, heart disease and cancer. These are the notorious Red Meat, Shellfish and Egg Yolks. You can also add in butter, lard and other drain cloggers. If food is to be the death of you, these are the ones that will cause it! Avoid these like the plague if you are aiming for the highest level of health possible.

Alcohol is an open issue, but it has some serious dependency and personality disorder risks. Some research indicates that one glass of wine daily (2 for men) may prove beneficial to the heart. This is due to substances in the wine other than alcohol. "Harder" alcoholic beverages are definitely not in the category of health food. They're good for cleaning the heads on your tape recorder, however.

Now for the big question! Can anyone really live this way? Ask some of the healthiest, thinnest, longest-living cultures in the history of human kind. Live it they do, and with gusto, vibrant health and joy! To say that this newer model of what constitutes a perfect diet for the human body is going to take some time for the American people to adjust to goes without saying. It will take lots of getting used to. But that's just the way it is. Personally, I find it a bit sad when I think about a prevailing attitude among some government health officials. That is that the American people are "not ready" to be told the truth. Well, I for one would rather be given the facts and have the option of making my own choices. I'm aware enough to do that and I believe that you are, too. Many new cookbooks, chefs and restaurants are reflecting this attitude by offering truly healthy fare. The more you demand it and support it by purchasing healthier foods, the more healthy foods you'll find available. Start referring to the New and Truly Improved Food Pyramid and know that it is the very best that you can do to get slender and healthy ... and to stay that way. Also, pay attention to portion sizes as defined by the THINNER WINNERS Basic Food Plan guidelines in Chapter 25 "What to Eat".

In A Nutshell

1) All foods fall into one or more of "The Big Three" categories: Protein, Carbohydrates & Fats.

2) 15-20% of your calories should come from protein.

3) Americans eat more than twice the amount of protein that they need for good health.

4) Vegetable protein is equivalent to meat protein and has no saturated fat or cholesterol.

5) There are 2 types of carbohydrates: Complex (starches) and Simple (sugars).

6) 65-75% of your diet should be carbohydrates (with no more than 10% simple).

7) Complex carbohydrates are mostly plant foods like grains, vegetables, beans and fruit.

8) Fats are essential for your health and should make up 10-20% of your total calories.

9) Only ⅓ or less of your total fat should be the saturated type (derived from meats and tropical oils).

10) Vitamins and minerals are essential for normal body functioning. You can get these substances through nutritionally adequate foods or by taking supplements.

11) Recommended Dietary Allowances (RDA's) are government guidelines advising you of your minimal nutrition needs. They currently emphasize avoiding disease rather than disease prevention.

12) Overweight people are under additional physical stress and require extra supplements of vitamins and minerals to maintain adequate levels of health.

13) There are certain supplements (thermogenics) you can safely take, if you are healthy and active, that can encourage your metabolism to increase and more quickly burn calories and supply more energy while losing weight. Be careful! Check with your health-provider.

14) The old "Four Food Groups" and the government's new "food pyramid" both fall short of adequately defining the way that foods impact your nutrition and health needs.

15) Consider "The New and Truly Improved Food Pyramid" as a more realistic guideline for healthful nutrition.

What to Eat   25

"Everything you see I owe to spaghetti."
Sophia Loren

Focus on Food Value

Every single day you need to satisfy your body's requirements for an array of essential nutrients. Plus you need to feel satisfied with the amount and type of food you eat. If you skimp in either of these areas you'll be left with a deep craving for food. If you find this happening, add a serving or two a day to your menu or vary your foods for variety, until you find a balance where you are satisfied with the way you feel ... both physically and psychologically. Never eat anything you don't like! Don't be concerned in the beginning if you think you're getting too many calories. In the early stages of your program they're of little importance to your overall health and thinness. In the past I have eaten literally thousands of calories a day of empty, nutrition-bereft "foods" and still been starving. My body *was* starving since I had added no beneficial nutrients to my system at all ... nothing it could use to help in the processes necessary for vital health. So first, let's get your body nourished and satisfied. Your focus now should be on food value. Ask,"What can this food do for my health?"

Below you'll find a description of the foods in each of the healthful food categories and suggestions for the number of servings to eat ... plus what makes up a serving. Start with the lowest number of servings. Use this as a guideline for your new eating style.

Fruits and Vegetables

It's hard to go wrong with this nutritious category of foods. Fruits and veggies are chock full of vitamins, minerals and trace nutrients, plus fiber and water. I use them a lot to "fill in the corners" that might still be empty in my stomach (or my mind!). Choose from this category first and as often as you need.

Select fresh food whenever possible, frozen if you can't get fresh and canned only occasionally ... if you must. Even then, choose canned varieties packed in their own juice or with reduced sodium. Rinse all canned veggies to reduce sodium content further. Wash all fruits and veggies thoroughly and scrub lightly with a soft brush (and "veggie wash" if you want) to remove any residues or dirt. Certified organic produce may not be as uniform or "perfect" in appearance as non-organic, but it has been grown without pesticides and chemicals that can build up in your body over time and cause health problems. Growing your own produce can be fun, rewarding and definitely tastier if you have the time, space and inclination.

Choose 2 or 3 servings of fruit a day and at least 4 servings of vegetables. Men can add up to two more servings of fruit and as many veggie servings as you want every day. What's a serving? A medium piece of fruit (not large or giant size) or 6 ounces of juice is usually about a serving. There are a few exceptions: bananas and dried fruits are very concentrated, so half of a medium banana makes a serving, and 2 small or one large piece of dried fruit is a serving. About two tablespoons of raisins is the correct amount. For berries, ½ cup is a serving ... except for strawberries of which you can have a full cup. Use common sense, but even if you go a bit large on fruits, it's alright because of their nutritional addition to your diet. For veggies, ½ cup cooked or 1 cup raw is a serving. So a dinner salad will fulfill your needs, as long as it has a variety of veggies in it ... not just iceberg lettuce and tomatoes. The more veggies you add, the better. They are vital, whole foods that add immeasurably to your body's vitality and satisfaction.

Try to make a "super salad" at least every other day with all your favorite raw veggies in it and keep it covered in the refrigerator. Fresh cut veggies should be eaten as soon as possible after you cut them to preserve nutrients. Use this salad for additions to lunch or a quick main meal dinner. I love my "salad-making" days because I get to completely cover every work surface in the kitchen with colorful veggies of every description. Then I have to "test" each variety, of course, as it's being prepared for addition to my salad bowl! I'm always on the lookout for new vegetables and often find exotic ones to try. It really has become a fun and healthy tradition. Veggies are your friends! Vegetables are just "rabbit food" you say? Now, now ... watch that attitude, and think "solutions". Cole slaw, V-8 juice, eggplant parmesan, carrot salad, soups, spaghetti sauce, chili, veggie omelets and quiche, salsa, tostadas, vegetarian pizza and pumpkin pie are all examples of "user friendly" veggies. Find your favorites and enjoy!

Breads and Cereals

This category of foods has certainly gotten a bad reputation among dieters as fattening. But happily that's far from the truth. Actually, as you learned in Chapter 21 "Get That Body Movin'", you absolutely need these high carbohydrate foods to burn off that extra fat you've been collecting! Yes, your dreams are about to come true! More breads and cereals than ever before are actually good for you! Hooray! Now become a wise and choosy buyer of foods in this group. Whole grains are always the most nutritious. Yes, angel food cake has less calories and fat than other kinds of cake, but the question is, what does it have that will nourish you? White flour, sugar and preservatives? Where's the nutrition? It's like eating a tasty bit of wood pulp as far as your body is concerned. Instead, get the most out of all the foods you choose here by sticking to whole foods, as close to the way they were grown as possible. The fewer the ingredients on the label, the better.

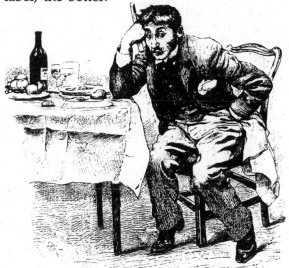

"You mean I can start eating the breadsticks again?"

Many companies are now responding to rising consumer awareness by offering more healthy varieties. Check the labels carefully however, especially with cereals. With all the zillions of colorful boxes of breakfast cereals on the shelves, you would think that more than a handful of them would be nutritious. But, no-o-o! I've read all the labels looking for the best ones, and for standard "big name" prepared cereals there really are only four or five of them that are health-promoting. I tend to stick to hot cereal because it isn't as adulterated with sugar and sodium. Also, health food sections and stores have much healthier versions of favorites such as shredded wheat, corn flakes and fat-free granola. They tend to be made with less white sugar, sodium, artificial colorings, flavorings or preservatives. But again, check the labels. Use the serving sizes given on the packages in general as a guideline. New labeling laws in effect as of May 1994 make it a lot easier to be realistic about serving sizes, too. Previously, some food manufacturers called their products "low calorie" but a recommended serving size would barely fill a thimble.

Experiment with different types of breads. Winners are whole wheat, rye, sour dough, raisin, pita pockets, whole wheat or corn tortillas (not white flour), English muffins and whole grain rolls. Muffins (especially the commercial type) tend to be loaded with fat, sugar and calories, so either make your own or save them for an occasional indulgence. Most crackers are also high in fat and sodium, so search out the healthier varieties such as crisp breads, flatbreads and rice cakes made with whole grains. Rice cakes have come a long way and now come in great flavors. Fat free whole grain crackers are now readily available.

Pasta, yes, pasta! Isn't it ironic that now that I'm thin I can enjoy pasta more than when I was fat? I love pasta and used to save it for a special occasion or thought I had blown it when I had a plate of spaghetti. Now I choose whole grain or vegetable pastas and top with a variety of yummy sauces (see Chapter 30 "Basic Recipes"). It is very satisfying and highly nutritious. Pasta also comes in a huge variety of different shapes and sizes which are always fun to play with in different dishes.

Rice is another good grain to use frequently. Buy the brown or wild varieties as they have more nutritional parts intact, such as the bran and germ. Instant varieties make them quick to prepare. Instant brown rice is the best of both worlds ... fast and nutritious.

In the breads and cereals group also include the starchy veggies such as corn, potatoes, yams, fresh peas and winter squashes. Potatoes are one of the greatest additions to a thin persons bag of tricks. They are high in nutrients and fiber, low in fat and sodium, very satisfying, economical, come in many tasty varieties and are a snap to microwave in under 5 minutes. They're also easy to grow at home even in buckets. Learn to use the right low and non-fat toppings and you can enjoy them often. Choose 4-6 servings from this group every day. Men can choose an additional 2 servings each day. As you become more fit and active, this is the group I would add to first. Carbohydrates are great fuel food.

Protein

Your body needs protein every day to build and rebuild cells. But it is now known that people don't need as much protein as previously believed. As a matter of fact, most Americans overeat on protein. Two servings a day is plenty for a woman ... with slightly larger servings for men. About ½ gram of protein per pound of body weight is suggested for non-overweight people. Use 45-60 grams for a 1200 calorie diet. Use 60-80 grams for a 1600 calorie diet. That's 15-20%. Your 2 servings will satisfy this need without counting grams.

There is still debate on the issue however ... groups such as the World Health Organization propose 20 grams as a minimum requirement. That's right! All we need is 20 grams. Other recent research has indicated that too much protein can cause a slow-down or blockage in the absorption of certain nutrients such as calcium and is not advised. Of course, certain activities such as very heavy weight-training, may call for more protein since the body is busy building muscle.

A serving is 2-3 ounces (cooked) of lean meat, poultry or fish (about the size of a deck of cards) ... or two ounces of cheese (preferably low-salt and low-fat varieties) ... or ½ cup of low or non-fat cottage or ricotta cheese ... or two eggs with yolks (or 6 egg whites only). If you like tofu, 4 ounces of the firm type, or 6 ounces of the soft variety makes a serving. Soy products like tofu can be high in fat however, so only choose them once a week or so. New low-fat tofu is beginning to appear in the market, so keep your eyes open and check this out. Dried beans, lentils and peas are good sources of protein, soluble and insoluble fiber as well, with 4 ounces (½ cup) cooked being a serving.

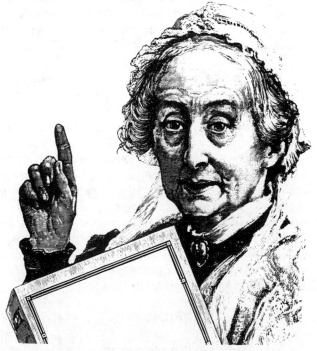

"Beans, beans ... the musical fruit ..."

It was once thought that beans had to be combined with a grain to be a "complete protein", but recent nutrition research now reveals that eating this way is not necessary. The amino acids needed to make the protein useful to your body can be stored for longer periods than previously believed. Eating a balance of foods provides enough amino acids for your body to get high quality protein from the nutrients that you take in during the day. So don't be overly concerned about this. As a matter of fact, a protein-deficient diet is almost impossible since our bodies need so little of it and can store and combine amino acids over a long period. That makes vegetable protein high quality protein, too, just like the traditional animal foods.

Some vegetables that are high in protein include broccoli, mushrooms, grains and cereal products. Textured vegetable protein (TVP) sounds unusual, but is really a great way to cut down on fat, cholesterol and animal products without giving up that hearty texture and flavor some people have become accustomed to. TVP comes in a variety of flavors such as beef and chicken, as well as a variety of textures such as ground, strips and chunks. It can be used in cooking just like meat ... in tacos, spaghetti sauce, stir-fry and stews. Be sure and check the label for sodium content and preservatives.

By far my favorite non-animal protein is a food called seitan (say-tan) or wheat-meat. It is extremely economical, comes in instant form (from Arrowhead Mills) and can be made easily at home. It can be shaped in the form of roasts, patties, balls, etc. I love it marinated and barbecued. These meat substitute products are a wonderful way for you to make the transition to a non-animal based diet. They are delicious, economical, healthy and help conserve the world's natural resources, as well as reduce the brutal treatment of farm animals in this country. Read either one of John Robbins' wonderful and enlightening books for a complete understanding of this subject and the impact that your food choices can make. They are Diet for A New America and May All Be Fed. The later includes a Recipe Section with some absolutely dynamite, total vegetarian dishes.

Some foods in the protein category are very high in undesirable fats and/or cholesterol. Therefore, you must limit their intake for your healthiest diet. Limit whole eggs to 3 per week (each contains up to 275 mg of cholesterol). You can enjoy egg whites as much as you want, however. Stretch your eggs by using one whole egg and 2-3 additional egg whites in an omelet. Or choose egg substitutes as often as you wish, since they're mostly egg whites. Cheese is also loaded with fat, sodium and calories so only choose 2 servings a week of regular cheese, or 3 servings if you pick low fat and low sodium varieties. For meats such as beef, pork, lamb, organ meats and shellfish limit your servings to 3-4 times a month, if you choose them at all.

All other fish can be chosen 2-3 times a week if you wish. White fish such as halibut, sole and cod are so low in calories and fat you can have 4-6 ounces as one serving. Check your food count book for fish in this category. Note: on your Daily Success Planner (see Chapter 18) there are 4-6 boxes for protein. Each box represents 1 ounce of cooked protein (or 1 egg, 1 ounce cheese, ¼ cup of cottage cheese, etc.) not total servings (which is 2 per day). It's easier to keep track this way if, for instance, you have 1 ounce of cheese for lunch, you can have 3 oz of turkey for dinner.

Dairy Products

Dairy products add vitamin D, calcium and protein to your diet, but since you can get these nutrients from other sources they are really not necessary. Just be sure you know the other sources of these nutrients and include them in your diet, if you choose not to eat dairy products. You can also take a supplement of calcium and vitamin D. As I mentioned before, a good paperback reference book on the nutrients contained in foods will prove very enlightening and useful here as elsewhere. Many people are intolerant of the lactose in dairy products, and are unable to digest them properly. After all, cow's milk is not intended by nature for human consumption, is it? If you don't include dairy products in your daily diet, add an extra ½ serving from the protein group and 1 serving from the bread/cereal group. Otherwise, 2 servings of non-fat milk, buttermilk or yogurt can be eaten daily. Non-fat yogurt (or the soy versions that are available), sweetened with fresh fruit or juice and a tablespoon or two of dry cereal thrown in for crunch, makes a fast, easy and yummy snack for kids and adults alike. Frozen non-fat or low-fat yogurt is not really a milk serving because of limited nutrition and lots of sugar. But I count it as a dairy serving about twice a week because I enjoy it so much (hey, I'm not perfect, okay!?). Canned evaporated skim milk is a thicker, creamier version of milk that can be used in cereal, coffee and recipes. It's similar to cream, but without the fat. Many non-animal based beverages are now available. These include creamy rice beverages, nut milks and soy products. My favorites are vanilla Rice Dream or carob soy lite. Nut and rice milks can easily be made economically at home.

Fats

Wow! Talk about a controversial subject in nutrition! Everything these days paints fats in the very worst possible picture nutritionally. But in reality, we all need a little fat for our bodies to function optimally. It aids in lubrication of joints and internal organs, hair and nail growth, and metabolism of certain nutrients. Now, note carefully that I said a little fat. Fat is still fat, and it doesn't make sense to eat a lot of it when that is exactly what you are trying to lose. So careful monitoring of your intake is important here.

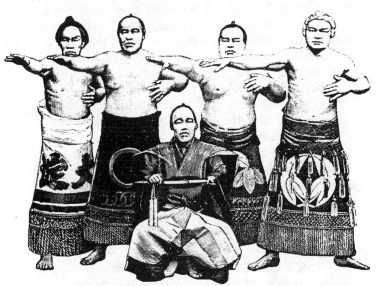

"The tofu is over there!"

I have included a great deal of additional information about fats and cholesterol in Chapter 32 "Fat and Cholesterol", so take a look there for additional information on this important subject. For right now, keep grams of fat to 13-26 per day if you are eating 1200 calories (women), or 18-36 grams if you are eating 1600 (men). This is between 10-20% of your caloric intake for the fat-losing stage. This is all you need to count ... fat grams. Look them up in your pocket fat-gram counter.

While you are in the "losing fat" stage of your program, consume no more than 2 servings a day of fat. A teaspoon (measuring spoon not cereal spoon!) of oil, margarine or mayonnaise is one serving ... or two teaspoons of diet margarine or mayo. Salad dressings are usually full of fat. As a matter of fact, they are the #1 source of fat in women's diets in the U.S. So choose the low-fat kind or even the non-fat kind. Better yet, make your own or use non-fat dressings and mayonnaise and avoid the problem.

Nuts, seeds and peanut butter are high in fat, too, so a small serving (1 tablespoon) only occasionally as an indulgence can be included ... but it is not recommended until you reach goal and stabilize on the THINNER WINNERS maintenance program. If you crave high fat foods, then have a small amount to avoid having the cravings turn into binges ... but if that's like "priming the pump", then avoid it for now. Even the new fat substitute foods can start a craving for more. To shut off your "fat tooth" avoid these, too.

Water

I feel so strongly about water being an essential nutrient that I have included an entire chapter on it (see Chapter 35 "Water—The Magic Potion"). Right now, I will just mention that water is an absolute necessity for thinness and good health. Work diligently on making it a habit to drink 6-8 eight ounce glasses of water a day minimum, and you will quickly begin to notice many health benefits. It also helps keep you filled up.

If you exercise a lot, or if it's hot, drink even more. I have found that for me, the optimum number of glasses per day is 10-12. Pay attention to how you feel and find the right amount for your own body. You should feel clear, clean and light in the morning if you have consumed enough water (and good foods!) the day before.

Additions

You'll probably want to use some foods not found on this list to spice up your daily fare. Some frills and fun foods can really help keep variety and interest from slipping into boring and bland. No need for that, since you can add about 120-160 calories a day, or about 10% of your calories, on anything else you want (low-fat preferred, of course). Some examples are cocoa powder for your coffee or ricotta dessert sauces such as the barbecue type jams, jellies (the new fruit-only ones are delicious) or chutneys honey or syrup occasionally for cooking, or on your French toast goodies such as cookies occasionally or even a glass (5 ounces) of wine or beer (limit to 3 drinks weekly). See Chapter 27 "Choosing Healthy Foods" for details on sugar and alcohol. Just look up any foods that you will be using in addition to the foods required in the program, and keep your calorie and fat intake within the limits. Watch fat closely. Pretty soon you'll know your favorites by heart and keeping track will be a lot easier. And every month or so, give yourself a "free day" where you can just relax and not count anything.

Cooking Methods

The healthiest cooking methods are baking, broiling, steaming, poaching, boiling, barbecuing (use foil between the charcoal and meat to protect from possible carcinogens) or grilling, using a pressure cooker, slow cooker or a microwave oven (a favorite for convenience and speed). You can sauté if you use a low-calorie cooking spray or a liquid such as broth, water, lemon juice, etc. instead of fat. Veggies are wonderful roasted. Deep frying in fat or oil is a definite taboo ... you'll end up eating more fat than food, since the food soaks it up while cooking. When baking meat, be sure to set it on a rack, so the excess fat can drip off. Special microwave plates are also available if you are cooking meats. Trim off all visible fat from your meat and poultry before cooking it. Don't make the mistake of cooking first, then removing the skin ... the fat will still soak into the food. You may use a small amount of oil to stir-fry or sauté poultry or veggies, but cook meats ahead of time by one of the methods that lets the fat drip off, then add it to the veggies after they're cooked.

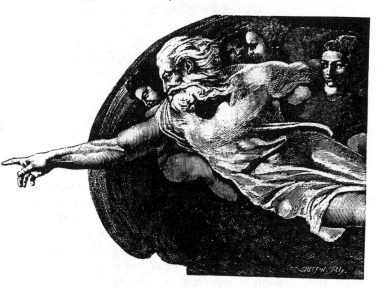

"Look! Non-fat ice cream!"

Let Common Sense Be Your Guide

That's it! Don't get fanatical about this. Just get used to some new ideas and techniques and let it flow, take it slow and use your common sense. This is a lifetime pattern you are developing. There are even a few foods that you can have without "keeping track" ... like spices, herbs and seasonings (see Chapter 34 "Sodium & Salt vs. Herbs & Spices"), splashes of lemon or lime juice, vinegars of all varieties horseradish (not the creamed kind), mustards (low salt) in reasonable amounts, soy or Worcestershire sauces (low sodium preferred) and herbal teas or decaf coffee (which come in a tremendous range of flavors).

A few foods that you will encounter may at first appear to defy your efforts to figure out what's in them. So use your best, most honorable judgment. (No, darling, a glass of wine can't be counted as a fruit! Nice try!) But a serving of coleslaw at your favorite eating joint is for sure going to have more than shredded cabbage in it ... usually a good dollop of some kind of fat for the dressing and maybe a bit of sugar, too. Don't deny yourself if you really want it ... just count it as your fat for the day, as well as a veggie. Let common sense guide you along.

For additional foods that you may wish to enjoy while eating out in restaurants and at parties, please refer to Chapter 36 "How to Survive Eating Away From Home".

In A Nutshell

1) Focus on food value, not calories. Ask what the food will provide your body nutritionally. Calories do count, but by following the suggested guidelines, both calories and fat will be in the healthy range.

2) Eat whole, fresh foods (as grown) whenever possible. Process very little.

3) Eat a minimum of 1200 calories per day for women and 1600 calories per day for men. Anything less than this may trigger a starvation response and lower your metabolism.

4) Daily recommendations: (Note: see the chapter text for suggested sizes of servings.)
You can easily keep track of your servings with the "serving boxes" on your Daily Success Planner.

* 65-75% carbohydrates, 15-20% protein, 10-20% fat
* Fruits - 2 servings for women, 4 for men
* Vegetables - 4 servings minimum
* Breads and cereals - 4 servings for women, 6 for men
* Protein - 2 servings or 45-60 grams (women) & 60-80 grams (men)
* Fat - 2 servings ... 13-26 grams (women), 18-36 grams (men)
* Dairy - 2 servings if desired. Optional.
* Water - 6 to 8 eight ounce glasses minimum, more if it's hot or you exercise and sweat a lot or are very overweight.
* Additions - 10% of total calories for fun or treats if desired (watch fats and sugar though).

5) Use cooking methods that focus on fat and salt reduction.

How to Eat   26

"To eat is human, to digest divine."
Mark Twain

Balance Weight-Loss with Satisfaction

If you're hungry or not satisfied, feel free to eat more of any of the healthful foods described in Chapter 25 "What To Eat". You'll still lose weight steadily even if you eat an extra serving or two of healthy low-fat foods such as fruit, beans, carbs or non-fat dairy. Just watch fat grams and sugar carefully . On the other hand, you must eat the required minimum amounts of the basics to establish a nutritious base upon which your body can firmly stand. If you try to eat a skimpy meal to save calories, you'll throw your body off balance and begin to crave certain nutrients or foods. You may begin to nibble or overeat at your next meal ... and this may even trigger a binge. Heaven forbid! When your body is well-nourished and satisfied you can forget about ever bingeing again. So eat!

At first the amount of food suggested in "What to Eat" may seem like a huge amount to you ... maybe even more than you are used to eating. However, it's the balance of nutrients and the type of food that's important and that will provide the basis for glowing health. I think the biggest mistake that I continued to make during The Fat Years was the tendency to "just get that weight off" as quickly as possible. I'd go hungry, try crazy shakes or liquid protein, anything to do it. And I'd usually ended up looking and feeling like a hollow-eyed, haunted hag by the time I did. My grandmother used to always say that she could tell when I was dieting by the circles under my eyes. That's not the way to permanent health and thinness. You've got to provide the nutrients that your body needs to do the work of losing the fat! Otherwise you'll end up malnourished, unhealthy and FAT! Do you see this? Are you ready to take the word of a 135 pound THINNER WINNER who finally saw this? Then follow me to Thinland, my friend.

The THINNER WINNERS plan provides approximately 15-20% protein, 65-75% carbohydrates and 10-20% fat. These percentages are recommended by many health professionals. They are the result of many years of dietary research and are the epitome of the very best nutrition you can provide for your one-and-only body. You can't do better.

Pace Your Eating During the Day

If you spread out your food during the day instead of stuffing yourself at one or two meals, and then starving the rest of the time, you will be less likely to start thinking about food, become ravenous and then eat everything in the refrigerator. Don't go for more than 4 or 5 hours without having something to eat. This will backfire every time. It does you no good to skip meals, probably some harm ... and may permanently slow your metabolism. The classic example of this is the person who skips or skimps on breakfast with the best intentions. "I'll just eat so little, I'll have to lose weight." Two things will then happen. First, their energy will drop as the morning goes on. They're usually starving by lunch or dinner and overeat. Also, if this practice is continued, your body begins to perceive this lack of food as a signal to begin conserving fuel for survival. In order to do this, your metabolism begins to slow down, burning fewer calories than if an adequate breakfast, providing energy and staying power, had been eaten. Studies show that people who skip breakfast burn fewer calories the rest of the day. So again, eat!

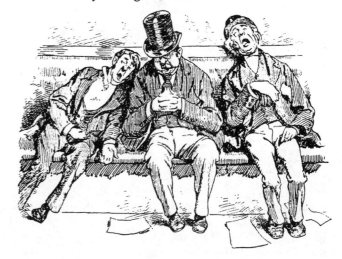

Waiting too long between meals can lead to fatigue.

Know yourself and be prepared. If late afternoon is the time you get hungry, then plan a satisfying snack or early dinner for that time. If this happens often, you're probably not eating enough for lunch. It may be a big change for you, but your goal should eventually be to eat a light, filling breakfast, a hearty main-meal lunch and light, satisfying dinner. You will find yourself with more energy throughout the day, sleeping better at night and waking up without that drugged, tired feeling of a food hangover. Studies have shown that people who eat at least 60% of their total food for the day by 2 P.M. are slimmer than their heavy-evening-meal counterparts. "Find out what winners do, then do it!"

Use the suggested meals in Chapter 29 "Sample Meals" as a starting point to arrange and create your own meal plans according to your style of eating. Note that not all breakfasts "fit" with all lunches and dinners. For instance, if you have 1 tablespoon of peanut butter (8 grams of fat) in your sandwich for lunch then you will have used up a large part of your fat for the day, and therefore wouldn't choose to have margarine on a roll or beef as part of your dinner.

Keep track of your servings on your Daily Success Planner as you eat them and you'll be fine. If you wait until the end of the day, the chance of eating something "by mistake" by forgetting exactly what you had all day will be increased. Plan well and write it down.

Plan and Eat Regular Meals

Plan and eat three meals and a snack every day for the fastest way to get rid of that fat for good!

Breakfast

Although everyone has their own style of eating, there are some universal principles that can prove beneficial to all. One of the most famous (and most valid) is the need for a good breakfast (as mentioned above). But what exactly is "good"? Some folks can eat lighter and do just fine for energy all day. Others need a solid, hearty meal to rev them up and keep them going. If you lack energy during the late morning, don't prop yourself up with a cup of coffee ... it's a jolt to your adrenal glands. Instead, choose a more substantial meal in the morning to carry you through. This could include some fruit or fruit juice for quick energy and a serving of bread or cereal for staying power until lunch, the main meal of the day. Cereal and bread contain some protein, but if you wish, you could include more protein such as milk or soy beverage, meat or meat substitute, or eggs. Don't be afraid to have a really hearty breakfast. Your body burns up calories faster in the morning than any other time of day. If you just can't stand the idea of eating anything first thing in the morning, then at the very least, have a

serving or two of juice or fruit. It will be lighter on your system and it will give your elimination cycle a little more time to complete itself. I personally wake up with desperate thoughts of devouring anything in my path so I haven't been able to take advantage of this calm, cool approach to breakfast yet. Just go with your own feelings ... don't force anything.

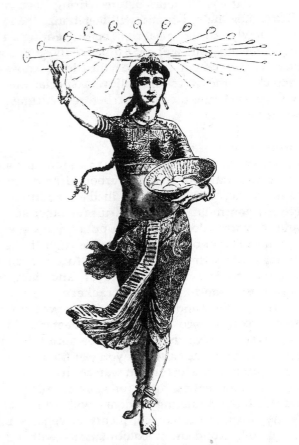

We all need to come up
with our own food strategies.

At mid-morning you can eat a fruit, veggie, grain, dairy or protein serving if you get hungry. But don't skip breakfast altogether since its been shown that by doing this, you tend to have lower energy for the rest of the day and you also tend to overeat at another meal ... usually late in the day when your metabolism is slowest. This is a killer for weight loss.

Lunch

Lunch should be hearty, your main meal of the day. Include some protein and at least one vegetable. Eat light in fat and sugar, especially if you need to stay alert in the afternoon. Fat is heavy food and will make you drowsy while your body digests. Lots of carbohydrate at lunch can be heavy and slow you down, too. So eat it moderately, 1-2 servings. Fruit is excellent.

Dinner

Dinner, or the last meal eaten before you go to bed, should be as light but satisfying as possible with one protein serving and two vegetable servings as your only "musts". If you continue to eat the traditional American heavy dinner, then at least eat early enough to get in some light activity before going to bed or parking on the sofa for hours. Try not to eat for at least 4 hours before retiring since your body is slowing down and will metabolize the food more slowly. A huge meal right before retiring is not only unhealthy but will tend to make those pounds stick to you longer. In case you didn't know it, Japanese Sumo wrestlers follow a special diet ... they eat a huge meal right before bedtime. So beware!

Evening Snacks

A light snack of yogurt or another dairy product, gelatin, or a light carbohydrate such as crackers, rice cakes or cereal in the evening is all right, if you must. But avoid fruit (or other simple carbohydrates) alone, since it supplies quick energy and may keep you awake or cause night hunger. Combine it with a carbohydrate to slow down absorption. Examples are toast and jam, or applesauce and graham crackers. Calcium-containing dairy foods or a hot drink would be a more relaxing choice. If you're a night eater and you don't want to give that up, then be sure to plan a snack into your menu which you can munch in the midnight hour. Most night eaters are breakfast skippers. Start eating more for your morning meal and this fat-encouraging tendency will fade.

Whenever you like, eat plenty of veggies, raw or cooked, alone or in combinations with other veggies. They are great vitamin, mineral and fiber-packed goodies. They also keep your system moving right along, keep you filled up, satisfy the urge to munch and crunch, and boost your fluid intake as they are mostly water.

After each meal, rest quietly for 5-10 minutes if possible. Sip a glass of cool water and allow the meal to settle. Then get up and take a short 5-15 minute walk. Get the mail, stroll around the neighborhood or your garden. Window shop for a few minutes or just keep moving doing housework or whatever. This helps the digestive process begin.

You Only Eat One Day at a Time

Planning your shopping ahead of time is the best way to make sure you're not left hanging some day without the right foods in the house. Just standing in the middle of the kitchen asking, "Now what should I have for dinner?" is an open invitation to fall back into the old ways of opening a box of macaroni and cheese or salty soup and crackers, and throwing in a couple of hot dogs or whatever the old fat-producing habit was around your kitchen. If you can't take the time to sit down and plan what you'll be having for the next several days, then at least plan ahead for one day at a time. That way at least you'll always know what's for dinner and you can eat your breakfast and lunch with that in mind.

Another advantage of taking the small amount of time to plan your meals and snacks is that you can look forward to that meal for hours. It's fun to anticipate popcorn (hot-air popped, of course!) at a Friday night movie pizza and beer on Saturday night or a home-cooked Sunday quiche with berry cobbler for dessert. If you haven't planned something you get excited about, then change it! Remember your Food Personality? (See Chapter 15 "Managing the Food-Mood Connection".) If fried chicken, mashed potatoes and gravy really turn you on, then find or convert a recipe that satisfies you, and plan it for dinner. Don't eat liver if you hate it! Food needs to be satisfying and fun. If it's not, then you won't continue with this plan or any other ... and you will remain fat, or on the unhealthy diet roller coaster. This is counter-productive and dangerous and will lead you straight down the road to poor health! So-o-o ... PLAN to eat something you love today ... and everyday! As you follow the THINNER WINNERS program, you'll find that each day will bring new successes and those important emotional rewards.

Free Days

Here's a method that really helped me stay sane (relatively) and on track for the year or so that it took me to lose the last and major part of my extra 137 pounds. Every month or so, I had a "free day" with food. That is, I didn't keep track of a blessed thing. I ate what I wanted, when I wanted it, and however much I wanted. No guilt, just sweet freedom. At first, I thought this would totally undo all the good I had accomplished over the previous weeks, but lo and behold I actually started to want more of the healthful foods and less of the fattening goodies. Oh, sure, I had a few doozies now and again, but when I began to be more in touch with just how awful I felt after a sugar overload or a salty binge, then slowly-but-surely I just didn't want or choose or crave those things any more. And actually I was glad to get back to regular eating the day after because it felt right and healthy.

I still do this at least once a month and it is a definite mental health day for me. Don't go totally berserk, but just relax and feel the flow of healthy choices you have been making. Take the day to look back in retrospect over your good work and changes. Take a moment and a deep breath while you enjoy the progress you're making. Notice if your food preferences or time to eat differ much from the parameters that you have set for yourself. Maybe you can work them into your regular weight control routine.

All work and no play is a drag. So have some fun with this. I think you'll be pleasantly surprised at the energy fluctuations you will experience after you do this for a few months. Sometimes pushing too hard sets up both mental and physical resistance. Just let go and let it be for a day, then begin again with a fresh perspective.

Atmosphere

Before you begin to experiment with all the fun and delicious recipes and meal plans that follow, let me just say a word here about how you can serve them for the greatest enjoyment. Think a moment about your favorite restaurant and what makes it your favorite (besides the food!). If you're like me, your top pick is probably more than just a plain room with a few tables and chairs. The owners have usually gone to quite a bit of trouble to design a pleasant, warm, interesting and inviting establishment. They've picked a color scheme and used accessories such as flowers, pictures and candles to create a certain mood. The waiters and waitresses may have appropriate and, often times, quite imaginative and amusing costumes. Some of my favorite eating spots are an absolute explosion of interesting pieces of art, odd objects and hodgepodge. Music is also very important in creating an enjoyable atmosphere.

A blaring radio or TV complete with the news or grating commercials is not very appetizing. Glaring overhead fluorescent bulbs don't create much of a romantic or soothing mood either.

These same principles hold true in your own home as well. After working so hard on a meal, give a little thought on how you will present it. A Mexican dish could be served on inexpensive pottery serving plates with a colorful flower or two such as geraniums on the table to set a festive mood. A single white flower or a rose is always elegant. Try playing appropriate music softly in the background.

Slow, relaxing music while dining has been shown to slow down eating speed as well. Ethnic meals are really fun to "accessorize" and even dressing up for the occasion could add to the event. At least once a week go all out and use all the suggestions here. But even on humdrum weekdays, use a little imagination to set the mood for the meal. Make it fun, and get the most satisfaction from your dining experience.

Similarly, learn to present the food on the serving plates in an appetizing way. Place a little sprig of parsley, fresh herb or an edible flower on the plate. Curl a veggie such as a carrot for a little color. Add a lemon or orange twist or slice. At the very least, sprinkle a dash of colorful contrasting spice, such as paprika or cinnamon, or some chopped parsley on the finished dish. This is very easy and really adds to the appeal of the dish. There are some terrific books on garnishes that are fun to make and appreciated by diners. Buy real cloth napkins in pretty designs to help set an attractive table. Use water goblets, placemats and a tablecloth if you have them.

Now, I know that as a nation, we are increasingly eating our evening meals in front of the television. I personally consider this a shame, as it wastes an opportunity to talk the day over with loved ones, share a meal without the news hammering away at us, and generally detracts from the enjoyment of the nourishment we are so fortunate to have. However, if you must do it, then at least fix up the coffee table or TV tray so it's not so bleak and for goodness sake, turn off the commercials and talk to the person you're with! Try to wean yourself away from this habit. Foods are metabolized more efficiently and completely when eaten in a congenial, pleasant, low-key atmosphere. Watching the nightly news just encourages poor digestion.

You will be surprised at how much more pleasant it is to eat in an environment that has received a little thought and planning. The meal just somehow tastes better when the setting is more interesting and warm and shows a little care. Be good to yourself, your family and guests! Make mealtime a special experience, relax and enjoy the atmosphere that you have created while savoring the healthy foods you have prepared. Bon Appetit!

In A Nutshell

1) Eat as much of the healthy, high fiber foods described in "What to Eat" as needed for your satisfaction.

2) Never eat anything you don't like!

3) Watch fat grams! They are very potent.

4) You will be eating 15-20% protein, 65-75% carbohydrate, and 10-20% fat. These amounts will help lead you to health and thinness.

5) By being well-nourished with this balance of foods, your cravings and many other indications of poor nutrition will fade away and you'll have more energy.

6) Plan and eat 3 meals and at least one snack daily. That's the fastest way to get rid of that fat for good.

7) Plan a Free Day at least once a month and don't keep track of anything. Use the time to relax and look back on your progress. Let go and lighten up the pressure. Start fresh tomorrow.

8) Planning ahead eliminates impulse eating and allows you to anticipate a favorite food or meal.

9) Food needs to be satisfying and fun. Devise healthier versions of your favorites.

10) Breakfast is the most important meal of the day for gearing up the metabolism.

11) Eat a light, filling breakfast , a hearty main meal lunch, and a light dinner. Rest for 5-10 minutes after meals, then go for a 5-15 minute light walk.

12) Create a pleasant atmosphere for better digestion, as well as a more satisfying meal experience.

13) Use meals to talk pleasantly and share experiences ... not to rehash the news or argue.

Choosing Healthy Foods   27

"Better to hunt in fields, for health unbought, than fee the doctor for a nauseous draught."
John Dryden

As you've learned in previous chapters, the world is just as full of fresh, natural, unadulterated foods as it is of the de-vitalized sort. After all, every processed food was fresh at one time. You will discover even more once you begin looking for and using them regularly. It's all a matter of focus, paying attention and of finding what you're looking for. Healthy, satisfying foods are all over the place, just waiting for you to seek them out.

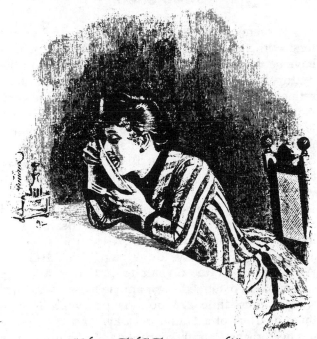

"Now THAT was good!"

Get The Most Out of Every Calorie

During the weight loss phase of your program, you will be eating a reduced amount of calories in order to lose your extra fat. In order to maximize your health at the same time, you must endeavor to get the very most nutritionally out of every calorie that goes into your mouth. This means eliminating or cutting down on any foods which are "borderline" nutritionally. Foods that have been reduced in their nutritional content by processing are in this category. Try for the very best ingredients in everything ... fresh, whole foods, as close to the way they were grown as possible, are superior. There is no room right now for stripped flours, empty sugar calories, excessive alcohol or fats

(saturated or hydrogenated). When you get yourself into great shape by following this program, then you can indulge by choosing these foods occasionally if you wish. But a healthy, strong body will know how to handle that night on the town. Start thinking of your food as super-charged fuel for your new streamlined body: a Ferrari, not an old clunker that will run on kerosene (and looks as if it won't make it to the next corner!).

Oils and Fats

There is clear evidence that saturated fats derived from animals, such as butter and lard, contribute greatly to the incidence of heart disease (see Chapter 32 "Fat and Cholesterol"). However, fats do supply your body with two substances that it cannot manufacture for itself: linoleic and linolenic acids. It also contributes to the functioning of certain organs, such as your gall bladder. So don't try to go totally fat free. Not only will you be a pretty boring person and cook, but you may lose a few friends, too! Use 2 servings of margarine or oils daily according to the THINNER WINNERS Food Plan. A serving is one measuring teaspoon of either oil or margarine. Remember though, most foods have fat in them, so stick to 10-20% total fat. For instance, if you choose to have 2 TBL of peanut butter in a sandwich for lunch, then you already have eaten 16 grams of fat in that one serving. No need to choose additional fat servings for that day.

Margarine has become a favorite alternative to butter because it is lower in saturated fat and cholesterol. However, you must choose your margarine wisely and use it carefully since butter and margarine have the same number of calories and fat grams. The margarine should consist of at least 3 times the unsaturated fat as saturated fat. That is, if there is 1 gram of saturated fat on the label per serving, then there should be at least 3 grams of unsaturated fat in the same serving. Buy margarine made from corn, safflower, or soybean oil. The soft tub-style of margarine is better, since the manufacturers of the stick-style margarine must further hydrogenate the product to give it solidity. The resulting "trans-fats" have been shown to be just as damaging in your body as saturated fat itself.

Check the labels the next time you are in the

grocery store and pick out a brand or two that fits the bill, then you'll always know automatically which one to reach for. Read the labels carefully since there is great variation in ingredients between brands. If you can tolerate butter, cholesterol-wise, it is a natural product without artificial colors, flavors and preservatives. However, use it sparingly. Diet margarine allows you to use 2 teaspoons for each serving. They are pumped up mostly with water and contain about half the calories of regular margarine. Surprisingly, they can be used in baking as well as cooking with good results. Promise has a new totally fat-free margarine. I like it, some people don't. Check it out for yourself.

Vegetable oils are a good alternative to solid shortenings and can be used successfully in many recipes including baked goods. These oils are extracted from seeds, nuts and vegetables, contain no cholesterol and are high in unsaturated fats or monounsaturated fats.

Various extraction methods affect the quality of the oils greatly, due to the heat used ... higher heat being more injurious to the oils. Buy cold-pressed and/or expeller-pressed oils available in the health food section of most supermarkets. Buy dark glass bottles, not clear, as light destroys nutrients. Oils are very susceptible to spoiling, so keep them in the refrigerator after opening. Discard if there is a rancid odor. The oils that harden in the refrigerator, such as olive and peanut, can be kept in a cool, dark cupboard for ease of use. Buy safflower, soybean, canola, corn, olive, peanut or sesame oils. The last three oils have specific and strong flavors of their own and should be used in recipes where this flavor is desired. I use safflower and canola oils for general purpose. Olive and canola oils, being mostly monounsaturated, are your healthiest choices. The amount of oil or margarine needed in cooking is surprisingly small. However, once you get used to the reduced amount, even that will seem to be too much at times.

Artificial butter substitutes such as Butter Buds and Molly McButter that are granulated and either sprinkled from a bottle like a spice or reconstituted into a liquid form can be a real treat since they contain only about 4 calories per serving. They come in various flavors such as cheese, bacon and sour cream. However, they contain some butter and buttermilk solids hence some saturated fat and, of course, dairy products, so are not suitable for the vegan vegetarian (those who consume no animal products at all). Also, watch the sodium content of these products and use sparingly.

Non-stick cooking sprays are either made from lecithin, a soy bean derivative, or are simply sprayed vegetable oils and contain no cholesterol.

They're very low in calories and now come in various flavors such as butter, olive oil and garlic. They 're excellent for stir-fries and sautéing vegetables, as well as for keeping foods from sticking to your baking pans and casseroles. I especially like the butter-flavor spray on air-popped popcorn. By first spraying lightly, the seasonings I sprinkle on top stick better. A light spray on pancakes or waffles gives them a shot of flavor. You can also spray a light coating on top of foods such as vegetables, chicken or fish before placing them in the oven to be baked. This helps keep them from drying out during baking. Sautéing in water, broth, wine or lemon juice are excellent low-fat alternatives to frying in oil and non-stick surfaces on your pans are a big help, too.

Sweeteners

It seems that practically no one can live for long without craving some form of sweet. Sweets have become a way of life ever since the turn of the century when improved processing methods made refined sugars widely available at reasonable cost. America's love affair with sugar has pushed our level of consumption, on average, to over 120 pounds per year for each of us. That's nearly one pound every 3 days! "I don't eat that much!" you say? Sugar is found in the most unlikely foods, as you will see.

Some people have chosen to eliminate refined sugar from their diets for reasons of health. That means others eat even more than the national average. One study done with children in Washington state revealed that the average consumption of refined sugar among these youngsters was an incredible 274 pounds per year! Nearly three-quarters of a pound per day. And that figure has been rising steadily. Early 1800's = 2 pounds per year average consumption. Late 1800's = 40 pounds per year. 1910 = 70 pounds. 1990 = 128 pounds of refined sugar consumed annually by the average person in the United States. We now eat more sugar in one week than our ancestors ate in a years time. This fact suggests not only the increased availability of refined sugar, but the addictive nature of the substance. It now takes more sugar to fill the need that a smaller amount did before. Dr. John Yudkin, a professor of Nutrition at London University in England, states in his book, Sweet and Dangerous, that sugar is, indeed, addictive. The more of it contained in the diet, the more is needed to satisfy the craving for sweets, just like drugs. Often, during the first week of a food plan which eliminates refined sugar, withdrawal headaches are reported. Many people mistake this as a symptom of not enough food and give up an otherwise good plan as a result. It has been suggested that if refined sugar was introduced today, it would not be approved by the FDA. It's too dangerous.

Sugar consumption has been scientifically linked to serious health problems including diabetes, heart disease, elevated triglyceride levels, obesity (which has many related health problems of its own), tooth decay, hyperactivity, depression and other mental disorders, hypoglycemia, allergies and cancer. Sugar chemistry in the body is very complex and these findings are constantly being challenged. But, to my mind, if I can choose a natural sweetener, whose effect on my health is known to be positive and is not in question, then the choice is clear. If the researchers discover later that sugar "just" causes cavities and that's all, then I may choose to imbibe occasionally and brush my teeth afterwards. For right now, with all the better alternatives, why take risks? You can hardly avoid all sugar, but cutting down drastically will improve your weight control efforts. Sugar affects your blood sugar levels and insulin sensitivity in ways that make it harder to burn fat. After dietary fat itself, sugar should be your next targeted food to eliminate.

Refined white sugar (sucrose) can be found in most prepackaged, canned and frozen foods available, although it is one of the least nutritious foods around. It contains absolutely no vitamins, minerals or fiber. As a result of having no fiber it is absorbed very quickly by the body and can cause blood sugar levels to rise and fall dramatically. This effect has been linked to dramatic mood swings, headaches, irritability and also fatigue when the body's blood sugar crashes through the floor after the sugar high.

Another problem with sugar over-consumption is that this non-food is very dense in calories. You can consume hundreds of calories worth of chocolate before being satisfied. One ounce of chocolate contains about 150 calories. An apple, high in fiber and around 80 calories, on the other hand is a much more nutritious choice. Refined sugar is a completely empty food and people who consume it on a regular basis may skip the more nutritious foods that could be adding to their health instead of tearing it down.

The obvious sugar-rich foods include table sugar, brown sugar, powdered sugar, drinks such as sweetened fruit juices and soda pop, jams, syrup, jellies, candy, cookies, cakes, pies, donuts, ice cream, presweetened cereals and canned fruit in syrup.

Finding all the rest of the refined sugar in your diet, in order to eliminate as much as possible, is not necessarily an easy task. About 65% of the sugar you consume is in unlikely sources. Some of the more surprising foods that contain sugar include commercially baked goods such as breads, rolls, muffins, and crackers; ketchup; salad dressings and mayonnaise; frozen fruit and sometimes vegetables; canned goods of all sorts including tomato products; spaghetti sauce; baked beans; pickled foods such as beets and bean salad; soups; sweetened yogurt; peanut butter; cured or pickled meats and fish; frozen dinners; flavored coffee, tea and hot cocoa mixes; and non-dairy creamers.

It seems you must become a trained investigator to discover all the sources of hidden refined sugar! Again, buy fresh and cook from scratch whenever possible. This is still the best way to make sure that some sugar doesn't get slipped into your diet by mistake. Make it a habit to read all labels for sugar content (as well as sodium, fat and calories!). A few of the names that refined sugar goes by are brown sugar, corn syrup, dextrose, fructose, glucose, lactose, maltose, malt syrup, molasses, and sucrose. If any of these ingredients are listed as one of the first three on a label, it would be better to pass that food up and look for or create a more healthful version.

There are many alternative sweeteners that can be used in different food preparation situations. Although some of these sweeteners do contain significant amounts of nutrients they can still affect your blood sugar in adverse ways if eaten in large amounts, so be careful! Use sugar as sparingly as possible and cut back gradually until you are eating only small amounts of refined sugars, if any, and mostly fruit, fruit juices and natural grain sweeteners. This will probably take some time as we are generally hooked on sugar, so be patient and just make improvements whenever you can. A cutting back program, similar to the one used to reduce salt intake, can be helpful and relatively painless. Start by reducing added sugar by about $\frac{1}{4}$ to $\frac{1}{3}$. When you get used to that, then cut back by another $\frac{1}{4}$ and so on.

The new food labels have made it a lot easier to see just how much sugar you're getting in each serving of the food in question. Check the label and you will see the sugar content of foods listed in terms of grams. It is recommended by health professionals that you get no more than 10% of your calories from sugars, so if you are eating 1200 calories that is 120 calories of sugar or 30 grams a day. If you're a man eating 1600 calories a day, then 160 of those calories can come from sugar, or 40 grams daily. Keep in mind that these are upper limits. There are no lower limits. In other words, you don't have to eat any at all, and less is better for all the reasons discussed.

What follows is a list of the more common sweeteners, so you can choose the appropriate form for your needs. Starting with the most refined and least desirable:

Sucrose - White table sugar. No vitamins, no minerals, no dietary fiber. Nothing but calories. Most refined result of processing sugar beet or sugar cane by pressing, chemically treating the juice and crystallizing by cooking. A series of extractions then produces several different products with white table sugar being the last. Widely used in processed foods.

Raw or turbinado sugar - This is the first extraction of processed beet or sugar cane and is 99% sucrose. Turbinado is even more highly refined than raw sugar.

Molasses - The second extraction of processing beet or sugar cane. Significant amounts of calcium and minerals and lowered amount of sucrose.

Black strap molasses - The final extraction of processed beet or sugar cane, therefore containing the least amount of sucrose and most nutrients such as calcium, iron and chromium.

Brown sugar - Made by adding small amounts of molasses or caramel coloring to white sugar. Small amounts of trace minerals but mostly sucrose.

Maple syrup - A natural sweetener made by boiling down the sap of the sugar maple tree. Although it is 66% sucrose, it contains significant amounts of calcium and trace minerals. Buy pure maple syrup without preservatives or additives. It has a wonderfully distinctive flavor. Containing about the same number of calories as sugar, it is much sweeter, so you can use less in cooking. Reduced-calorie versions are really just sucrose or glucose syrups with maple flavoring, usually artificial.

Honey - Long a favorite with the health crowd. This tasty sweetener, when used in refined form, is actually almost identical in nutrition to sucrose and acts the same in the body. Honey may contain small amounts of trace minerals, however. Unrefined honey also contains bee pollen which is very nutritious. Since it is so concentrated it can contribute to obesity and blood sugar instability if abused. And since it is so sticky, it clings to teeth and contributes even more than sucrose to cavities. Buy unheated and unfiltered natural honey to preserve nutrients. It 's about twice as sweet as sucrose, but has only 25% more calories ... used wisely, you can reduce total calories in cooking. It has a lovely, unique taste and comes in a variety of flavors, indicating the origin of the pollen, such as clover, orange, blackberry, etc. Some vegans do not eat honey as it is an animal product.

Sucanat - The name stands for "sugar cane natural", thus su-ca-nat. Made from the juice of the sugar cane plant, only the fiber and water are removed. All of the nutrients are retained, including many minerals, calcium, B and E vitamins. Think of it as whole grain sugar. It looks like a granulated brown sugar and can be purchased in health food stores and health food sections of larger supermarkets. Used measure for measure like sugar in cooking, it imparts a slightly stronger flavor. One of my favorites.

FruitSource - Brand name of another natural sweetener sold in health food stores or health food sections of larger supermarkets. It is made from rice syrup and grape juice concentrate. You can buy it in liquid or granulated form and use it like sugar or syrup respectively.

Grain sweeteners - Natural sweeteners made from various grains such as barley, sorghum, rice and corn. The grain is sprouted, allowed to ferment and the resulting liquid is cooked down to a syrup. Significantly more nutritious than white sugar and each grain produces a different level of sweetness and a unique taste. I use many of these syrups in my recipes and you can find them in your health food section or store under the names of rice syrup, barley malt, sorghum molasses, amasake and pure corn syrup (not Karo which is made from refined cornstarch).

Fruit - These gems are the ideal way to satisfy your sweet tooth, but you have to know how to use them in recipes. Sometimes an apple just won't cut it! Contains varying significant amounts of nutrients and usually a large amount of fiber which slows down the absorption of sugars in your body and satisfies by filling you up. Some of the sweetest fruits are bananas, apples, pears and grapes. These can be used in various forms in recipes calling for sweetness. Baking brings out the sweetness of some fruits, also. Ripe fruit is the sweeter, but contains no more calories than unripe fruit! Place fruit in a paper bag with a few holes in it and ripen for a few days to increase sweetness. Buy organic if you can and wash all fruit thoroughly with a soft brush in mild veggie soap and water, then rinse to reduce pesticide residues.

Dried fruit is highly concentrated and can be combined with other foods to make them sweeter (such as hot cereal or carrot salad). Buy the highly nutritious, unsulfered varieties and use sparingly, so you don't upset blood sugar levels and calorie consumption. Date sugar (ground dates in granulated form) is very sweet and can be used like sugar.

Fruit juices - Again, significant amounts of nutrients and a concentrated sweetener. Fresh pressed juices are best since more nutrients and fiber are retained. Use within 20 minutes of juicing for maximum nutrition. However, fresh frozen may also be used. Concentrates are ideal forms when needing a very sweet taste and can be kept conveniently in the freezer. I use them often in baking. Drink undiluted juice sparingly since it is highly concentrated and may effect your blood sugar abruptly.

Vegetables - Yes, even veggies can be a source of sweetness when used properly. Carrots, beets and yams are examples of vegetables that are surprisingly sweet when used in certain recipes such as pies, cakes and salads. Combining them with dried fruits, fruit juices or grain sweeteners is also very effective.

Since there are so many varieties of sweeteners there is no reason to depend on the empty calories and possible health hazards of white sugar, right?! Experiment and soon you will find your favorite natural sweeteners. I love hot cereal on a chilly winter morning made with fruit juice replacing some of the water, dried fruit cooked into it, garnished with a chopped banana and drizzled with pure maple syrup! Who needs sugar?

Flours

If you have been accustomed to eating and cooking with only highly refined white flour, then you're in for a treat! The nutritional content of whole grain flours is far superior to refined flours and the full-bodied texture and rich flavor of a whole grain bread is so wonderful that it will be hard to return to the insubstantial quality of white flour. Any baked good such as pie crusts, cakes, cookies, coffee cakes and quick breads are much more satisfying when whole grain flours are used.

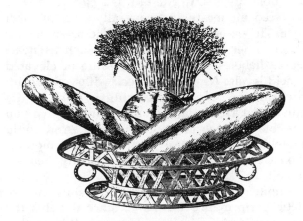

When you first begin to experiment, the heavier texture and flavor may overwhelm your taste buds so I suggest mixing the heavier flours with a lighter flour such as unbleached white. There is even a new product called "white wheat flour" with all the nutrition of whole wheat and a texture close to white flour when baked. Use it in all foods where a lighter texture is desired. It's available from the King Arthur Flour Company.

Whole grain flours contain all the elements of the grain such as the bran and the germ (which contains oil). Because of the increased bran content it would be wise to introduce these whole grains into your diet gradually, as the increased fiber may effect your digestive tract (see Chapter 33 "Fiber is Your Friend"). Because of the oil content, be sure to refrigerate all flour to preserve freshness. Buy high-fat flours such as soy and peanut (and also wheat germ) from a refrigerated case. However, freezing them will destroy the vitamin E.

There are many flours to experiment with and each one gives a distinctive flavor and texture to the finished product. Oat flour, rice flour, soy flour (high protein and fat content ... defatted soy flour is available), wonderful fragrant whole wheat flour, barley flour and amaranth flour are all excellent alternatives to plain old refined white flour. I'm sure white flour started out as a good idea, but now that we know better nutritionally, there really is no excuse to continue eating a substance that has had all of the nutrients stripped away and then a few synthetic vitamins pumped back in as an attempt to "enrich" the sad product. The superior nutritional content alone is plenty to cause a person to begin adding whole grains to their diet, but what really hooks most people is the marvelous taste, aroma and texture of these whole foods. Once you get to know whole grain flours, you'll be hooked.

Caffeine

The bad news about caffeine

Just about as many health problems have been pinned on caffeine as have been associated with white sugar. Interesting, isn't it, how they seem to go hand in hand? (One lump or two? Coffee and donuts.) Everything from cardiovascular disease, raising of LDL (bad) cholesterol levels, certain cancers, severe headaches such as migraines, sleep disorders, breast disease, birth defects, miscarriage, infertility, osteoporosis, glaucoma, mood swings and indigestion have been documented in laboratory studies. Then other studies come along and successfully refute those previous findings. It can be very confusing!

One problem lies in the fact that we're all individuals and as such we each react to this powerful drug in differing degrees. A person's size is one factor that determines the extent of the effects. A child, for instance will be affected just as much by a small cola as a man may be by 3 cups of coffee. Some people are just more susceptible to certain maladies, such as headaches and indigestion than others. Pregnant or lactating women may pass the caffeine on to their far more sensitive offspring. Even men who use caffeine regularly may affect the new fetus by passing it along in their sperm. Anyone who does not use caffeine at all or who has not had any in several days will be much more affected than someone who is used to a regular dose. And it seems that other risk factors for health problems including poor diets, lack of exercise, type-A personalities using inadequate or no stress-reduction methods and smoking are often present in heavy caffeine users. Certainly these factors could significantly affect health and research results in unpredictable ways, causing variable and contradictory conclusions.

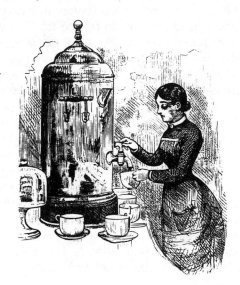

Woman overboard on the S. S. Espresso!

Two properties of caffeine that are not desirable for weight loss are its diuretic action, causing you to need even more water to make up for the lost amount in your system (remember, your body needs and uses the water you drink to help it run smoothly) and substances called caffeols that can cause hunger. But I will outsmart those party pooper caffeols in just a moment.

By the way, research on decaffeinated coffee is not as complete as that on caffeinated. But if you opt for decaf because of the substantially lowered caffeine amount, it seems that the water processed kind is the best choice since it doesn't use chemical solvents with questionable health safety during the decaffeination process. The other 700 (!) substances in coffee, however, may still cause health problems such as irritated digestive tract or interference with the absorption of certain minerals such as iron and calcium.

The good news about caffeine

What is caffeine and what does it do in your body? Caffeine is a natural substance, one of a group of compounds called methylxanthines, found in over 60 cultivated plants and trees. However, it is considered a psychoactive drug since it directly stimulates neurotransmitters (the "chemical messengers" that transmit messages between nerve cells) such as norepinephrin and dopamine in the brain. These actions produce the well-known effects of heightened alertness and shortened reaction times. The ability to think clearer and connect thoughts and ideas more easily makes caffeine useful for studying and taking tests as long as you don't go overboard. What?! I can hear some of you screaming all the way to Oregon! Yes, there are some benefits to caffeine consumption, just like other useful drugs, as long as it is done intelligently and not abused.

One of caffeine's most relevant and interesting uses is its ability to briefly increase resting metabolism. Higher metabolism means more calories burned. This I like. As reported in the American Journal of Clinical Nutrition, researchers at the University of Geneva tested people who had never been overweight and ones who had been overweight but were now thin (that's me, and you too as soon as you lose the weight). A single cup of coffee (100 mg of caffeine) caused them all to increase calories burned by 3-4% over the next 2½ hours. Doesn't sound like much, but when they had a cup every 2 hours for 12 hours, the total calories burned increased by as much as 11%. That could be 130 calories a day! And following a meal, the formerly fat increased their heat production even more than the never-fat ones.

I don't recommend drinking that much coffee considering all the other health risks that you could possibly bring on. But 1-2 cups a day is considered moderate and generally safe for most people. The exceptions are those who are pregnant or have other medical conditions such as heart disease, diabetes, high blood pressure or elevated uric acid levels. As always, check with your health professional before changing your habits significantly! This small amount will still give you a possible increase in calorie-burning. And could definitely be significant over the course of months. A boost for the sluggish, yet basically healthy metabolism.

Another benefit of caffeine is the enhancing of athletic performance for some, since it helps the body break down fats for energy use. Why is that good? With the fat being used first, it saves the glycogen which is usually used first, for later. Then later in the workout, there is still some glycogen left and thus you can perform your exercise longer. And of course, when you are looking to lose fat, longer and slower exercise does the trick better than anything. In a sense, you will be just like an endurance athlete when you work up to exercising an hour at a stretch. It won't do any good for shorter workouts though. And for some people, it doesn't make any difference at all. Individual differences become even more important when you put them together with two variables, caffeine and exercise.

So how much caffeine is in common drinks, foods and other substances? As I mentioned above, a 6 ounce cup of coffee generally contains 100 mg of caffeine. But here again is a case of averages. For instance, a rounded teaspoon of instant coffee has about 55-100 mg and drip or brewed has 80-175 mg. The wide variation is because of the type of coffee, fineness of the grind and type of brewing filter and method. Decaffeinated coffee contains about 5 mg, tea (brewed 3 minutes) 30 mg but brewed 5 minutes 70-100 mg, cola drinks 30-45 mg.

Contrary to popular belief, chocolate and hot cocoa don't have very much caffeine at all unless you eat a couple of pounds, in which case you have more to worry about than the 7-10 mg of caffeine per ounce. Bittersweet chocolate has about 35 mg per ounce though. Chocolate cake or coffee-flavored yogurt could have significant amounts ... in the range of 25-45 mg.

You may be surprised to find out that certain medications have quite a bit of caffeine. Take two Excedrin and you'll also get 130 mg! Anacin or Midol have 64 mg per two tabs. And of course you would expect a big dose, 200 mg for two tablets of over-the-counter medications to either stay awake or lose water. Diet pills are heavily loaded with caffeine. Check the labels carefully.

As in most things, it's good old moderation that's key to healthy, wise choices with caffeine. If you have any of the symptoms or conditions discussed above, then caffeine may not be for you. The human body does not need it at all to survive, so if you don't imbibe, then there is no reason to start. If you drink more than 5 cups a day you're running the risk for potential health problems down the line. But 1-2 cups a day is moderate and there is no reason to believe it compromises health if your system tolerates it and you don't have any existing conditions. Use your common sense. I have a mug in the morning (80% decaf) because I enjoy the taste and it gets me going in a pleasant way. More than that and I am worthless and grouchy. I have another before a long morning workout and find the time goes quicker and I don't get tired. Often in a restaurant or even at home, I enjoy a cup, usually half decaf-half regular, after a meal. That's how I outsmart those caffeols I mentioned earlier. After, or with a meal, it doesn't matter whether caffeols try to make me hungry, because I'm already eating or full! So there, ha ha! And during a workout, my endorphins are flowing and I'm again not hungry, so their effect is limited. Experiment for yourself and maybe you can also use caffeine to your advantage while enjoying the wonderful taste and aroma of roasted coffee beans.

In A Nutshell

1) Get the most nutrition out of every morsel you eat!

2) Buy properly produced vegetable oils and store them correctly. Buy "acceptable" margarine and use substitutes where possible to save calories, fat and cholesterol.

3) Eliminate as much empty refined sugar as possible by checking labels and limiting obvious sources.

4) Experiment and use a variety of natural sweeteners instead of sugar.

5) Use a variety of properly produced and stored whole grain flours and cereals instead of devitalized white flour.

6) Caffeine can cause many health problems. It can also be used for possible enhanced calorie burning and athletic endurance. Know yourself and be moderate. Check with your health professional first before adding any caffeine to your diet.

7) Question all ingredients and go for the most nutritious choice each time you have an opportunity.

8) Small changes add up to big nutritional benefits!

The THINNER WINNERS Kitchen   28

"I will make a palace fit for you and me. Of green days in forest and blue days at sea. I will make my kitchen ... "
Robert Louis Stevenson

You probably have many of the foods and items listed below, but just in case you're starting from scratch, here are some basic staples that will help you get started. Remember to respect your tastes and keep on hand those items that are your particular favorite flavors or types. For instance if you just love chocolate (anybody else out there besides me?) and you can handle having it around right now, then be sure to keep the ingredients on hand to whip up something that will satisfy that chocolate urge ... a healthy version, of course! Keep a variety of foods on hand so that if you have a hankering for a certain dish you won't be caught with your cupboard bare and end up eating something that doesn't really satisfy you.

Shopping Tips
Health Begins in the Supermarket

Before you even set foot inside your local market, there are a few things you need to do. First of all, make a shopping list for yourself. I'm sure you've heard this tip before, because it's a very valid one. A lot of the goodies that are brought into the house are a reaction to the packaging, display and marketing of the product. It just looks so great that you must have it. Impulse buying. But you will not fall prey to this ploy any longer, right? You're going to the store well prepared with a list of the items you need from the food plan you have made for the week. Shopping will still be fun ... and a lot less caloric. When I want to buy a goodie nowadays, I head for the houseware or kitchenware section, office supplies, cosmetics, books or magazines, floral section or any other non-food section now available in our superstores. I may indulge my need to bring home something unique and new to eat in the produce section or the reduced-calorie foods section or the health-food section. Don't go roaming around the bakery, cookie, chip, candy or deli sections hoping to find that special no-calorie health goodie. It just won't happen.

Another condition to be aware of in the typical grocery store is the layout of the store itself. Generally, the fresh produce, fish, meats, dairy and bread sections are arranged around the perimeter of the store. These are the sections that you will be visiting most since the foods here are the least processed. Buying fresh and cooking from scratch is the best way to insure the least amount of additives such as sugar, sodium and artificial ingredients. As soon as you get into the aisles, beware ... danger lurks! That's where almost all of the processed foods are found. The canned goods, frozen goodies, row upon row of cookies, crackers, candy, alcohol, sodas, snack foods, tobacco products and more that you just as well could buy fresh, if at all, most of the time. A few convenience items and staples are all right, but get in the habit of sticking to the outside walls most of the time and you'll do much better.

Of course, never go to the grocery store when you're hungry. Everything will look good to you and more of it will end up in your shopping cart. Also, try to shop during a less hurried time of the day and week than Saturday morning or 5 P.M. on weekdays. This will allow you a more relaxed, uncrowded visit and a much more enjoyable shopping experience. I love to just hang around reading labels, checking out new products and communing with the lovely vibrations of all that gorgeous food. Take your time and enjoy it. Food is your friend after all ... just be sure your food friends aren't deadbeats.

Following these suggestions will raise your awareness of the grocery store environment and keep you from buying those items that you may regret later. Stick to them and happy shopping!

Here are some basic health-promoting foods you can begin to stock in your refrigerator and pantry:

These are some of my kitchen standards. I'm sure you'll discover your own favorites as you explore the supermarkets with new, healthier goals in mind. Watch salt, fat, sugar, and artificial ingredients when choosing. Let me know what you find that's good.

Berries - fresh or frozen ... strawberries, blueberries, raspberries, etc.

Beverages - WATER!, a variety of herbal teas (orange, lemon, mint, Celestial Seasonings varieties), flavored mineral waters (raspberry, mango, lemon, orange, lime, etc.), flavored coffees (mostly decaffeinated if possible) in a variety of flavors such as chocolate brandy, Irish cream mint, vanilla cream, hazelnut, etc., low sodium club soda. If you choose to drink sodas, pick no-caffeine, no-sugar, low-sodium varieties. Natural soft drinks are available, but they also have sweeteners and calories.

Breads (whole grain) - bagels, corn or whole wheat tortillas (with no lard), pita pockets, reduced calorie breads (wheat, oat, cinnamon, rye, 7-grain, buns, etc.). There are many good brands ... read the ingredients. French or Italian baguettes, rolls, English muffins, crumpets.

Butter substitutes - Molly McButter (regular, sour cream, cheese, bacon flavor), Butter Buds, no-stick butter spray, refrigerated butter spray.

Cereals - dry cereals such as amaranth flakes, Fiber One, Nutrigrain, shredded wheat, Grapenuts, puffed varieties, Healthy O's, fat-free granola, (favorite brands are Health Valley, Barbara's, Erewhon, Bob's). Hot cereals such as Zoom, Wheatena, Cream of Wheat, oat bran, cream of rice, cream of rye, oatmeal, Roman Meal, etc.).

Cheese - As a general rule cheese is high in fat and sodium but in moderate amounts it's a standard in many recipes. Use grated parmesan cheese or low-fat varieties.

Chips - health food variety (Skinny Munchies, Barbara's no-salt pretzels), homemade varieties (pita, potato, tortilla), Guiltless Gourmet, Rice Bites, No-Fries.

Dressings - reduced calorie and fat-free versions of mayonnaise & whipped salad dressing, no-oil salad dressings, no-fat sour cream (I use this on everything!)

Eggs - use whites only, or egg substitutes.

Extracts and Flavorings - coffee, vanilla, almond, orange, banana, rum, chocolate, lemon, butter, brandy, peppermint, mint, etc. Try for natural.

Flour - whole wheat flour (regular and pastry) or whole grains if you grind your own, specialty flours such as buckwheat or rice, arrowroot, cornstarch, baking powder (low-sodium), baking soda, buttermilk powder, cocoa or carob powder.

Frozen foods - keep a wide variety in stock, including complete dinners and lunches in healthy versions (check the sodium and fat contents on the label carefully), desserts, frozen yogurt, frozen fruits and juices, breads can be frozen (bagels,

tortillas, pita bread, etc.), vegetables (spinach, corn, peas, pearl onions, artichoke hearts and many combinations are available ... these are a boon when you're rushed, or looking for out-of-season vegetables), frozen egg substitute (Egg Beaters, Second Nature, etc.), Ore-Ida hash browns, vegetarian sausage and Garden Burgers (Wholesome and Hearty Foods).

Fruit - Fresh! Try them all.

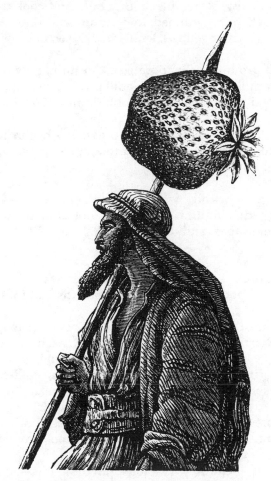

Early vegetarian returning from the hunt.

Fruit (water or juice packed) - apple slices or pie cherries in pie filling section, peaches, pears, pineapple, etc.

Fruits and juice concentrates - apple, orange, pineapple, etc.

Grains - barley, oats and oat bran, millet, corn meal, polenta, popcorn (you can grind popcorn to make your own corn meal), whole wheat.

Herbs and Spices - parsley, dill, basil, mint, cilantro, garlic powder (not salt!), onion powder, black pepper, cayenne pepper (red), chili powder, oregano, curry, cumin, minced onions, bay leaves, marjoram, thyme, cinnamon, nutmeg, ginger (see Chapter 34 "Sodium & Salt vs. Herbs & Spices"). Herbs and spices (blends) - salt-free herb blends (Mrs. Dash, Parsley Patch, etc.), filé gumbo, pumpkin pie spice, homemade varieties.

Jams - all fruit, of course.

Legumes - beans such as garbanzo, kidney, lima, pinto, navy, white, black. Buy bulk and cook them yourself, or buy canned, low-sodium and rinse. Split peas (green or yellow), lentils (red, green or brown).

Milk products - Evaporated skim milk, powdered skim milk, Rice Dream (vanilla, carob or regular), almond milk, lite soy milk , buttermilk (1%).

Oils (cold-pressed, expeller-pressed) - health food section, safflower, soy, canola, peanut, sesame, olive, hot sesame oil.

Pasta - whole wheat or vegetable lasagna, spaghetti, linguini, angel hair, hot chili flavored. More shapes and flavors than I could list in a month.

Potatoes - baked, mashed, Barbara's instant mashed potatoes, Ore-Ida hash browns and fries.

Reduced calorie foods such as syrup (maple, blueberry, etc.), flavored gelatins, hard candies, gum,   sugar substitutes such as Equal or Sweet One (if tolerated),margarine, cookies, cold-cuts, cheese, dairy products, hot cocoa, bread, frozen desserts, ice-cream, mayonnaise , salad dressings ... almost everything comes in a reduced calorie and often reduced fat version these days. Look around!

Relish - chutney (various flavors), low-sodium pickle relish.

Rice - brown, wild, special blends, instant, basmati.

Sauces - Low-sodium soy sauce, teriyaki sauce, hoisin sauce (for marinades, stir fry), Tabasco sauce, Worcestershire sauce (lower in sodium than soy, very flavorful), Wright's smoke flavoring, barbecue sauce, steak sauce, seafood cocktail sauce, tartar sauce (non-fat), Oriental stir-fry sauces such as peanut or hot chili (use just a touch for flavor).

Seasonings - see Herbs and Spices above.

Seeds - sesame, poppy, caraway, pumpkin, etc.

Soups - bouillon cubes or powder (low sodium varieties), Health Valley canned veggie soups.

Spices - see Herbs and Spices above.

Sprays (non-stick cooking type) - regular, butter-flavor, olive oil flavor, garlic flavor, canola.

Spreads - stone ground mustard (low sodium available), regular mustard (various flavors), non-fat mayonnaise, ketchup (low sodium and sugar), horseradish (not creamed).

Stock (defatted) - Pritikan, homemade, low-sodium cubes or powders.

Sweeteners such as frozen concentrated apple and orange juice, honey, grain sweeteners (barley syrup, rice syrup, etc. found in the health food section), fructose, maple syrup, date sugar, jams and all-fruit preserves, Sucanat (natural cane sugar) or FruitSource (natural fruit sugar).

Syrups - Maple and blueberry (lo-cal varieties), butter flavor.

Thickeners - arrowroot, cornstarch, mashed potatoes or sweet potatoes, agar, flaxseed gel, nut butters, lecithin, bean liquid.

Tomato products such as tomato sauce (Del Monte or Hunt's low-salt versions), paste, puree, whole canned, no-oil spaghetti sauce, salsa (all reduced-sodium varieties if possible). Pure & Simple no-salt salsa. S&W 50% less salt stewed tomatoes.

Vegetables - Fresh! Some basic ones to keep around for recipes would be celery, onions (yellow or brown, green, red), garlic, lemons, tomatoes, ginger if you like Chinese food, peppers (green, red, chili, yellow, purple), potatoes, squash, broccoli, carrots, mushrooms, etc.

Vegetables (low sodium canned and bottled) corn, beans, S & W lo-salt garbanzo, kidney and black beans, (Eden).

Vinegars (flavored) - rice, herb, basalmic, fruit, wine vinegar (red, white), apple cider.

Wine - tenderizes, flavors and moistens. Try for sulfite-free.

Noteworthy brands
with multiple health-oriented products

Health Valley Foods - chili, soup, granola bars, cookies, cereal, many excellent products.
Healthy Choice - frozen meals.
Life Choice - frozen meals.
Ore-Ida - hash browns, fries.
Pritikan - spaghetti sauce, salad dressings and marinades, broth, dip mix, frozen foods.
Weight Watchers - defatted peanuts (regular and honey roast), shake mixes, crisp bread, popcorn, individual servings of chips, puffs, frozen foods.
Wholesome & Hearty - Garden Burgers , Mexi-Burgers, Garden Sausage.

Handy Contraptions
to Make Kitchen Life Easier

Heavy **cookware with lids** - enamel-coated cast iron is nice, or non-stick. Include a skillet with a lid and a griddle.

Food processor or blender - The food processor really helps the chopping/shredding chores go faster.

Indoor grill - non-stick.

Mini food processor - I have really found this to be useful when chopping small amounts of onion, other vegetables or herbs. Also it is perfect for making just one or two servings of ricotta-based dip or one serving of frozen banana ice cream.

Garlic press - If you like garlic as I do. I find the Zyliss press excellent. Terra cotta garlic/onion roaster.

Glass baking dishes - assorted sizes such as 8x8, 9x13, loaf.

A good set of **knives and a cutting board** (wood for veggies, plastic for meats).

Set of standard **measuring cups and spoons.**

Microwave oven or toaster oven - (very handy, but a conventional oven will do nicely).

Muffin tin, baking (cookie) sheet and pizza pan - non-stick if possible.

Sandwich griller - non-stick.

A small **food scale that measures in ounces** - a must in the beginning, so you can get used to the right portion sizes and what they look like.

Nice **serving dishes** to attractively serve your creations.

Vegetable steamer basket - (the microwave also does a nice job of steaming, too).

In A Nutshell

1) Plan your supermarket strategy in advance ... make a list.

2) Stock up on basic foods that will be ready to help you prepare healthy meals and snacks.

3) Substitute healthier foods when you can. My favorites are listed.

4) A few well-chosen contraptions can help the preparation and serving of foods go faster, easier and more enjoyably.

Sample Meals   29

"Let us keep the feast ... with the bread of sincerity and truth."
The Bible

Meal Suggestions

Please let me emphasize, the following meal suggestions are just that, suggestions. They are not set in stone, although you may follow them as written if you wish. From my experience, I know that as soon as Friday night fettucine comes along, the suggested meal plan goes out the window. This, in itself, is not bad (see Chapter 5 "Motivation and the Success Mindset", especially "Balance"). However, the psychological state of "going off" the plan, usually accompanied with a what-the-heck attitude encourages you to overeat and order the cheesecake, too. Self-esteem plummets and for the next few days you're off in Binge-Land somewhere, feeling like you'll always be fat and what's the use of trying anyway. To avoid this occurrence, please think of these meal plans as guidelines only. Learn from my experience and don't waste as many years as I did trying to stick rigorously to someone else's plan. If you order and eat Fettucine Alfredo (with its creamy, high-fat sauce), then just enjoy it and count it the best (and most honest!) way you can towards your daily servings. If you're over your daily limits, then cut back for a few days so it averages out. Similarly, feel free to substitute your favorite foods instead of the ones suggested if they don't appeal to you. Be sure to keep them in the same categories, of course, such as a fruit for a fruit and a protein for a protein, etc. On the other hand, the basic structure of the suggested meals is a good example of the balance for which you should be striving. Only in this way will you get a variety of foods and nutrients to satisfy both your emotional and physical needs. So with that out of the way, on to the food!

• See Chapter 30 "Basic Recipes to Get You Started" for recipes of foods with this symbol (*).
• Additional servings of the same or similar foods may be added for men as needed.
• See Chapter 26 "How to Eat" for suggested servings per day and serving sizes . Use the guidelines until you get a feel for how much food satisfies you while still losing weight at a healthy rate (1 to 1½ pounds. per week). Never overstuff, but don't go away hungry either.

Breakfasts

Magic Cream Dream Cereal *
Evaporated skim milk, rice or soy beverage
Fresh blueberries
Decaf coffee or herbal tea or beverage of your choice

Toast - Whole grain
Topped with fat-free margarine, cinnamon and a
    sprinkle of Sucanat (whole natural sugar cane) or Equal
Creme Caramel non-fat yogurt
    (mixed with psyllium or bran if desired)
Sliced fresh strawberries
Beverage

Scrambled egg whites with onions, green peppers and mushrooms
Whole wheat bagel with fat-free cream cheese and all-fruit jam
Fresh mixed-vegetable juice (or low-sodium if bottled)
Beverage

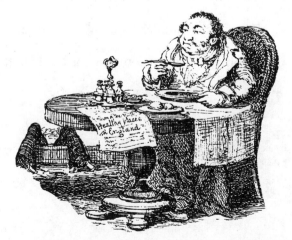

"Now that's what I call good eating!"

Whole Wheat Buttermilk Pancakes * (with light maple syrup) or Easy Fruit Topping*
Vegetarian low-fat sausage patty
Fresh cantaloupe
Beverage

Pita Pastries with Spiced Apples and Ricotta Cheese *
Beverage

Whole grain corn flake cereal (or other grain of your choice)
Lemon non-fat yogurt
Fresh blueberries (or frozen blueberries thawed)
Beverage

Cheese Toast (whole grain toast broiled with low or non-fat cheddar cheese)
Fresh tomato juice or low-sodium V-8
Beverage

Whole grain raisin English muffin, split and toasted
Top with low or non-fat ricotta cheese, sweetened if desired
Raisins mixed into the cheese
Beverage

Whole grain shredded wheat cereal
Skim milk, rice or soy beverage
Fresh-squeezed orange juice, 6 ounces, or sliced orange
Beverage

Cinnamon-raisin bagel, toasted (with fat-free margarine or all-fruit orange marmalade)
Fresh pineapple chunks
Non or low-fat cottage cheese
Beverage

Oat Bran Raisin Muffin*, or homemade healthy muffin
Fresh papaya chunks
Non-fat vanilla yogurt topping
Reduced-calorie hot cocoa or homemade non-dairy cocoa

Instant French Toast *
Sliced banana or fresh strawberries
Beverage

Spanish Omelet made with egg whites or egg substitute, non-fat cheddar cheese and salsa
Hash brown potatoes (Ore-Ida or homemade)
Sliced orange or juice
Beverage

Lunches

Pasta Salad (cooked pasta, chopped mixed veggies such as cherry tomato halves, red onion, broccoli, green
     pepper, celery or cauliflower). Serve in butter lettuce bowl.
Plain non-fat yogurt, sour cream or ricotta cheese plus herbs/spices for dressing
Fresh or frozen grapes

Tuna Melt (water-pack tuna on reduced-calorie or regular rye toast add sliced tomatoes, dill and low-fat
     cheddar cheese. Broil, or grill in non-stick sandwich griller ... a great invention!)
Onion-flavored natural potato crisps, individual bag (diet section of grocery store) or homemade Chips*
Versatile Vegetable Soup*

Tacos (sauté onion, garlic, green and red pepper add mashed kidney beans, diced green chilies, chili seasoning stuff into taco shells)
Shredded lettuce, sprouts, chopped tomatoes, salsa (low salt or homemade), 3 sliced black olives. Shredded low-fat cheddar cheese
Plain non-fat yogurt or non-fat sour cream
Reduced-calorie chocolate pudding

Turkey Sandwich (reduced-calorie or regular sourdough bread spread with all-fruit cranberry relish, fat-free mayo, lettuce, tomato, white meat turkey breast slices or vegetarian turkey)
Steamed cauliflower and broccoli florets with cheese-flavored sprinkles
Low-calorie or regular cranberry or cran-apple juice

Hearty Chili* (or Health Valley is excellent)
Pita Chips * or non-fat crackers
Green salad with chopped raw veggies (topped with no-oil Ranch dressing)
Milk, rice or soy beverage

Hamburger or Garden Burger (reduced-calorie or regular whole grain hamburger bun spread with fat-free 1000 Island dressing, tomato and red onion slice, lettuce, ground lean beef or turkey or vegetable-bean patty)
Homemade Fries (slice potato, sprinkle with onion powder, bake until crisp in single layer on baking sheet turning once)
Creamy Coleslaw*
Chocolate shake (reduced calorie)

Creamy Garlic Pasta* with pasta of your choice
Mixed steamed veggies (mix into pasta)
Iceberg lettuce wedge (topped with no-oil Creamy Italian dressing)
Cappuccino frozen yogurt or Cocoa-Banana Cream Fluff*

Spaghetti Squash and Salsa (fresh or no-salt) - heated, sprinkled with parmesan cheese
Babe Rosie Bar *
Sparkling cherry-flavored mineral water

Nutty Surprise Sandwich (Mix 1 TBL peanut butter with non-fat cottage or ricotta cheese and raisins spread on reduced-calorie or regular whole wheat toast, top with alfalfa sprouts and second slice of toast)
Jicama and carrot sticks
Reduced-calorie orange shake

Baked Potato (or microwaved) - Topped with non or low-fat cottage or ricotta cheese or yogurt, reduced-fat cheddar cheese (shredded), steamed broccoli florets and green onions sprinkled on top or stuffed with chili
Fresh pear slices
Peach diet soda

Homemade Split-Pea Soup or Warm-Hearted Lentil Soup*
Chili Cornbread * - topped with diet or regular margarine (Note: good cornbread does not need a spread!)
Mixed green salad with no-oil Russian dressing
Baked apple with cinnamon, nutmeg & topped with non-fat vanilla yogurt

Seafood Salad - tuna (or shellfish if your diet allows) and chopped tomato on salad greens
Non-fat plain yogurt mixed with non-fat tartar sauce or cocktail sauce
Whole grain breadsticks
Vegetable bouillon (low salt)
Sliced kiwi fruit and banana

Dinners

Stir-fry - made with carrots, broccoli, mushrooms, onion and garlic tossed with lemon juice, low-sodium soy
        sauce, fresh grated ginger and veggie broth, spices. ½ tsp sesame oil over top when done to season.
Brown rice
Fresh mandarin orange or orange diet gelatin or both

Pizza Parlor Veggie Pizza (made with low-fat mozzarella or order with either no cheese or
        "light on the cheese")
Salad bar with garbanzo and kidney beans (no-oil Italian dressing or vinegar or take your own dressing)
Sliced pear or other fresh fruit from salad bar

Baked halibut topped with lemon yogurt sauce
Steamed spinach with bacon sprinkles
Quick Orange-Mint Rice *
Reduced-calorie lemon gelatin with whipped topping

Bean and Cheese Burrito (mashed kidney or pinto beans, low-fat cheddar cheese, tomato, lettuce, green onions
        rolled in whole wheat tortilla and heated)
Sliced jicama with lime juice on fresh salad greens
Vanilla frozen yogurt or tofutti with Easy Hot Fruit Topping (Papaya)*

Simple Saucepan Soufflé with onions and green and/or red pepper, low-fat cheddar cheese (shredded)
Reduced calorie or regular whole grain toast with raspberry all-fruit jam
Baked banana with nutmeg and vanilla yogurt

Roast Turkey or Seitan*
Roast potatoes, carrots and onions seasoned with rosemary
Chunky Cranapple Sauce* on fresh salad greens
Fresh strawberries in reduced-calorie strawberry gelatin with whipped topping or low-fat pumpkin pie (use the
        recipe on the can, but practice your recipe conversion technique by substituting low and non-fat ingredients)

Whole wheat pasta with low-sodium and low-fat chunky spaghetti sauce, sprinkled with parmesan cheese
Garden salad with sun-dried tomatoes (no-oil Italian dressing)
Garlic toast with diet margarine or wonderful roasted garlic spread on top
Non or low-fat cheesecake (made with ricotta or yogurt cheese)

Barbecued chicken breast or vegetarian chicken patty (remove skin, spoon on barbecue sauce, grill or bake)
Corn on the cob, spray with butter-flavored cooking spray
Roasted whole baby zucchini and summer squash
Sliced tomatoes with basil dressing and olive oil drizzle
Fresh pineapple chunks sprinkled with wheat germ and vanilla yogurt

Chef's Salad - made with mixed greens, sliced tomatoes and assorted veggies, sliced turkey, turkey ham or
        seitan chunks, reduced fat Swiss cheese. Topped with no-oil Vinaigrette or honey Dijon dressing
Your favorite low-fat muffin (try a new recipe!)
Spiced and sliced hot apple topped with vanilla non-fat yogurt and maple syrup

Macaroni and cheese (whole wheat macaroni, cubed low-fat regular or soy cheddar cheese, evaporated milk or
        soy beverage, seasonings and steamed veggies like broccoli, peas or pearl onions)
        Try "veg-a-roni" recipe in Chapter 31 "Converting Your Favorite Recipes".
Baked tomato half with parmesan cheese
Spinach salad with olive oil, basalmic vinegar and bacon bits
Coconut Cream Fluff *

Garbanzo Bean Hummus * (stuffed into whole wheat pita pocket with sprouts, sliced tomato, non-fat creamy
dressing if you like)
Steamed summer squash, asparagus and mushrooms with fresh herbs
Sliced nectarine or fresh mixed fruit and fat-free cookies

Smoked Salmon Spread * (or vegetarian version) thinned to dip consistency, (use non or low-fat cottage or
ricotta cheese and yogurt as a base, add canned or fresh salmon, spices and herbs of your choice such as dill,
onion, garlic, Tabasco and liquid smoke)
Assorted raw veggies for dipping such as carrots, jicama, Chinese pea pods, cauliflower, green beans,
asparagus, etc. and whole grain crackers
Homemade tomato soup or gazpacho
Hot Easy Fruit Topping (Blueberry)* with non-fat granola on top

(Note: You can always save your dessert for a snack later if you're too full to finish!)

Snacks

To snack or not to snack, that is the question! I
find that if I plan for a snack, then it's there if and
when I need it. It's better than being caught without
a plan and it makes me feel so in control when I
have that "safety net" snack waiting. Experiment
with your favorites and develop a few old reliable
snacks to help out in a pinch. Try something new
every so often to avoid boredom and just reaching for
that apple and yogurt again.

Snacks can be just about anything in the
healthy foods categories. The same foods you're
eating now: fruits and vegetables, low-fat protein
choices and all kinds of complex carbohydrates. But
that's like saying a car is made of metal, glass and
rubber. You have to get creative to make something
useful! Same with snacks. Take that vegetable and
make it into pumpkin pudding or that fruit and
make frozen banana ice-cream. I usually keep my
snacks to around 100-150 calories so the serving is
small, but snacks are just meant to take the edge off
your hunger. They are not main meals, but are mini-
meals instead. Eat snacks because if you get too
hungry you're more likely to overeat at the next
meal. Also, by snacking throughout the day, you
keep your blood sugar levels stable and have a
steadier source of energy so you'll stay more active.

Below are some of the basic snacks. Enjoy
creating your own satisfying versions tailored to
your tastes and desires at the time.

Fruit

Fresh apples, bananas, peaches, strawberries
or other fresh berries, papaya, fresh pineapple,
melon, cherries and especially cut-up mixed fruit
are my favorites. Add a little vanilla or other
creamy yogurt on top and sprinkle with fat-free
granola. Make a yogurt-based dip for fruit slices
or whir together in a blender to make a refreshing
fruit smoothie.

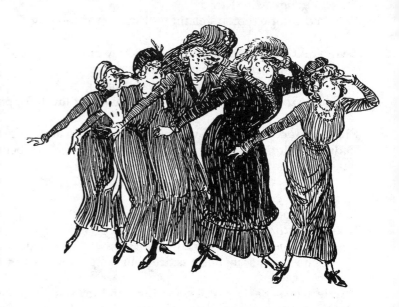

"Where did she put those low-fat brownies?"

Frozen fruit is refreshing and can be eaten
whole (such as grapes) or made into "ice cream" or
Cream Fluffs* (such as bananas or strawberries).
Frozen all-fruit popsicles can be bought or
homemade easily. Or try fruit sorbet or sherbet.

Don't forget to try cooked fruit, too. The classic
is baked apples or pears or applesauce. You can
sauté bananas or put together a fruit cup, then zap it
in the microwave for 1-2 minutes for a satisfying
snack. Top with yogurt or milk, granola, bran or
other cereal for crunch.

Dried fruit such as raisins, dates and figs are
very concentrated in sugar, so I think of them as
natural candy and only have them occasionally ...
or sometimes in very small amounts mixed with
other foods (such as sprinkled in a salad, a fresh
fruit cup or a curry dish). Dried fruit chips such as
apple and peach now come in individual serving
bags making them easy to take to work or traveling
and also insure that you get just one serving.

Juice packs or individual servings (like

applesauce) are another example. Fruit is the simplest of the complex carbohydrates, so it can effect your blood sugar levels very quickly. I suggest eating fruit along with yogurt, milk or other light protein or with a carbohydrate such as cereal, crackers or rice cakes. Fruit Newton's or other cookies sweetened with fruit only are good examples.

Vegetables

Keep some veggies handy in the refrigerator to munch. If you cut them up ahead of time, though, they may lose nutrients. So I use the smaller or even baby varieties such as baby carrots and cherry tomatoes. Some that don't need much preparation are celery, zucchini circles, red and green peppers, asparagus spears, radishes, broccoli florets, snow peas, green beans, low-sodium or sweet pickles and jicama.

Make a quickie veggie dip in your mini food processor from non-fat ricotta, plain yogurt and herbs or spices of your choice.

Salad greens are now being offered pre-washed and spun dry (very convenient for a quickie salad). Serve with non-fat dressing, a few extra veggies on top and maybe a few beans such as garbanzo or kidney. Salad bars are terrific places to get your veggie fix. You know to leave off the goopy dressings and fatty potato and pasta salads.

Fresh or bottled low-sodium tomato or mixed vegetable juice is a handy way to drink your veggie nutrients (although the fiber isn't as high as whole veggies).

Keep your favorite vegetable soup in individual containers in the freezer. Add whole grain crackers for a hearty snack. Soups now come in individual containers, dried or regular (watch the sodium content). Add water to the dry ones and heat in the micro. Half a bag of frozen combination veggies heated in the microwave with a topping of salsa is one of my favorites.

I also really love spaghetti squash. If you haven't tried it, you are in for a great treat. Look for a big, yellow squash in the store (pierce and cook in the microwave for 10-12 minutes on high, split in half, scoop out seeds). Use a fork to separate the strands inside so that it looks like spaghetti. I top mine with spaghetti sauce and a sprinkling of parmesan or salsa and Tabasco. Excellent fiber and beta-carotene, too.

Pumpkin Pudding* is another one of my reliable stand-bys. Also leftover stir-fry veggies.

Dairy Foods and Protein

Flavored yogurt is a great snack and the new flavors mean you can have a great variety of tastes. Banana cream, caramel, lemon, vanilla custard, cappuccino, tropical fruit, cherry vanilla and all sorts of fresh fruit flavors are available. Also different styles of yogurt (such as fruit mixed in, fruit on the bottom, granola packs to add and rich custard style). I usually add cereal for crunch. On the road, these individual cups are a great snack or addition to lunch. Fat-free pudding is easy, quick and also available in individual serving sizes. Watch your sugar grams. Cream Fluffs* are quick and filling or try fruit shakes.

Frozen non-fat yogurt is a great treat and is almost everywhere now. It's high-sugar usually, so limit this treat to 2-3 times a week and have with a carb if possible such as cereal or a rice cake.

Frozen dairy bars (non-fat) come in great flavors (such as chocolate mousse or orange-vanilla) and are a satisfying 30 calorie snack.

Fat-free cheese comes in one ounce sticks and slices and can be taken to work for a protein snack. Whole-grain crackers and cheese is good. Melt cheese on a rice cake or in a corn tortilla in the micro. Add a little salsa or chopped green chilies for zing. I also like low-fat ricotta cheese flavored with almond and cocoa powder with an Equal for an instant chocolate cheesecake taste. It's good on a honey-nut rice cake, too. Stuff celery with ricotta or cottage cheese (add a little peanut butter for flavor). Or make a dip to dunk veggies or fruit in.

Grains, Breads and Cereals

Fat-free crackers of all kinds are available. Ry-Vita or any rye-type is satisfying, flavorful and high in fiber. I used to hate diet crackers, but now there's a lot of variety and I love them topped with fat-free cheese slices or spread, dipped into ricotta or eggplant dip or served with soup or chili. Akmak is great!

Rice cakes have come a long way from the old cardboard days, too. They now come in flavors such as teriyaki, popcorn, honey nut and sesame to name a few. The big ones are great for topping or the mini ones for snacking and dipping.

Make your own Chips* or choose one of the new fat-free varieties such as cheese puffs or tortilla.

Air-popped popcorn is a special favorite of mine. As it shoots out of the popper I spray lightly with butter-flavored cooking spray and immediately sprinkle on herbs, spices, parmesan cheese or brewer's yeast (for a cheesy flavor). Microwave popcorn is usually too high in salt and fat still, but there are a few brands, such as Weight Watchers, that make individual microwave servings without salt or fat.

Dry "cold" cereals eaten without milk make a tasty, crunchy snack and I often eat it after a workout. And cereal and milk, either hot or cold can be eaten for under 150 calories and no fat. A favorite night-time snack for me.

Fat-free granola bars, cookies, muffins and toaster pastries are now available in a wide variety of flavors. Keep homemade Oat Bran Muffins* ready in the freezer for a snack. Heat in the micro briefly or it just takes 10 minutes to thaw at room temperature. Animal crackers, ginger snaps, graham crackers, fig and fruit bars and vanilla wafers are just some varieties that are lower in fat. Watch the sugar content on some of the commercial brands and fast-food ones, though.

A corn tortilla or taco shell makes an easy base for a quick snack. Stuff them with low-fat refried beans or cheese and salad veggies, top with salsa.

Pretzels are low fat and tasty, but get the low-salt variety.

Miscellaneous

Individual packets of defatted peanuts, regular or honey roasted are great, although 7 grams of fat all at once is an indulgence. However, they have saved me from skipping lunch during really busy on-the-road can't-stop days. Small shrimp cocktails can also tide you over. A slice of fat-free turkey or bologna on crackers, or just rolled up with a veggie stick or pickle slice inside, is easy finger food. Hummus or fat-free chili or other beans such as split pea or lentil soup are satisfying. Try with pita chips or other crackers.

Variety is a key factor here and as you can see, I eat! I consider this one of my "top secrets" for weight loss and maintenance. Deprivation just has not and will not ever work. Again, if you starve, you will always be overfat for the many reasons explained in this book. So eat! And enjoy.

In your Personal Journal or workbook, on the top of 4 separate pages, write the following headings: My Favorite Breakfasts, My Favorite Lunches, My Favorite Dinners, and My Favorite Snacks. Whenever you hit on a particularly wonderful meal, jot it down on the appropriate page. Pretty soon you will have a valuable collection of your favorite meals that you can turn to whenever you're in a hurry or your mind goes blank. Even if you only use these periodically, you'll be amazed at how many dishes you may have forgotten if you hadn't jotted them down.

Basic Recipes to Get You Started   30

"There is no sincerer love than the love of food."
George Bernard Shaw

Who out there doesn't love food? What, no hands? Just as I suspected. Let's face it, everybody who's alive loves to eat! After all, food is how we maintain our energy and health (as well as sanity at times). And it just plain old tastes great at all the right times, too. Bon appetit! It's natural and healthy to love to eat and to love food that tastes great. So I'd like to share with you some of my favorite recipes to do just that.

I literally have thousands of terrific recipes that people have shared with me and I have developed over the past 6 years since I've been at goal. Since I know that many of you have limited time in the kitchen, either by choice or because of busy schedules, I have chosen my simplest and quickest recipes for the most part, some of them are even in the "instant" category.

This section is by no means meant to be complete in its use of foods. There aren't a lot of "how to cook chicken the skinny way" recipes. I feel there are so many good recipe books out there (see Bibliography) that it would just be redundant to repeat them here. What I've done instead is try to give you a few basic recipes and, more importantly, basic techniques for getting your creative juices going and sparking ideas. Then you can begin to experiment and create your own favorites out of healthier ingredients and with healthier methods.

These recipes show that you can use foods in unordinary ways with surprisingly good results. There are chocolate pastries made with ricotta cheese (but without the fat and sugar), muffins without the oil, bean spreads, veggie sandwiches, satisfying soups and chili, creamy salad dressings and dips (without the fatty sour cream), rich pasta dishes and special desserts and snacks using non-fat dairy products and fruit in new ways. It's this kind of thinking that can lead you to new heights of anything-but-boring meals and snacks while losing weight healthfully. Then you can stay healthy and thin by using all your new "tricks" like I do. I really have to admit, though, sometimes I feel like I'm cheating because these foods taste so great! I can still have my favorites like chips and dip, pizza and pasta, pancakes and muffins, Mexican food, "candy" and milkshakes! Sound too good to be true? Try them out yourself and then get going as ideas come to you through experimenting. I know you'll find, like many do nowadays, that great tasting food doesn't have to be loaded down with unhealthy ingredients.

If our smart mothers and grandmothers knew what we're privileged to know about health today, you can bet they would have embraced the "lighter cooking" not only because of taste but out of love for their families. After all, isn't good health, including a healthy weight, a blessing for a lifetime provided in part by the wonderful food that we eat? Yes! So get busy and change those old heavy family favorites into something Mom would have been proud to serve. You'll soon see that a clever THINNER WINNER cook doesn't need to sacrifice taste to do just that!

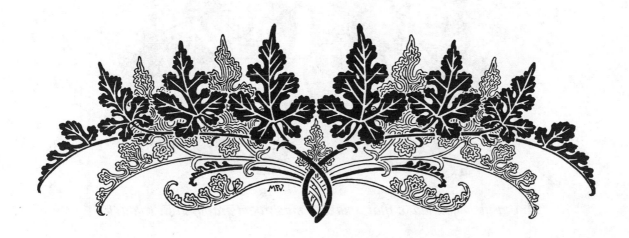

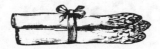

Breakfast and Brunch

Instant French Toast; Magic Cream Dream Cereal; Easy Hot Fruit Topping; Pita Pastries; Potato Pancakes; Oat Bran Raisin Muffins; Whole Wheat Buttermilk Pancakes; Simple Saucepan Soufflé

Breads and Sandwiches

Hummus; Chili Corn Bread; Grilled Cheese and Friends; Veggie Crunch Burrito

Soups, Salads and Dressings

Versatile Vegetable Soup; Warm-Hearted Lentil Soup; Salads; Basic Buttermilk Dressing; Creamy Italian Dressing; Creamy Coleslaw

Appetizers and Snacks

Stuffed Mushrooms; Savory Spinach Appetizers; Ricotta Onion Dip; Chips

Pasta, Pizza and Grains

Simply Lasagna; Creamy Garlic Pasta Sauce; Tomato Sauce with Roasted Peppers and Eggplant; Zucchini Crust Pizza; Pizza Pie; Quick Orange-Mint Rice; Veggie Bean Polenta

Other Main Dishes

Hearty Chili; Rolled, Stuffed and Breaded Things; Veggie Curry; Stir-Sauté Dishes; Seitan (wheat meat)

Sauces and Gravies

Chunky Cranapple Sauce; Onion Gravy ; Mushroom Gravy; Assorted Marinades

Desserts and Sweets

Cream Fluffs; Babe Rosie Bar; Roseanna Bananas; Instant Pumpkin Pudding; Orange-Cocoa Truffles

NOTE: All protein, carbohydrate, fat and fiber figures are expressed in grams. All sodium figures are expressed in milligrams.

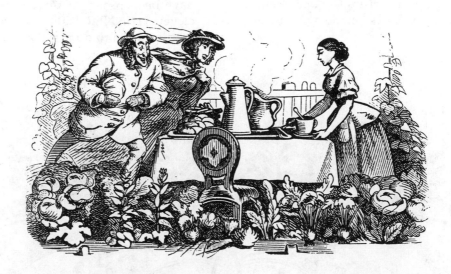

"Mm-m-m ... you made that amazing mushroom gravy, didn't you?!"

Breakfast and Brunch

Instant French Toast

Serve this morning favorite with Hot Fruit Topping* or warmed applesauce sprinkled with cinnamon. Great with fresh berries in season, too. For a unique twist, cook the bread on a waffle iron for waffle French toast or make a pocket in one slice and stuff with banana or ricotta!

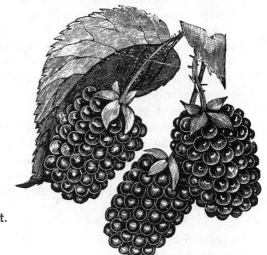

4 slices reduced-calorie bread (full-size) or 2 slices regular bread
½ cup egg substitute or 4 egg whites
Cinnamon and nutmeg to taste
½ tsp vanilla
2 TBL skim, soy milk, rice milk (vanilla is yummy) or orange juice

Beat together last four ingredients in a shallow bowl.
Heat a 12" non-stick skillet or griddle until water droplets bounce
    on the surface using medium low heat. Spray with butter-flavored
    non-stick spray just before adding bread slices.

Dip bread briefly into egg mixture coating both sides thoroughly
    but do not soak diet bread as this type of bread will not hold up to it.
Lightly brown both sides.

Serves 2   Per serving: cal 115, pro 12, carb 16.5, fat 0, sod 305, fiber 1
****

Magic Cream Dream Cereal

The high-fiber psyllium husk in this recipe doubles the amount of cereal you get without adding calories or fat! Very rich and satisfying. Be sure to drink at least 16 ounces of tea or water along with this dish as the psyllium tends to absorb water in your body. Two of my favorites are Hot Blueberry Topping with almond-flavored ricotta cheese or pear and raisin combination with light butter-flavored maple syrup as the sweetener.

2 svgs of your favorite hot cereal, prepared as directed with water or skim, soy or rice milk for a richer texture
    (creamy wheat or rice, oat bran or oatmeal, etc.)
1 cup water
2 heaping teaspoons pure psyllium husk, not seed (find it at health food stores)
Cinnamon and sweetener to taste (maple or rice syrup, fruit juice concentrate, Equal, etc.)
½ cup part-skim or fat-free ricotta cheese
½ tsp natural flavoring (vanilla, almond, etc.)
Butter-flavored sprinkles (optional)
2 svgs Easy Hot Fruit Topping* or fruit of your choice (banana, applesauce, etc.)

Place psyllium in a one cup measuring cup. Add water and stir to combine. Set aside. Just as the cereal is finished cooking, add the psyllium mixture and stir thoroughly to eliminate lumps. Continue cooking on medium low heat, stirring occasionally until thickened, about 3-5 additional minutes. If you are using the microwave, stir the mixture into finished cereal and cook an additional 1 minute. Meanwhile, measure ricotta cheese into the same measuring cup. Add flavoring, sweetener and cinnamon. Mix well.

Divide cereal equally into 2 cereal bowls. Sprinkle with more cinnamon, sweetener and sprinkles (if used). Make a slight depression in the center of each serving of cereal. Place half of the cheese mixture in the depression. Top each with Easy Hot Fruit Topping or warmed fruit of your choice. Cold chopped fruit or raisins can be used if you're in a hurry. Enjoy!

Serves 2   Per serving (w/ cream of wheat, skim milk, Equal and blueberry topping):
            cal 279, pro 13, carb 56, fat 2.2, sod 80, fiber 2.2

Easy Hot Fruit Topping

Use these easy, thick and versatile sauces for topping Pita Pastries, pancakes, French Toast, waffles or hot cereal in the morning. Also great over pudding, frozen desserts, cake, yogurt or ... !! For each serving:

½ cup fruit (fresh, frozen or canned in juice)
    use the fruit juice as the liquid
1 tsp arrowroot blended with 1 TBL of water until smooth
1 TBL frozen apple juice concentrate
    mixed with 3 TBL water or ¼ cup juice
Sweetener of your choice to taste (optional)

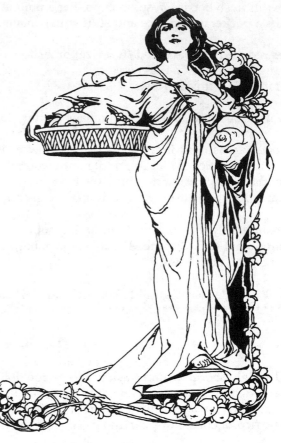

Place the fruit in a small saucepan with the apple juice
    concentrate-water mixture.
Heat over medium almost to a boil.
Reduce to a simmer and stir in the arrowroot mixture.
Continue simmering and stirring until the mixture thickens,
    about 2 minutes. Add more liquid for more sauce,
    adjusting arrowroot to thicken, if desired.
Remove from heat and cool slightly before adding Equal
    (if you choose).

Suggested fruit:
1 small chopped apple
½ chopped banana
½ cup chopped canned peaches, pears
    or crushed pineapple (yummy!)
½ cup fresh or frozen berries
    (blueberries and strawberries are good)
½ cup cubed papaya
½ cup canned apricots
    (water or juice packed with all fruits)
Use a mixture of two fruits such as bananas and raisins,
    apples and raisins, rhubarb and strawberries,
    bananas and pears, etc.

Serves 1   Per serving (with crushed pineapple): cal 110, pro 0, carb 26, fat 0, sod 3, fiber 2
****

Pita Pastries

These rich and creamy pastries take the place of the morning Danish or donut, but with a much healthier effect. They are very quick to prepare and can be made ahead and refrigerated, then heated or eaten cold for a quick snack or breakfast.

1 small whole wheat pita pocket per serving
¼ cup part-skim or fat-free ricotta cheese per serving
½ tsp flavoring of your choice - almond, vanilla, cocoa or carob powder, etc..
Sweetener of your choice to taste (maple or rice syrup, fruit juice, Equal, etc.)
Easy Topping or filling (see below) of your choice or Hot Fruit Topping

To make open faced pastries, split the pita by cutting all around the edge with a sharp knife and separating the two halves. Mix together the cheese, flavoring and sweetener. Spread the mixture evenly on the inside surfaces of the pita halves. Top with fruit topping. Serve cold or broil for a few minutes and serve warm.

To make stuffed pita pastries, cut around the edge of the pita only about ⅓ of the way. Mix the cheese mixture with the fruit and stuff it into the pita. Wrap in aluminum foil for a warm pastry and bake for about 8-10 minutes in a 350°F oven.

To make rolled pita pastries, cut completely around edge as with open-faced pastries. Spread each half with filling and topping and roll up. Serve cold or wrap in aluminum foil and heat in oven for 8-10 minutes. Cinnamon flavored ricotta and raisins are good with this style or try cocoa powder and sweetener in the ricotta for a chocolate pastry! Sprinkle with toasted almonds for a special indulgence.

Some Easy Toppings and fillings:
Chop or mash ½ banana, flavor with cinnamon and vanilla or almond and sweetener.
    Mix with cheese and use in stuffed pita.
Chop a small fresh apple, seeded and cored. Flavor with cinnamon, vanilla and sweetener.
    Mix with cheese and use in stuffed pita.
Flavor ½ cup of any canned fruit (water or juice packed) such as peaches, pears, apples or pineapple.
    Spoon on top of open-faced pitas or mix with cheese and stuff inside.

Per serving (with banana and Equal): cal 184, pro 10.1, carb 29, fat 3, sod 190, fiber 1.5

****

Potato Pancakes

Fabulous and filling snack, lunch or side dish. Low fat, sodium and calories high fiber, vitamins and minerals. Potatoes are winners!

1½ pounds of potatoes, scrubbed, peeled if you wish and shredded
½ onion, grated
2 TBL fresh parsley, chopped
¼ cup whole wheat pastry flour
2 TBL water

Lightly spray a non-stick griddle or large skillet and heat to medium.
Place all ingredients in a medium bowl and mix thoroughly.
Spoon mixture onto hot surface making 8 pancakes. Flatten the pancakes slightly. You can also cook 4 pancakes
    at a time, warming the first batch on an oven-proof plate in a 200°F oven while the second batch cooks.
Cook for 10 minutes, then turn and cook another 10 minutes until crispy brown.
Spray each side with butter-flavored cooking spray for more flavor and crispiness if desired.
Serve with homemade or natural applesauce and/or fat-free sour cream.

Serves 4   Per serving: cal 132, pro 4.3, carb 29, fat 0.3, sod 9, fiber 3

****

Oat Bran Raisin Muffins

These are great for snacks and quick breakfasts. Warm in micro for fresh-baked fragrance.

2 cups oat bran
⅓ cup unbleached flour
½ tsp baking soda
½ tsp cinnamon
¼ tsp baking powder
¼tsp allspice
1¼ cups skim milk or rice milk
½ cup plus 2 TBL apple butter or other all-fruit preserves
2 egg whites, lightly beaten
¾ cup raisins
Chopped fresh fruit to top each muffin before baking (optional)

Preheat oven to 350°F.
In a large bowl, combine the oat bran, flour, baking soda, cinnamon, baking powder and allspice.
In a small bowl, whisk together the milk, preserves and egg whites.

Pour the liquid ingredients over the flour mixture.
Stir with a rubber spatula to moisten the flour gently. Carefully fold in the raisins. The batter will be wet.
Spray 12 muffin cups or use paper liners. Divide batter evenly into cups.
Top with small amount of chopped fresh fruit if desired.
Bake for 22 minutes or until brown and firm.

Makes 12 muffins.   Per muffin: cal 126, pro 5, carb 12, fat 1.5, sod 87, fiber 4
****

Whole Wheat Buttermilk Pancakes

Everyone loves pancakes! Here's a delicious, light healthy version you will use often.

1 cup whole wheat pastry flour
¼cup wheat germ or bran
½ tsp baking soda
1½ tsp Sucanat or brown sugar
¼ cup egg substitute
1½ cups buttermilk (1%)
2 tsp canola oil (optional)

Stir together the first four ingredients in a medium bowl.
In a small bowl, combine egg substitute and buttermilk, then add to dry ingredients and briefly just to mix.
Stir in oil if used.
Cook on heated non-stick griddle using about ⅓ cup batter per pancake. Turn when bubbles rise to the surface and
    pop. Cook pancakes without oil a little longer.
These are also great with blueberries mixed into the batter.

Makes 8. Per pancake (w/ oil & wheat germ): cal 102, pro 6, carb 15, fat 2.6, sod 107, fib 1.1
        Per pancake (w/o oil & bran used): cal 80, pro 6, carb 15, fat 0.6, sod 107, fiber 1.1
****

Simple Saucepan Soufflé

I make this yummy dish when I want an extremely low calorie, high protein and surprisingly satisfying light lunch, breakfast, dessert or snack. Fun to make, too! I like to have cinnamon toast with this version.

6 egg whites
1 cup chopped fresh strawberries or ½ cup blueberries or other fruit
½ chopped banana
1 TBL frozen apple juice concentrate
 Ground spice such as cinnamon, nutmeg or cloves

Beat egg whites on high with electric mixer until stiff peaks form.
Spray a 3 quart saucepan with non-stick spray and add fruit and juice. Cook over medium heat until the fruit is
    softened. Spoon the egg whites gently onto the fruit and spread to the edges of the pan. Cover and cook on
    low heat about 4-6 minutes until at least doubled in size. It's best not to peek while cooking.
Remove lid and invert a plate over the top of the pan. Turn pan over carefully to invert the soufflé onto the
    plate. Spoon any remaining mixture over the hot soufflé. Sprinkle with ground spice.

Serves 2   Per serving: cal 110, pro 11, carb 16.5, fat 0.5, sod 150, fiber 2
Variations:
* Sprinkle non-fat granola or other cereal into fruit before adding egg whites or sprinkle on top.
* Many varieties of fruit can be used such as papaya, apples or raisins.
* Try this with veggies also such as onions and mushrooms. Makes a great light omelet. Sprinkle with low fat and sodium shredded cheese.

Breads and Sandwiches

Hummus

This luscious dish of Middle Eastern origin features garbanzo beans, also known as chickpeas. Hummus can be stuffed into a warm pita pocket, used as a dip for veggies, spread on crackers for appetizers, or simply mounded on fresh greens for a light, cool salad main meal. Once your family discovers its rich and satisfying texture they will consider it a treat whenever you make it. Easy to prepare, economical and keeps well, too!

3 cups homemade cooked garbanzo beans or 2 15-oz cans
     low sodium garbanzo beans, drained and rinsed
4 cloves garlic, crushed
Juice of 1 lemon, about ¼ cup
¼ cup water or low-sodium vegetable broth
2 TBL parsley, minced
1 TBL olive oil (optional)
1 TBL sesame seeds, toasted (optional)
1 tsp low sodium soy sauce
Cayenne pepper to taste
Freshly ground pepper to taste

Toast raw sesame seeds, if used, by placing them
    in a foil dish and then in a medium oven until
    lightly browned. Watch closely, as they tend
    to burn. The seeds can be omitted, but they add
    a taste distinctive to hummus.
Place the beans in a food processor.
Add the remaining ingredients and pulse to mix.
Add more liquid, if necessary, as you process.
Then run the machine continuously for 1-2 full minutes until you get a smooth consistency. Adjust the seasonings.

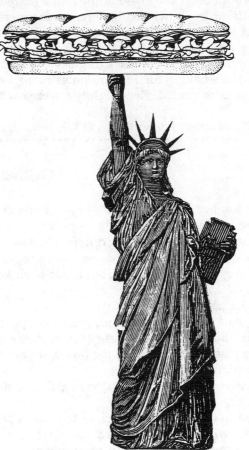

"Freedom from boring sandwiches!"

Makes about 3½ cups.
Nutritional information per ⅓ cup: cal 78, pro 3.6, carb 12.8, fat 1.2, sod 17, fiber 4

****

Chili Corn Bread

Made without oil or egg yolks, this yummy cornbread is surprisingly moist and wonderfully fragrant served warm! I like it with Warm-Hearted Lentil Soup or Hearty Chili.

1½ cup sifted cornmeal
¾ cup whole-wheat pastry flour or finely ground corn flour
4 tsp chili powder
1½ tsp cumin
1 tsp coriander
1 tsp baking soda
1 TBL baking powder (low sodium preferred)
1 small can (4 ounces) green chilies, chopped
1 small onion, finely chopped
¾ cup apple juice concentrate (or less if you prefer)
¾ cup 1% buttermilk
¼ cup low sodium tomato sauce

3 egg whites
Preheat oven to 400°F.
In a medium bowl stir together the first 7 ingredients, mixing well.
In a small mixing bowl, combine remaining ingredients, except egg whites, mixing well again.
Add wet ingredients to dry ones and stir just to combine.
Beat egg whites until soft peaks form and fold carefully into batter.
Spoon into a sprayed non-stick or glass 9x9 baking dish. Cover with foil and bake for 20 minutes. Remove foil and
    continue baking for 15-20 minutes more. Remove from oven and cover with foil until cooled enough to cut.
Serve warm or cooled. Keep tightly covered with foil.

Makes 12 servings. Per serving: cal 129, pro 4.2, carb 26.8, fat 0.5, sod 53, fiber 2
****

Grilled Cheese and Friends

A nice, hot sandwich and a bowl of homemade soup is the perfect answer for lunch on a chilly day. There are as many versions of this popular sandwich as there are appetites! Experiment with your favorite combinations or try something different just for fun. Now you can have grilled sandwiches anytime because, using these healthier cooking techniques, they are no longer on the "too fatty" list. A new-fangled appliance called a sandwich griller is great here, but a non-stick skillet does the job nicely, also.

Here's the basic technique:
On a slice of your favorite bread, spread or spoon your choice of vegetable filling and seasonings.
Top with sliced or grated cheese of your choice and another slice of bread. You may very lightly spread some
    acceptable margarine on the bread, if your diet allows, although they are just wonderful without the
    addition of the fat.
Heat a non-stick skillet or sandwich griller to medium-low heat and spray with butter-flavored non-stick
    spray.
Place sandwich in griller and close the top as per directions for appliance. Or place sandwich in skillet and
    press with a spatula several times while browning.
Remove sandwich briefly and respray skillet.
Brown the other side and melt the cheese, pressing again with spatula to flatten.

Some suggested fillings to get you started:
Sliced tomatoes, sprouts, dill, red onion and cheddar on whole grain bread
Sautéed onion, broccoli, basil, pepper and Swiss on rye
Sautéed shredded zucchini, green pepper, garlic and parmesan on sourdough
Low-sodium sauerkraut, tomatoes, mustard and cheddar on pumpernickel
Mashed veggie-bean spread, cilantro, lime juice and hot-pepper Monterey Jack on split corn bread
Drained chopped spinach, red onion, nutmeg and feta cheese on 7-grain
Thinly sliced apple, raisins, sprouts and Jarlsberg on cinnamon-raisin bread
Lettuce, pineapple ring, dates and fat-free cream cheese on French bread
Cottage cheese, peanut butter (small amount just to flavor!), raisins and sprouts on whole wheat
Fat-free cream cheese mixed with green onions, dill, radishes on rye
Seitan slices, red onion and blue cheese on sourdough

Of course, follow all the THINNER WINNERS principles in choosing the highest quality, natural ingredients with the lowest fat and sodium contents available. Soy cheese won't melt quite as well, but will still taste great inside these grilled beauties.
****

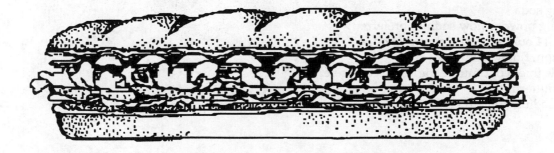

Veggie Crunch Burrito

The combination of steamed and raw, crunchy veggies in this juicy burrito is absolutely fabulous. Great to pack on picnics and outings, colorful enough for Fourth of July!

4 whole wheat tortillas, heated until soft
4 cups broccoli florets, sliced thin and steamed
2 cups cauliflower, small pieces, steamed
2 carrots, shredded
½ cup yellow summer squash, shredded
½ cup red cabbage, finely chopped
1 medium onion, halved and sliced
¼ cup natural barbecue sauce
 4 TBL fat-free mayonnaise or salad dressing or honey mustard
1 dill pickle (low-sodium), slivered
4 cups mixed well-chopped greens (lettuce, sprouts)
Salt-free herb seasoning to taste
Garlic powder to taste (optional)
Freshly ground pepper to taste

To keep tortillas warm while preparing the filling, wrap them in a damp towel and place on an oven-proof plate in an oven set on low heat.
Place the broccoli, cauliflower, carrots, squash and cabbage in a medium bowl and toss well to combine. Set aside.
Heat a small sprayed non-stick skillet over medium, then add the onions and stir-sauté until soft, about 4-5 minutes. Add the barbecue sauce and continue stirring until well coated. Do not overcook. Remove from heat. (These are great on all kinds of sandwiches!)

To assemble:
Place the four tortillas on the damp towel on a flat work surface.
To prepare the burritos for traveling, place a large sheet of plastic wrap under the tortilla.
Spread 1 TBL fat-free spread on each tortilla.
Top with ¼ of the greens, ¼ of the pickles and sprinkle on any seasonings.
Divide the veggie mixture evenly into the four tortillas, then top each with ¼ of the onion mixture.
Fold up one end to close, then roll to enclose filling or use your favorite rolling technique.
Serve immediately or wrap tightly in plastic wrap and refrigerate.

Serves 4   Per serving: cal 248, pro 8, carb 39, sod 512, fiber 7, fat 4.7 (3g for the tortillas and 1g for the barbecue sauce. If you find fat-free versions of these, then there will be less fat. Let me know!)
****

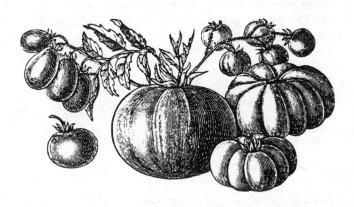

Soups, Salads and Dressings

Versatile Vegetable Soup

A good basic soup that can be changed to suit your individual tastes or the availability of vegetables. Toss in leftover cooked grains, rice, noodles, beans or vegetables the last five minutes to just heat them through without overcooking them. A fresh salad and some good bread makes a satisfying meal. Or just heat a cupful for a nutritious, low calorie snack anytime.

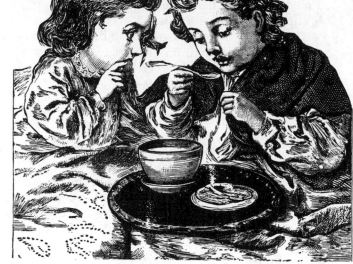

2 quarts water or homemade vegetable broth
2 cups low sodium tomato or mixed vegetable juice
2 TBL low sodium soy or Worcestershire sauce (reg. or veg.)
2 medium onions, chopped
2-4 cloves of garlic, crushed (optional)
2-4 carrots, sliced
1 large leek, split, rinsed well and sliced
1 green pepper, chopped
3 tomatoes, chopped
2 cups frozen okra
1 zucchini, halved lengthwise and sliced
2 cups green beans, fresh or frozen, cut in one inch pieces
2 potatoes, peeled and cut into cubes
1 cup corn kernels, fresh or frozen
1 tsp each basil, thyme and oregano
½ tsp each marjoram, dill and cumin
2 bay leaves
¼ cup chopped fresh parsley
Freshly ground pepper to taste

*"Did you know that people
who eat soup eat less calories?"*

Place all ingredients in a large soup pot.
Bring to a boil, then reduce heat and simmer,
    partially covered, for about 45 minutes.
Remove bay leaves before serving.

Serves 8-10, about 16 cups total. Per cup: cal 67, pro 2.3, carb 14.8, fat 0.3, sod 40, fiber 3
****

Warm-hearted Lentil Soup

This savory, satisfying rib-sticker takes only minutes to put together and then simmers away with a delicious aroma while you make Chili Corn Bread or put together a salad and warm whole wheat French bread for a grateful family! Healthfully high in fiber, too!

1 cup dry lentils, rinsed
5 cups defatted canned (low sodium) or homemade stock or water
1 medium onion, finely chopped
1 carrot, finely chopped
1 stalk celery, finely chopped
1 clove garlic, minced
1 medium green pepper, finely chopped
1 small potato, peeled & diced
2 cups tomato sauce (low sodium)
½ tsp each curry powder and basil
Freshly ground pepper to taste

Combine the first 6 ingredients in a large pot and bring to a boil.

Lower heat and simmer, covered, about 30 minutes.
Add the remaining ingredients, stir, recover and continue to simmer about 15 minutes until potatoes are done.

Serves 4-6   Eight cups total. Per cup: cal 127, pro 7.4, carb 24.7, fat 0.4, sod 35, fiber 5
****

Salads

The subject of salads is such an individual one. Everyone has their favorites and the varieties are virtually endless. Since a large salad eaten every day is a great way to get healthy nutrients and fiber, manage weight and have something to order in restaurants that they usually can't mess up, spend some time experimenting with ingredients. Come up with at least one basic everyday salad for yourself and a couple of fancier ones for variety. A mixed green salad is a good place to start. Below I list some fresh ingredients to get you started. Buy the freshest vegetables available, those that are seasonal. If tomatoes don't grow year round where you live, then don't buy the supermarket mushy ones just out of habit. Try beets or turnips or jicama or kale or something that is in season. Keep a big, covered salad bowl in the refrigerator and always have a fresh munchy snack ready.

I never had a salad until I was about 13 years old and when I did I wasn't too fond of them. They were diet food and I never ate them unless I was on a diet. Now I've really grown to love them and I'll even order salad as a preferred dish in a restaurant! I guess they are an acquired taste, like fine wine. So keep trying!

Greens:
Experiment with the many flavors and textures available such as red, green and butter lettuce, fresh spinach, cabbage varieties, kale, endive, arugula, romaine, fresh herbs such as parsley, basil, dill, watercress, mint, cilantro or chives, etc. Bags of prewashed greens are a time saver.

Vegetables:
Don't just stop at tomatoes and cucumber! Branch out to keep your taste buds hopping. Try jicama, mushrooms (many different varieties), shredded carrots or fresh beets, peppers (green, red and yellow), chili peppers, onions of all types (green, red, yellow, brown), radishes, sun chokes, grated fresh ginger, celery, green beans, sprouts of all varieties (easy to grow at home), shallots, garlic, fresh peas, summer squashes, turnips, asparagus, etc.

Frozen or canned:
For convenience, keep some of these on hand. Be sure to rinse all canned vegetables two or three time to remove excess sodium. Buy low sodium when available. Thaw or microwave briefly, then add to the salad bowl. Frozen peas, corn, green beans, cauliflower, broccoli, mixed vegetable combinations, artichoke hearts, water chestnuts, hearts of palm, roasted peppers (not in oil), pimento, capers, diced green chilies, marinated vegetable mixtures (again, not in oil), etc.

More:
Raisins, currants, fresh chopped fruit such as apples, oranges, figs, kiwi, sun-dried tomatoes (soak in hot water for a few minutes to soften up. Don't get the kind in oil), a few beans (garbanzo, kidney, black or white), rice, pasta, anything leftover, etc.

Now, you have no excuse for a plain, old boring salad night after night! But what about the dressing?!
****

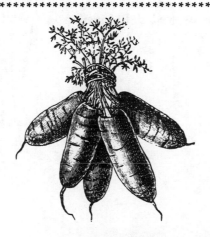

Salad Dressings

Most bottled dressings are full of either fat, sodium, artificial colorings, flavorings and/or preservatives. There are a few exceptions, such as the Pritikan line, and certainly more are coming to the market very swiftly as demand rises, so keep your eyes open at the supermarket. However, dressings are very easy and economical to make at home and you can tailor them exactly to your tastes. Try out the basics below and add as you get more proficient.

For a burst of flavor when you don't have any time or want no extra calories at all, try a tablespoon of basalmic vinegar or a squeeze of fresh lemon juice. Grind on fresh pepper, dust with chopped fresh or dried herbs and voilá! Or for a super fast and very tasty creamy dressing, simply mix plain non-fat yogurt with an equal amount of salsa. Add an Equal if you want a sweet Thousand Island-type taste.

Keep in mind that most people use about 4-5 tablespoons of dressing! Especially the creamy kind because it is thicker. That's really a killer at salad bars where they rarely have low-cal or low-fat dressings. So either measure yours or figure about 4 tablespoons per serving.

Basic Buttermilk Dressing

½ cup salt free tomato sauce
1 cup skim or low fat buttermilk
¼ cup basalmic or flavored vinegar
1 tsp basil
1 TBL chopped parsley or 1 tsp parsley flakes
1 clove garlic, crushed or ½ tsp garlic powder

Blend or whisk thoroughly.
Store in airtight container in refrigerator.
Shake or stir before serving.

Makes 1¾ cups.
Per tablespoon: cal 4, pro 0.2, carb 0.5, fat 0, sod 0.8, fiber 0

****

Creamy Italian Dressing

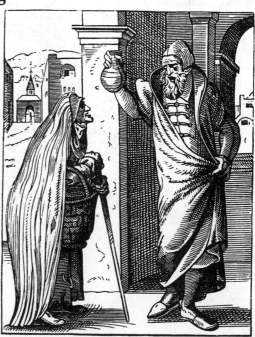

1 cup low-sodium fat-free or 1% cottage cheese,
    ricotta cheese or tofu (8 ounces)
½ cup plain nonfat yogurt
¼ cup onion, chopped
1 clove garlic, crushed
1 TBL fresh lemon juice
1 TBL low-sodium stone-ground mustard
1 TBL fresh parsley, chopped
1 tsp basil
1 tsp oregano

Combine all ingredients in a food processor and process
    until smooth, scraping down the sides as needed. Refrigerate.

Makes 1½ cups.
Per tablespoon: cal 11, pro 1.4, carb 0.7, fat 0.1, sod 13, fiber 0

"Psssst. Wanna buy some low-sodium Italian dressing? Secret recipe!"

Creamy Coleslaw

Coleslaw is almost an American institution! Every family seems to have it's favorite ingredients, but most have been weighed down in the past with heavy mayonnaise or sour cream. With the introduction of non-fat versions of these ingredients we can once again enjoy the creamy coleslaw of yesteryear! Feel free to add or subtract ingredients according to your taste.

Coleslaw is usually a salad with shredded cabbage in it. However, there are many tasty variations of this popular dish and just about any shredded vegetable or fruit combination can be used. Keep the dressings light, such as the sweet one below, with non-fat dressings and you've got a cold, crisp winner every time.

1½ cups grated red cabbage
1½ cups grated green cabbage
½ cup grated carrot
2 TBL cider vinegar
2 TBL rice syrup or honey
2 tsp poppy seeds
¼ cup fat-free sour cream
½ cup fat-free mayonnaise
1 Granny Smith apple, grated
½ cup raisins

Soak the grated vegetables in cold water in the refrigerator for 30 minutes.
Meanwhile, combine remaining ingredients except the apple and raisins and whisk until smooth.
Spin the chilled vegetables in a salad spinner until very dry.
In medium bowl, toss all ingredients together thoroughly. Chill covered for several hours or overnight to
    blend flavors.

Serves 4-6   Per ¼ recipe: cal 152, fat 0.7, sod 284, fiber 1.7
****

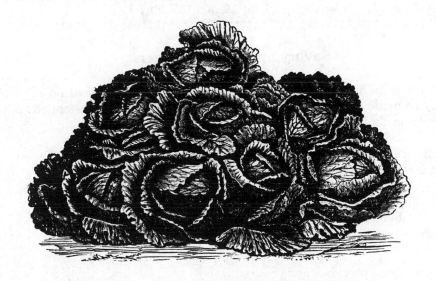

Appetizers and Snacks

Stuffed Mushrooms

Simply wonderful and quick to prepare, these savory delights can be served as appetizers or as a side dish.

8-12 giant white mushrooms (as many as will fit in an 8 x 8 glass baking dish in a single layer)
½ cup chopped onion (green or white)
3 cloves garlic, crushed
½ red pepper, chopped fine or one 2-oz jar of pimento, chopped
1 slice fresh whole grain bread, made into fine crumbs in the food processor
1 TBL parmesan cheese (optional)
1 tsp Liquid Smoke
1 tsp light soy sauce
1 tsp basil
Cayenne pepper to taste
Freshly ground pepper to taste

Preheat oven to 350°F.
Remove stems from mushrooms, rinse briefly and set aside. Wipe mushroom caps gently with a damp paper towel to clean and set aside. Finely mince the mushroom stems.
In a medium non-stick skillet sprayed lightly with olive oil spray, sauté the onion, garlic, mushroom stems and red pepper (if used) 1-2 minutes until soft. Add pimento (if used), bread crumbs, cheese (if used) and seasonings. Heat briefly, stirring to mix thoroughly. Remove from heat.
With a spoon, pack each mushroom cap with the mixture. There should be a smooth, rounded mound of the mixture in each cap. Place the caps in a lightly sprayed 8 x 8 glass baking dish. Cover and bake for 25 minutes.

Serves 4   Per serving: cal 62, pro 3.8, carb 10.4, fat 0.9, sod 145, fiber 3
****

Savory Spinach Appetizers

This quick, delectable combination is always a healthful hit at any party or as an unusual addition to a lunch plate. It can easily be made from ingredients on hand if you keep a box of chopped spinach in your freezer or use fresh spinach for super flavor.

1 10 ounce box frozen chopped spinach, thawed & well-drained, not squeezed
½ cup onion, finely minced
¼ cup egg substitute, lightly beaten
1½ slices whole-grain bread, toasted then crumbed in food processor
1 TBL parmesan cheese, grated
¼ tsp each garlic powder, thyme, sage and nutmeg

Preheat oven to 350°F.
In a medium bowl, combine the first 3 ingredients, mixing well.
Add remaining ingredients and mix thoroughly.
Shape mixture into 16 equal balls. Wet hands with a little water if it sticks to your hands.
Place balls in a sprayed baking dish and bake uncovered about 18-20 minutes until lightly browned.

Makes 4 servings   Per serving: cal 60, pro 6, carb 7.5, fat 1.0 , sod 149, fiber 3

Ricotta Onion Dip

Use ricotta cheese as a creamy base for dips, spreads and sauces of all kinds. It is very bland in taste and takes well to any added seasonings. Here's a tangy dip for your next gathering.

1 cup nonfat ricotta cheese
2 cloves garlic, crushed
2 TBL nonfat mayonnaise (optional)
2 TBL nonfat plain yogurt
1 TBL Worcestershire sauce
2 tsp onion powder
1 tsp low-sodium soy sauce
1 tsp honey
3 TBL dehydrated onions

Place all ingredients except dehydrated onions in a food processor and process until smooth, scraping down sides
    at least once.
Transfer to storage container with lid. Add onions and stir well to combine. Cover and refrigerate overnight to
    combine flavors.

Makes about 1½ cups. Per ½ cup: cal 40, pro 9.5, carb 4, fat 0, sod 129, fiber 0
****

Low-fat Chips

Nothing like a good crunch now and then to satisfy that crunchy, munchy urge! If carrots and other raw veggies just aren't doing the trick, try one of these fun-to-make, healthful and satisfying recipes! Check the individual packages for nutritional information as it varies with the brand. They are usually less than 1 gram of fat per whole pita, whole tortilla or whole potato!

Pita Chips
Whole wheat pita
Non-stick butter or garlic flavored cooking spray
Garlic powder, onion powder, dried herbs, etc.
Parmesan cheese, grated (optional)

Split the pitas in half by cutting all the way around the edges with a sharp knife. Lightly spray the inside surfaces. Sprinkle on your choice of seasonings. Cut each round into 6 wedges. Place wedges on baking sheet and bake at 375°F about 10 minutes until browned and crispy. Store in an airtight container. About 7 calories each.

Tortilla Chips
Corn tortillas made without added oil (check the label)
Garlic powder, onion powder, paprika, chili powder, etc.

Score each tortilla into 8 wedges with a sharp knife leaving about 1 inch to the edge. Spray and sprinkle with your choice of seasonings. Place entire tortilla directly on oven rack or baking sheet. Brown one side then turn and brown the other in a 375-400°F oven. Break tortillas into chips. About 7 calories each.

Potato Chips
Potatoes, scrubbed

Using the thinnest slicing blade of your food processor, slice potatoes. Place slices in a bowl of ice water for about 20 minutes, then pat dry with paper towels. Place in a single layer on a non-stick baking sheet. Spray and sprinkle as above if you wish. Bake at 375°F until browned slightly and crispy. 30 chips is about 80 calories.

****

Pasta, Pizza and Grains

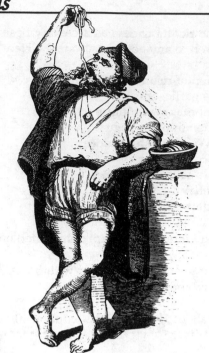

Pasta Presto!

Pasta is a wonderful high energy, high complex carbohydrate food good for active people like you. Naturally low in sodium, fat and cholesterol as well as calories, it is a great choice for those watching their health as well as their waistlines. Choose whole grain varieties and chunky vegetable toppings for added fiber benefit. Filling and tasty, all this good nutrition and it cooks in 8-12 minutes making it a great fast food, too. Finer pasta, such as angel hair, cooks in only 1-2 minutes!

Pasta comes in dozens of varieties from wide lasagna to the finest angel hair. Vary the sauces according to your taste and the time you have to prepare them. Serve with a fresh tossed green vegetable salad perhaps with a few garbanzo or kidney beans, non-fat salad dressing and crusty Italian bread (plain or spread with non-fat margarine or olive oil-flavored cooking spray and garlic powder, then toasted under the broiler). Buono Gusto! Here are a few recipes to get you started with pasta ... a superfood!

"Everything you see I owe to spaghetti ... and Sophia Loren."

Simply Lasagna

Lasagna can be made so many ways -- feel free to add your favorite ingredients to this basic recipe. The great joy here is the uncooked noodles that save you an extra step during preparation. Using bottled spaghetti sauce, frozen chopped spinach and pre-shredded mozzarella also saves time and work when you don't have the luxury of spending all day in the kitchen.

Filling:
16 ounces low-fat or non-fat ricotta cheese
4 egg whites, lightly beaten
1 10 ounce package chopped spinach, thawed and squeezed to remove excess water
2 TBL fresh parsley, chopped
1½ tsp oregano
1 tsp basil
½ tsp garlic powder
Freshly ground pepper to taste
12 whole grain lasagna noodles (16 ounces), uncooked
3 cups low-fat low-sodium chunky spaghetti sauce or homemade
2 medium zucchini, thinly sliced
4 ounces fat-free mozzarella cheese, shredded
2 TBL parmesan cheese, grated

Preheat oven to 350°F.
Combine the filling ingredients in a medium bowl or food processor until smooth.
Spray a 13 x 9 glass baking dish with olive oil non-stick spray.
Spread ¾ cup sauce evenly over the bottom. Place 4 lasagna noodles over the sauce, breaking them to fit if
    necessary. Spread ½ cup sauce over the noodles. Arrange ½ the zucchini slices along the seams of the
    noodles. Spread on ½ of the filling. Sprinkle on ½ the mozzarella cheese.
Again, layer noodles, sauce, zucchini, filling and mozzarella.
Finish with noodles, remaining sauce (about 1 cup) and parmesan cheese.
Cover and bake 1 hour. Remove cover and bake 20 minutes longer until pasta is tender.
Serves 10   Per serving: cal 264, pro 15.7, carb 49, fat 2.7, sod 158, fiber 4

Creamy Garlic Pasta Sauce

Luscious, low-fat and quick. Use tofu if you do not eat dairy products simply heat gently in a saucepan. Also good over vegetables or baked potatoes.

Another quick, low-fat and also high-fiber pasta sauce can be made by pureeing white (cannelini) or other beans with some broth in a food processor and adding herbs and spices to season.

1 16-ounce container low-fat or fat-free ricotta cheese
1/4 cup evaporated skim milk
6 cloves garlic, crushed
1 TBL low-sodium soy sauce
2 TBL fresh parsley, chopped
1/2 tsp white pepper

Place all ingredients in a food processor and process until very smooth, scraping down sides at least once.
    Add more milk if a thinner consistency is desired.
Pour into the top of a double boiler or in a metal mixing bowl. Place over the bottom of a double boiler or over a
    medium pot of simmering water.
Heat gently until bubbles just begin to form around the outside edges.
Stir gently until heated through.
Do not boil.
Remove from heat and ladle over hot pasta.

Serves 4   Per serving (w/ low-fat cheese): cal 105, pro 13, carb 6, fat 4 , sod 248, fiber 0
****

Tomato Sauce With Roasted Peppers And Eggplant

Prepare the eggplant and peppers earlier in the day or the day before. Peel and store in a covered container in the refrigerator and you'll have a super quick pasta dish ready to assemble. Roasting vegetables is so easy and gives them a smoky, substantial taste with an extra dimension of flavor.

1 medium eggplant
2 bell peppers, green, red or one of each
2 cups low-sodium tomato sauce
4 cloves garlic, minced or crushed
2 TBL capers, drained and chopped lightly. These tasty additions are found in the condiments section.
2 tsp oregano or 3-4 TBL chopped fresh
1 tsp basil or 1-2 TBL chopped fresh
Dash of cayenne pepper or red pepper flakes
Freshly ground pepper to taste

Place whole pricked eggplant and peppers on a baking sheet in a preheated 450°F oven.
Roast until soft, about 40 minutes, turning occasionally.
Slip or peel skins off the peppers, seed and dice, then set aside.
Allow the eggplant to cool slightly then peel it carefully and dice the pulp.
In a large non-stick skillet, warm the tomato sauce over medium heat.
Add the remaining ingredients and heat thoroughly.
Adjust the seasonings to taste adding more pepper (red or black) or a touch of honey if tomato sauce is bitter.
Serve over hot pasta of your choice.

Serves 4   Per serving: 70 cal, fat 0.8, sod 50, fiber 4

Zucchini Crust Pizza

All out of bread servings for the day? Try this satisfying, unique pizza! Add more toppings too! Crumbled garden or soy sausage makes it heartier. Made on a cookie sheet, servings look huge!

½ cup egg substitute
¼ tsp each onion and garlic powders
4 cups shredded zucchini, about 4 medium (squeeze out moisture)
4 ounces shredded fat-free mozzarella cheese
4 ounces shredded fat-free cheddar cheese
2 tsp olive oil (optional)
½ cup each chopped onion and green bell pepper
½ cup sliced mushrooms
2 garlic cloves, minced
1 ⅓ cup low-sodium spaghetti sauce or tomato sauce
1 tsp oregano leaves
½ tsp Italian seasoning
⅛ tsp pepper
4 tsp parmesan cheese, grated

Preheat oven to 400°F.
Beat together first 3 ingredients. Add zucchini and half of each cheese , mixing well.
Spray a cookie sheet or two 14 inch round pizza pans with non-stick spray.
Press zucchini mixture into pan or pans and bake until set and slightly browned, 8-10 minutes.
Meanwhile, in a non-stick medium skillet heat oil, if used, over medium heat and sauté veggies until softened, about 5 minutes.
Add sauce and seasonings and cook, stirring occasionally about 5 more minutes.
Spread veggie mixture evenly over crust.
Top with remaining cheeses and sprinkle with parmesan.
Bake 15-20 minutes until lightly browned.

Serves 4   Per serving (w/ oil): cal 201, pro 24, carb 19, fat 3.8, sod 495, fiber 2.5
****

Quick Orange-Mint Rice

A fast and colorful dish to use up that leftover rice!

¾ cup each diced celery and onion
2 cups cooked brown rice
¼ cup orange juice
2 tsp fresh mint, chopped (or 1 tsp dried)
1½ tsp onion powder
1 orange, cut in half and sliced into half circles (10-12 half circles altogether)

Preheat oven to 350°F.
Boil 3 TBL water over medium-low heat in a medium non-stick skillet.
Add onion and celery and sauté until veggies are softened and water has evaporated.
Add rice and heat another 2 minutes, stirring to break up clumps.
Add orange juice, stirring and cooking another 1-2 minutes.
Stir in seasonings.
Press into a sprayed 1 quart glass baking dish.
Stand the half orange slices around the inside edge of the dish pressing down into rice mixture.
Cover and bake for 15 minutes.

Serves 4   Per serving: cal 155, pro 3, carb 33, fat 0, sod 20, fiber 2.2
****

Veggie-Bean Polenta

Polenta (coarsely ground corn grits) is used in this versatile northern Italian dish. You'll find it in health food sections or bulk bins. Cornmeal will not do either in flavor or texture. You can serve this satisfying dish either warm or cold with a variety of sauces or a sprinkling of cheese. It keeps well in the refrigerator and makes a nice, light lunch, too.

1 cup carrots, diced
1 cup onions, diced
½ cup celery, diced
½ cup green pepper, diced
½ cup red bell pepper, diced (optional)
3 cloves garlic, crushed
1½ tsp basil
1 tsp cumin
½ tsp freshly ground pepper
Dash of ground fennel seed
1 tomato, seeded and chopped
4 cups water
2 cups polenta (whole grain corn, not corn meal)
1 cup cooked kidney beans, homemade or low sodium canned (rinsed)
3 cups low sodium tomato sauce, spaghetti sauce or Italian sauce

Spray a large pot with olive oil spray.
Sauté all the veggies and seasonings on medium-low heat for 8-10 minutes until soft.
Add the chopped tomato and water. Stir and bring to a simmer.
Slowly pour the polenta into the pot in a slow, steady stream while stirring constantly to prevent lumping.
Add the kidney beans and mix well.
Simmer over low heat for 20-25 minutes, stirring frequently to prevent sticking.
Spray a 9 x 13 glass baking dish with olive oil spray.
Turn the polenta into the dish and pack evenly, smoothing the surface.
Cover and chill until set, several hours.
To serve, cut into 8 portions (a triangle shape is traditional) and top each portion with ½ cup of sauce of your
    choice.
Heat the individual dish in a microwave for 2-3 minutes if you want to serve it hot.

Serves 8   Per serving: cal 165, pro 5.9, carb 32, fat 0.9, sod 38, fiber 2.8
****

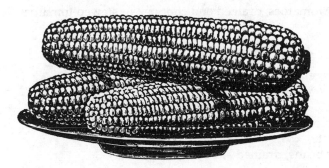

Pizza Pie

Super quick to prepare, use this basic crust recipe and top with your favorites such as mushrooms, extra veggies, a few olives, fat-free or low-fat cheese, pineapple tidbits, fresh thinly sliced tomato ... the works! Crumbled garden sausage or soy sausage is a favorite hearty choice.

Crust:
¾ cup whole wheat flour
½ cup skim milk
½ cup egg substitute
1 tsp oregano leaves

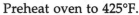

Topping:
½ cup each diced onion and green pepper
½ tsp garlic powder
Freshly ground pepper to taste
1 ⅓ cups low-sodium tomato sauce or spaghetti sauce
6 ounces fat-free mozzarella cheese, shredded

Preheat oven to 425°F.
In a small bow, beat together crust ingredients.
Spread evenly in a sprayed 14" deep dish pizza pan or 13 x 9 inch glass baking dish.
Sprinkle evenly with the toppings and seasonings (not the sauce or cheese yet).
Bake 20 minutes. Remove from oven. Now top with sauce and sprinkle with cheese. I like to sprinkle on some
     basil or other seasonings under the sauce first. If you sprinkle it on top, it may cook too much and get bitter.
Bake until slightly browned and cheese is melted, about 10-15 minutes.
Serves 4   Per serving: cal 218, pro 21, carb 30, fat 1.3, sod 386, fiber 4.6
****

Other Main Dishes

Hearty Chili

Spicy and filling, try this with cool fat-free sour cream (ah, the wonders of science!) and Chili Corn Bread*
on a cold winter's evening!

14 ounces (½ box) cooked Seitan*, ground in food processor or crumbled, or ground turkey breast
2 medium onions, chopped
2-4 cloves garlic, crushed
3 15-oz cans low sodium whole tomatoes, drained and chopped or stewed tomatoes (low-sod)
2 cups low sodium tomato sauce
2 cups water
3 TBL chili powder
2 TBL Worcestershire sauce, vegetarian or regular
2 TBL vinegar
4 bay leaves
½ tsp each cinnamon and allspice
¼ tsp cayenne pepper (or to taste)
1 15-oz can low sodium kidney beans, drained and rinsed (optional)

Heat a sprayed Dutch oven over medium heat. Add seitan or turkey breast, onion and garlic.
Sauté, stirring occasionally until browned, about 5 minutes. Add remaining ingredients and stir well to combine.
Reduce heat to low and simmer for about 30 minutes until chili is thick. For thicker chili, combine 3 TBL water
     with 1 TBL of arrowroot until smooth and stir into simmering chili.
Stir constantly and continue to cook until mixture thickens, about 4-5 minutes. Remove bay leaves before serving.
Serves 6   Per serving (w/beans & seitan): cal 255, pro 21, carb 41, fat 1, sod 170, fiber 4.5

Rolled, Stuffed and Breaded Things

No, this isn't how you feel after the holidays! The idea here is to find something flat (fish filet, seitan slice, pounded poultry breast, tortilla, lasagna noodle, thin eggplant slices or cabbage leaves, etc.) or hollow (green pepper, scooped out zucchini, pie shell, etc.). Then concoct something yummy to roll up in it or stuff into it or bread it with! Add a veggie-based low-fat sauce to finish if you want.

There are actually so many possibilities that I will just list some suggestions for you. They are all fast, simple and impressive enough for company. Experiment with your favorite ingredients and personal tastes.

Pot Pies	Calzone (stuffed pastry)	Stuffed Potato Shells
Crust Pies	Breaded Poultry or Seitan	Lasagna Rolls
Wonton Ravioli	Stuffed Peppers or sweet onions	Eggplant Rolls
Eggplant Parmesan	Veggie Tacos or Burritos	Stuffed Pasta Shells
Stuffed Poultry or Seitan	Stuffed Zucchini Boats	Stuffed Tofu
Cabbage Rolls	Steamed Stuffed Dumplings	Fish Rolls
Sushi Rolls	Layered or stuffed phyllo (thin, no-fat pastry sheets)	

Basically, you can roll, stuff or bread almost anything! Be creative with leftovers.

****

Veggie Curry

Here is yet another versatile dish that can be prepared with a wide variety of different vegetables. This version uses eggplant, green peppers, carrots and onions primarily. Other veggies that would be good include cauliflower, green beans, mushrooms, potatoes or fresh peas.

Serve over hot instant or regular brown rice with homemade whole wheat chapatis (Indian flat bread) or heated pita. Another traditional dish served with curry is Dal, which is a very simple and tasty thick bean sauce usually made with yellow split peas. Fresh fruit such as pineapple, papaya or mango goes well with this dish. And a simple salad of chopped cucumbers in yogurt dressing with chopped fresh or dried mint and green onions cools the curry and is a traditional accompaniment in Indian cooking. It takes a bit longer to make the entire meal, but is well worth the effort and you can make it a fun family affair. This is one of my favorites.

1 TBL turmeric
1 TBL whole wheat pastry flour
1 medium eggplant, cubed
4 medium carrots, cut into julienne strips
2 green peppers, sliced into strips
2 medium onions, chopped
1½ TBL curry powder
2 large tomatoes, chopped or low sodium canned tomatoes (2 cups)
1½ tsp ground coriander
¼ cup raisins

Whisk together the turmeric and flour in a medium bowl.
Add the eggplant, carrots and peppers and toss to coat lightly.
In a large non-stick skillet, bring 1 cup water or low sodium vegetable broth to a boil and add the vegetables.
Return to boil, then reduce heat and stir-sauté for 3-4 minutes. Remove vegetables from the skillet and set aside.
Add ½ cup water or broth to the skillet along with the onion.
Stir sauté for 3-4 minutes.
Add the curry powder and stir sauté for another 2-3 minutes.
Stir in the tomatoes, coriander, vegetable mixture, raisins (if used) and another ½ cup water or broth.
Bring to a boil, lower heat and simmer, covered, for 25 minutes.
Stir occasionally to prevent sticking and add more water or broth if needed.

Serves 4   Per serving: cal 138, pro 3.2, carb 33, fat 0.6, sod 30, fiber 6.5
****

Stir-Sauté Dishes

No commentary on fast, healthful cooking would be complete without mentioning the versatile stir-sauté, traditionally called "stir-fry". Since cooking oils can be damaged and rendered unhealthful at high temperatures, lower the heat and sauté instead of frying the food.

Simply heat the non-stick wok or skillet over medium for 1-2 minutes. Then spray the pan briefly with a flavored non-stick spray or add about 1 tsp of oil to the pan if your diet allows. Remember hot pan, then add oil. Peanut oil is traditionally used for lightness, taste and the ability to resist burning at high temperatures. However, canola, safflower or even olive oil can be used with good results since you will sauté, not fry the food.

Next, add the veggies (the firmer ones first) and stir constantly for about 4-5 minutes, turning and flipping the veggies to cook all sides. Add softer veggies next, again stirring and turning for about 4-5 minutes. Cooking liquid can be added at any time to avoid burning. Broth, water, wine, lemon juice and small amounts of low sodium soy are some choices. Add seasonings and very soft veggies last, continue to cook and stir until heated thoroughly. Flavorful sesame oil should be added last or drizzled over the top before serving, since it is meant to season only, not to cook. It adds a great, distinctive taste.

You can cover the pan briefly to steam the whole dish for a few minutes also. Your choice of protein may be added at the appropriate time. Cooked meats, tofu or seitan chunks. Raw meats or poultry should be stir-sautéed separately before beginning the veggie cooking. Don't overcook! Slightly crisp veggies add to the freshness of the dish. The secret to easy stir-sauté is to have all your ingredients ready and at hand before beginning to cook.

Some favorites veggies:
> carrots, onions, mushrooms, broccoli, flowers and peeled stalks, cauliflower, zucchini, winter squash or yam, summer squash, bamboo shoots, chili peppers, chinese pea pods, green, red and yellow bell peppers, green or yellow beans, jicama or water chestnuts, corn, cabbage - white, red or Napa (Chinese), bok choy, turnips or parsnips, asparagus, spinach or other dark greens, whole garlic cloves, anything you like!

Protein:
> tofu (firm, cubed), seitan (sliced thin or cubed), textured vegetable protein, cooked beans
> chicken or turkey breast (bite-size pieces sautéed in lemon juice first)
> fresh shrimp, crab or lobster chunks (if diet allows), your choice!

Some favorite seasonings:
> garlic (minced, whole, crushed, even powder), ginger (fresh grated or powder)
> red pepper flakes or cayenne, Hoisin sauce (small amount to flavor --it's high in sodium)
> sesame oil - hot chili or regular
> soy sauce - low sodium
> Braggs Amino (available at health food stores)
> powdered kelp, coriander, powdered mustard, lemon juice

The above seasonings are traditional oriental seasonings. Why not try a different version such as a Mexican stir-sauté with chili, cumin, onion and garlic? Use suitable veggies such as firm tomatoes, corn, chilies or beans. Or an Indian Curry stir-sauté could be seasoned with curry and coriander. Use veggies such as peas, potatoes, eggplant, green peppers, etc.

Thicken the mixture if you wish by mixing 1 TBL of arrowroot or cornstarch with 2 TBL of water in a small cup and stirring the mixture slowly into the almost finished dish while still cooking. Continue cooking and stirring until the mixture thickens and clears. One TBL of powdered thickener will thicken about 1 cup of liquid.

Some fruits can be added also although they tend to break down quickly, so add them at the end of the cooking time. Some good choices are fresh or canned pineapple, apples, raisins or papaya.

Most of all, experiment and have fun with this technique and be sure to have the kids or other family members join in, either by watching and rooting from the sidelines or chopping and stirring and adding seasonings, too. This is a great, fun cooking experience with a rich history for the whole family, creating a joyful meal for body and soul!

* *

Seitan (Wheat Meat)

Seitan (say-tan) is a wheat-based protein alternative with a texture similar to meat or fowl. It is very versatile and being somewhat bland, takes on the flavors of the broth or the seasonings added to the seitan itself. It is high in protein, cholesterol free, nearly fat and sodium free, low in calories and has 2 gm of fiber per serving, something no meat can boast. Not only that, it is very economical and can be prepared in many different forms, such as slices, chunks or "roasts". It is well worth experimenting with this super food, in spite of it's unusual name. Use it just like meat in sandwiches, soups and stews, pasta dishes, ground for meatballs or loaves, or marinate and grill.

Make seitan with gluten flour as below or Arrowhead Mills offers a boxed Seitan Quick Mix which I highly recommend with recipes and instructions available in health food stores. Once you try it, I'm sure it will be a regular in your kitchen, too.

1½ cups gluten flour
¼ tsp finely minced fresh herbs (thyme, sage, oregano, etc.)
Freshly ground black pepper
2 TBL low-sodium soy sauce
1 cup chopped onion
1 cup chopped carrot
½ tsp whole black peppercorns
2 bay leaves

Combine the flour, herbs and ground black pepper in a large bowl.
Stir together the soy sauce and 1 cup water in a small bowl and add slowly to the flour mixture, stirring with a
   wooden spoon until it forms a ball.
Turn the dough out on a clean surface dusted with a little more gluten flour.
Knead for 3-5 minutes.
Now hold the dough under cold running water and stretch the dough using your fingers to work out and rinse
   away any bran and starch.
Form into a 2 inch diameter roll and slice thinly into ¼" slices.
In a large pot, add the remaining ingredients with 3 quarts water and bring to a boil.
Gently lower the slices one at a time into the simmering broth.
Lower the heat and simmer gently for 20 minutes. The slices will rise to the top and puff up a lot.
Remove the slices with a slotted spoon.
Slice into strips if desired.
Place in a storage container with lid and cover with the broth.
Refrigerate for up to one week.
Makes four cups.

Per ½ cup: cal 104, fat 0.6, sod 150 mg (from broth), fiber 2g
****

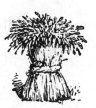

Sauces and Gravies

Chunky Cranapple Sauce

This luscious sauce can also be used over hot cereal, frozen desserts or pudding, or to accompany meats as well as the Holiday Turkey or Seitan Roast.

2 cups raw cranberries, frozen or fresh
½ cup frozen apple juice concentrate
½ cup water
5 medium apples, peeled and chopped
3 TBL reduced sugar pectin
1 TBL arrowroot
1 TBL vanilla
¼ tsp lemon extract (opt) or a squeeze of fresh lemon juice

Place the first 3 ingredients in a Dutch oven and bring to a boil over medium high heat.
Add the apples and pectin.
Reduce heat to medium low and simmer, uncovered for 8-10 minutes stirring occasionally.
Mix the arrowroot with 2 TBL water and add to the mixture along with the flavorings.
Stir constantly for about 2 minutes or until the mixture thickens.
Taste for sweetness as cranberries can vary in tartness.
Add natural liquid sweetener or more apple juice if desired.
Serve warm or chilled.

Makes about 4 cups. Per ½ cup: cal 109. pro 0.4, carb 27.7, fat 0.3, sod 3

To make a jelled Cranapple Sauce:
1.   Increase apple juice to ¾ cup
2.   Increase water to 1 ¼ cups
3.   Omit arrowroot mixture
4.   Sprinkle 2 envelopes plus 1 tsp unflavored gelatin over ½ cup of cold water. Add to the apple cranberry mixture after cooking, stirring well to dissolve.
5.   Pour into 1 quart mold and chill until firm. Unmold onto a lettuce-lined plate and garnish with fresh fruit such as orange slices or grapes.

****

Onion Gravy

This thick and delicious recipe is very low in calories and tasty. This is one of the recipes most requested at the holidays and goes well with turkey or seitan roast and mashed potatoes.

1½ tsp dried minced onion
1½ cup defatted turkey, chicken or vegetable stock or water, divided
1 TBL low sodium soy sauce
1½ TBL arrowroot or cornstarch
1½ TBL whole wheat pastry flour
6 TBL nonfat dry milk

Toast the onions by placing them in an aluminum foil pie tin and then in a hot oven for just a few minutes until
        toasted. Place in a saucepan with ¾ cup of the stock and the soy sauce.
In a small bowl, combine the last 3 ingredients and blend in the remaining stock with a whisk.
Bring the contents of the saucepan to a boil, then stir in the flour mixture.
Reduce heat to low and simmer, stirring constantly until thickened, about 3 minutes.

Makes about 1½ cups. Per ¼ cup: 28 cal, 0.1g fat, 105 mg sod

Mushroom Gravy

1 onion, minced
3 cups mushrooms, thinly sliced
1 TBL sesame oil
2½ cups water, divided
¼ cup low sodium soy sauce
½ cup whole wheat pastry flour
¼ cup nutritional yeast flakes (in the health food section or health food store)

In a medium heavy pot, sauté the onions and mushrooms in the sesame oil until soft, about 5 minutes.
Add 2 cups of the water and the soy sauce.
Bring to a boil, lower heat and simmer for about 5 minutes until the vegetables are tender.
In a small bowl, whisk together the flour and yeast, then add ½ cup water and stir until smooth.
Add the flour mixture to the mushrooms, whisking to mix.
Simmer for 5-10 minutes, whisking often until mixture is desired consistency.

Makes about 4 cups. Per ¼ cup: 20 cal, 1g fat, 75 mg sod
****

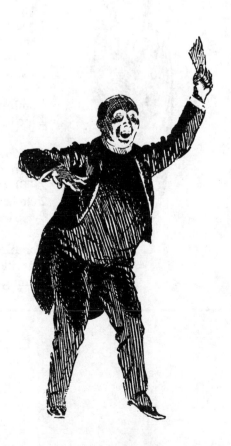

"Eureka! I found the secret recipe for low-sodium mushroom gravy."

Marinades

Marinades are a great way to add complex flavors to foods. They also serve to keep the foods moist and to tenderize tougher cuts of meat. Here are several concoctions for different types of foods. Use your imagination and personal taste preferences to custom blend your own marinades. Start with a simple mixture of wine, broth, juice, and a variety of herbs and spices. As you get more experienced, expand your mixtures. Creativity will be well rewarded!

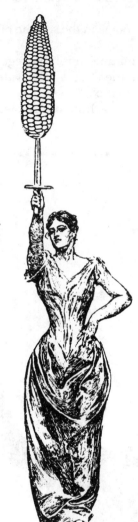

Tofu Marinade
1 tsp lemon zest
½ cup fresh mint, chopped
4 cloves garlic, crushed or minced
1 serrano pepper, seeded and minced
2 TBL cilantro, chopped
2 TBL fresh ginger root, chopped
3 scallions, chopped
1 TBL Sucanat or brown sugar
Juice of 1 lime
¼ cup non-fat yogurt
2 TBL low-sodium soy sauce

Process all ingredients in food processor. Marinate tofu chunks 4-6 hours.

Honey-Ginger Marinade
2 TBL scallions, minced
2 TBL low-sodium soy sauce
1 TBL honey
1 TBL fresh ginger, grated
1 tsp fresh lime juice
2 cloves garlic, crushed

Combine all ingredients. Marinate 2 inch chunks of white meat for at least 30 minutes in refrigerator.

Seafood Marinade #1
1 cup pineapple juice
1 TBL low-sodium soy sauce
1 TBL white wine
1 TBL garlic powder
1 TBL fresh ginger, grated

Combine all ingredients. Marinate 1½ inch chunks of white fish overnight in refrigerator

Vegetable Marinade and Sauce
½ bunch fresh thyme
Dash of cayenne pepper
Zest of 1 lemon
½ tsp freshly ground pepper
10 cloves garlic, crushed
Juice of 2 lemons
⅓ cup vegetable broth
¾ cup tomato sauce

Strip thyme from stems, reserving stems for the grill. Process all ingredients except tomato sauce in food processor. Marinate cut-up veggies for 15 minutes. Heat marinade and tomato sauce insmall saucepan. Serve with veggies over pasta.

Spanish Marinade
½ cup fresh orange juice
¼ cup tomato juice
2 tsp olive oil
1½ lemon juice
1 tsp oregano
½ tsp each paprika and cumin
Freshly ground pepper to taste

Combine all ingredients. Marinate 2 inch chunks overnight in refrigerator.

Seafood Marinade #2
¼ cup fresh lemon juice
2 TBL chopped parsley
2 cloves garlic, minced or crushed
½ tsp oregano

Combine all ingredients. Marinate white fish fillets for 1 hour in refrigerator, turning occasionally.

* *

Desserts and Sweets

Cream Fluffs

This versatile recipe can be flavored to your own tastes and available ingredients. Experiment with what you have and you may just come up with your favorite one. That's how I discovered some of the best and most unusual combinations! Some favorite Cream Fluff combinations: Bananas and pineapple, Strawberries and almond flavoring, Applesauce and bananas, Blueberries and Chocolate, Yogurt and Bananas and on and on ... !! These are worth some experimentation as they are basically just skim milk and fresh fruit, excellent healthy snack foods. Most of the Cream Fluffs are around 100 calories per large and satisfying serving!

Basic recipe for 2 servings:
1 cup skim milk or ½ c evaporated skim milk or ⅓ c powdered skim milk with additional liquid such as water or
    fruit juice or 1 envelope of reduced calorie shake mix
1 cup frozen fruit
½ - 1 tsp flavoring
sweetener of your choice

It is very important that all ingredients are very cold and also the bowl and blade of the food processor itself. Place everything in the freezer for 15-30 minutes before making your Cream Fluff. Place all ingredients in the food processor and process by pulsing until mixed then on highest setting for 2-4 minutes. The longer you process, the fluffier this will get. Serve immediately as these do not keep. Add more frozen fruit if you want a thicker consistency.

Berry Cream Fluff
    1 cup skim milk
    1 cup frozen blueberries or strawberries or cranberries
    ½ tsp vanilla or almond flavoring
    2 pkts Equal or use fruit juice concentrate or natural liquid
        sweetener as part of the liquid

Chocolate-Banana Cream Fluff
    1 cup skim milk
    1 frozen banana - cut into chunks before freezing
    2 tsp cocoa or carob powder - unsweetened
    ½ tsp vanilla
    ½ tsp rum, chocolate or banana flavoring
     sweetener to taste as above

For an easy and quick Chocolate-Banana Cream Fluff substitute 1 envelope of reduced calorie fudge shake mix for the cocoa, flavoring and sweetener. Add a few more banana slices or frozen strawberries for a thicker Fluff.
This is a favorite treat.

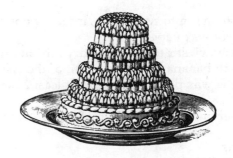

"Coconut" Cream Fluff
    ⅓-½ cup canned evaporated skim milk, chilled
    2 carrots, 1 banana and 1 orange - peeled, seeded,
        cut into chunks and frozen
    ½ tsp orange flavoring
    2-3 drops of coconut flavoring
    sweetener to taste as above

Babe Rosie Bar

When I want a candy bar, I usually reach for fruit or dried fruit. But sometimes, a chocolate-peanut butter treat is in order! The new sports bars found in the health food section have really improved and offer good flavor with minimal fat, but are high in simple sugars. So unless you are an athlete, they can be too sugary. This version has protein, whole grain and fruit.

A satisfying confection which is a variation of an OLD SECRET neighborhood recipe. Actually I used to make this up when I was a kid and eat it by the bowlful! It still satisfies my urge for a candy bar and I have it for a quick lunch (or even breakfast) on the run as well as snacktime.

It is high in fat because of the peanut butter, although the new reduced-fat peanut butter helps. But still, use it sparingly as an occasional indulgence. Or slice it into pieces and have one or two at a time. Be sure to eat lower-fat foods the rest of the day so your overall fat grams stay within your range.

For each serving:
1 TBL reduced-fat peanut butter (I prefer chunky)
2 TBL hot black decaffeinated coffee or hot water
1 envelope diet hot cocoa mix or chocolate fudge shake mix
¼ cup dry oatmeal (¾ ounce)
2 TBL raisins

Place the coffee or water and peanut butter in a small bowl and stir until blended.
Add the envelope of mix and stir again.
Add the oatmeal and raisins combining everything thoroughly.
Turn mixture out onto a sheet of waxed paper and mold into a bar about 5-6" long.
Wet hands with a little water if the mixture is too sticky.
Wrap in the waxed paper and freeze for at least several hours, if you can wait.
Thaw for about ten minutes before eating. Cut into 8 pieces if you don't want to eat the whole bar all at once.

Serves 1   Per whole bar: cal 255, pro 10, carb 40.5, fat 8, sod 275, fiber 3.5
              Per 2 pieces: cal 64, pro 2.5, carb 10.1, fat 2, sod 69, fiber 0.9

****

Roseanna Bananas

These yummy snacks remind me of childhood trips to the fair or carnival, but are a much healthier variety! Kids love them and they are fun to make.

2 ripe bananas, peeled
1 envelope diet hot cocoa mix or diet chocolate fudge shake mix
¼ cup water
¼ cup fat-free granola
wooden popsicle sticks

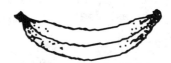

Cut the bananas into two halves, insert a popsicle stick into the bottom of each one and place each half on a
    piece of wax paper.
In a small bowl, stir together the dry mix and the water until smooth.
Spread each banana half with 1 TBL of the chocolate, then roll in 1 TBL of the granola.
Wrap in the wax paper and freeze at least 2 hours.

Makes 4 servings. Per serving: cal 80. pro 2.1, carb 19.4, fat 0.3, sod 67, fiber 1.9

Variations:
1. Roll the coated bananas in toasted wheat germ, another crushed cereal, defatted chopped peanuts
    (Weight Watchers makes honey-roasted and regular), nuts or seeds if your diet allows
2. Cut the bananas into bite-size pieces before coating and freezing in individual paper candy cups

****

Instant Pumpkin Pudding

Yes, this is an old trick, but very effective in filling up an empty tummy in an emergency. Low in fat, sodium and calories and high in fiber and beta-carotene a perfect snack or dessert.

¾ cup canned pumpkin (plain, not the pumpkin pie type)
½ tsp vanilla
½ tsp pumpkin pie spice
1 tsp light maple syrup, Sucanat or sweetener of your choice (optional)
1 TBL raisins (optional)

Place pumpkin in a microwave-safe bowl. Add the other ingredients, stirring to mix well.
If you are using maple syrup, you could drizzle it over the top after the pudding is cooked. If you are using Equal
    for the sweetener, add it after you have cooked it.
Cover with plastic wrap and cook in the microwave on HIGH for 1½ minutes.
Serve plain or with whole grain graham crackers (kind of tastes like pumpkin pie), a sprinkling of fat-free
    granola or fiber cereal, a tablespoon of skim milk or carob or vanilla rice milk or yogurt. I especially like to
    stick a frozen chocolate mousse bar or orange vanilla frozen bar right in the middle. It melts nicely and adds
    creamy flavor for only 30 calories.

Serves 1   Per srvg (w/ raisins & syrup): cal 95, pro 3.3, carb 24, fat 0.4, sod 48, fiber 7.5
****

Orange Cocoa Truffles

Another treat for the sweet tooth. I served these as Halloween treats and everyone loved them. You can vary the flavor with different juice and extracts. Mocha with decaf coffee is great, too.

6 TBL fat-free plain cream cheese
1½ TBL frozen orange juice concentrate
½ tsp each vanilla and orange extracts
14 graham cracker squares rolled into crumbs
1½ packets sugar-free chocolate fudge shake mix or hot cocoa mix

In small bowl, beat together first three ingredients until creamy.
In medium bowl, whisk together cocoa and crumbs.
Pour cream cheese mixture into crumb mixture and stir slowly until creamed and well combined. Add a little
    water if necessary.
Knead briefly with moistened hands to thoroughly mix.
Form into a ball.
Divide ball into fourths.
From each fourth, roll 6 small balls.
Roll small balls in additional crumbs or unsweetened cocoa powder.
Place on a small plate or in individual candy papers to serve.
Refrigerate to store.

Makes 24   Per truffle: cal 25 , fat 0.4 , sod 58

Variation:
Use 3 TBL plain cocoa powder instead of mix for
    a bittersweet truffle. Sweeten if desired.
Try different flavors such as Peach-Mint.

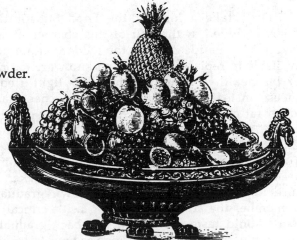

Last but not least ...
a simple bowl of fruit is always delicious.

Converting Your Favorite Recipes   31

"The more things change, the more they are the same."
Alphonse Karr

Aunt Fanny's Old Favorites are Full of Fat

We all have our very favorite recipes and foods that may be hard to live totally without: Aunt Bessie's Two-Ton Fruitcake, Uncle Dewey's Gooey Chewy Bars, or Cousin Edna's Stockyard Pizza with Extra Cheeze Pleeze. But wait! You don't have to give up your favorites after all. You can have your cake (even Grandma Mabel's Monstrous Mud Pie) and eat it too! In this chapter you will find practical suggestions for converting your old-style fat, calorie and sodium laden recipes into more healthful varieties. Many chefs are doing this nowadays as they have found out that the taste is hardly ever compromised and actually can improve in some recipes. The butter, sugar, whole eggs and cream are just not needed to turn out first rate, absolutely delicious and healthful dishes. They are passé, darling. New, healthier versions of classic cookbooks such as Betty Crocker and Better Homes and Gardens now include information on food values and lighter versions of old favorites. So get with it and start living the thin life in the way that many others are discovering ... and do it without depriving your taste buds one bit!

Weaning Yourself Off the Worst Offenders

First, take a look at the Food Substitution Chart included at the end of this chapter. It will give you some ideas about the foods that are now available to replace the ones you know are too rich to be healthy. Examples include: light ricotta cheese instead of cream cheese in a cheesecake, lower fat cheese instead of full fat, fruit canned in juice instead of heavy syrup. Also, be sure to read Chapter 34 "Sodium & Salt vs. Herbs & Spices". You will find plenty of options for tasty seasonings besides habitually reaching for the salt shaker. Be sure to cut your taste for salt down gradually (remember the attitude of EASE? ... it's critical) or foods could taste flat. By cutting back gradually, you will hardly notice the change as your taste buds become more accustomed to the reduction.

Follow the desensitization schedule in "Sodium and Salt" to gradually cut down salt without feeling deprived. The same is true for other ingredients. If the dish just isn't sweet enough or rich enough to satisfy you, then either decide to give yourself some time to adjust or add a bit more sweetener or rich stuff back until you get used to it. Then cut back again later if you still need to. Fats are actually quite easy to reduce without compromising the taste. The light, fresh taste of food comes through without being obliterated in oily grease.

You also need to develop lighter cooking methods to save on fat and calories. For instance, using broth, wine, water or cooking spray for sautéing instead of using butter or oil. Baking breaded chicken instead of deep-frying. Steaming vegetables instead of boiling away all the vitamins (if you do boil, be sure to save the liquid for soups or gravies). For further discussion of cooking methods see Chapter 25 "What to Eat".

How Many Servings?

Begin converting an old recipe by first determining how many servings in the entire dish. You can then determine the amount of each ingredient each serving will have. One-half cup of canned fruit, for instance, equals one serving. Generally, follow the package guidelines for serving size or check your reference book on food values. If you have 2 cups of fruit in 4 servings, then each serving will have one fruit.

Converting is really very simple and you'll be pleasantly surprised how many of your old favorites you will still be able to enjoy. Once you get good at this, there is practically no limit to the recipes that you can convert (well, maybe not Mabel's Mud Pie). But you can get pretty close! Go ahead and buy that magazine with the holiday recipes so attractively shown on the cover. Now you'll be able to enjoy them on your terms and stay thin at the same time!

Below, I've converted a recipe to a healthier version to show the basic principles. When you see how simple it is, you'll wonder why you didn't think of it yourself! Don't be afraid to experiment.

Meat-a-Roni (Original Recipe) Serves 4

4 cups cooked macaroni
1 pound ground beef
2 tablespoons butter
2 tablespoons flour
1 tsp salt
2 cups whole milk
1½ c Cheddar cheese, shredded
1½ c Monterey Jack cheese, shredded
¼ c parmesan cheese, grated
2 tsp parsley flakes

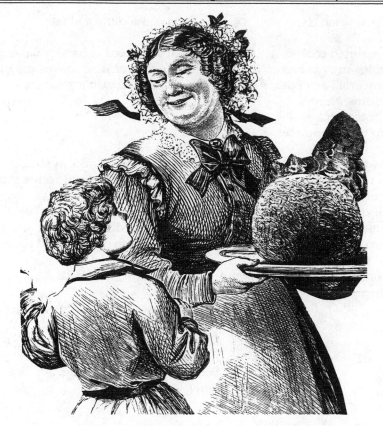

"It's your Uncle's favorite dinner on his bowling night."

Veg-a-Roni (Converted Recipe) Serves 4

Use this instead:	Why?
3 cups whole grain macaroni	¾ cup of macaroni equals 1½ servings of grain. You could increase to 4 cups cooked macaroni and count as 2 grain servings but the extra vegetables add enough bulk to compensate for the reduced macaroni. Try it out. Whole grain macaroni is also a healthier choice for fiber and vitamins.
8 ounces cooked Seitan* or ground turkey breast	This amount will still count as 2 protein servings each, even with reduction in meat. Ground turkey breast can save even more fat. * In Chapter 30 "Basic Recipes".
2 tablespoons diet margarine	Especially used in recipes, the taste difference is not noticeable between butter and margarine. Diet is half the calories and saturated fat of regular. You could try using a bit less, too. Fat-free available, also.
½ tsp salt (optional)	Eventually you can eliminate the salt altogether when you train your taste buds to be more sensitive. The cheese will provide plenty of sodium.
2 TBL whole wheat pastry flour	More nutrients and fiber.
2 cups low-fat or skim milk	Again, incorporated in a recipe, the taste difference is negligible and the fat and calorie savings are substantial.
4 ounces (shredded) each of reduced-calorie, fat and sodium cheddar and jack cheese	Two ounces of reduced calorie cheese is one protein serving. That would be one more protein serving per portion for the cheese. Try part fat-free cheese to further reduce fat, but it melts differently. Experiment here.

2 TBL parmesan cheese   Reduced sodium and fat.

2 cups assorted cooked   Two teaspoons of parsley flakes just wasn't enough veggies.
vegetables such as broccoli,   This addition also makes the dish very filling, with added
cauliflower, red pepper,   fiber and nutrients galore.
mushrooms, carrots,
green beans, etc.,
cut into bite-size pieces

As you can see, the converted version is much lower in fat and calories without compromising on the basic nature of the dish: rich, creamy and filling. In the original recipe the ground beef was browned in a skillet and used in the recipe without even draining off the fat. Of course you have learned to cook your beef or turkey so the fat will drip off while cooking! The "after" figures include turkey breast, but using the Seitan will decrease the fat, cholesterol and sodium further. I find that with the cheese and vegetables, the addition of meat or seitan is not even needed. Actually the converted dish is so filling that it serves six instead of just four.

Look at what you're eating!

	BEFORE	**AFTER!**	
	(¼ recipe)	(¼ recipe)	(⅙ recipe)
Calories	1044.	356	237
Cholesterol	174 mg	79 mg	53 mg
Fat	69 g	4.8 g	3.2 g
Sodium	1405 mg	506 mg	337 mg
Fiber	1.7 g	5.1 g	3.4 g

If at First You Don't Succeed

Keep experimenting with your favorite recipes until you have them trimmed down to THINNER WINNERS proportions. With all the great new reduced-fat, sodium and calorie foods available, it is a cinch and really eye-opening fun. The more you look for the healthier alternatives, the more of them there seem to be! Twenty-five years ago, diet and health foods available in the markets consisted of cans of meal replacements and maybe a vile-tasting diet soda or two! Nowadays, consumer demand has produced a huge variety of great-tasting healthier foods to put to work in your kitchen. In the Food Substitution Chart you will find suggested replacements for the old heavy foods. Many health-oriented magazines have regular features with recipe conversions as their topics. You can learn a lot, practice your skills and pick up tips for foods and techniques. Lighten up your recipes and you will have another key to lightening up your body without missing the tastiness that you want and deserve.

The Food Substitution Chart lists quite a few ideas to help get you started. There is a good reason why each of these alternate foods are suggested. Many of the foods that we seek substitutions for are either high in sodium, fat, cholesterol, sugar, or they contain artificial chemicals, preservatives, colorings or flavorings ... all the things we need to avoid or limit for optimum health! For the increasing number of vegetarians foods of animal origin have alternatives suggested on the chart, also. To increase your success rate of replacing the less healthful foods in your diet, make a point to appreciate the taste of the alternate foods in and of themselves. Nothing will exactly duplicate a pat of real butter, either on your bread or in your arteries. But the taste of margarine or other flavorings can be delicious also. Comparing one taste to the other will only disappoint you and is not really fair to the alternate food. The classic example of this is trying to substitute carob for chocolate. Carob just doesn't taste at all like chocolate! But carob has its own rich, full taste that is quite good and satisfying in many recipes.

My goal here is to point out ways in which you may be able to improve your health through more intelligent food choices. However, the choice is yours. You are an individual traveling your own unique nutritional road. Your responsibility to yourself will best be served by knowing your needs and clearly defining your nutritional goals. If a vegetarian diet is not what you choose to follow right now then that is your choice. Perhaps your goal is simply to reduce your blood pressure or weight to a more healthful level. Follow your own path ... and better health to you, whatever you choose. In all cases, the substitution foods have been chosen for their superior nutritional content compared to their customary counterparts. Now here are some of the best choices in each category.

Food Substitution Chart

Substitute healthier foods for the nutritional question marks you want to replace in your diet. Here are just some of the foods available that can be used instead of the listed target items that may not be as healthy as you would like. Add your own favorite discoveries and any new foods that might come along in the future.

Alcohol - mixed spritzers, coolers, light wine, mineral water with a twist of lemon or lime, fruit or vegetable juice, sodas, club soda/seltzer.

Bacon - bacon bits, health food varieties, vegetable protein versions, Canadian bacon.

Beef - lean cuts (loin or round), use healthy cooking methods (broil or grill), ground turkey breast, mix beef and turkey, vegetable protein versions, seitan.

Bread - reduced calorie, pita, homemade, buns, rolls, whole grains, rice or corn cakes, use recipes that stretch your bread (like pumpkin muffins, magic cereal, magic-crust pizza, etc.).

Butter - Molly McButter, Butter Buds, butter flavored cooking spray (refrigerated or spray can), margarine and diet margarine(soft tub), whipped, butter flavoring, water or broth, non-stick cookware .

Cake - many healthier and diet varieties in the frozen food section, new fat-free varieties (read labels), home baked carrot, zucchini, spice, pumpkin, cupcakes, muffins.

Candy - fruit, dried fruit (like dates, figs and papaya), carob, health food varieties, recipes such as "Babe Rosie Bar"*, frozen grapes or banana slices, Sorbee.

Canned foods - low-salt varieties, canned in juice, fresh or frozen, rinse foods thoroughly three times to remove excess sodium.

Chips - homemade tortilla, pita or potato, low-salt varieties, popcorn, raw vegetables, health store varieties, whole grain crackers, rice or popcorn cakes, whole grain pretzels, ready-to-eat cereals, dried fruit and veggie slices (banana chips, carrot chips - home made).

Cheesecake - ricotta cheese (fat-free or part-skim), yogurt cheese, non-fat or low-fat cottage cheese, fat-free cream cheese or sour cream, frozen dietary varieties, homemade recipes, gelatin as thickener, non-bake recipe can use nutrasweet for sweetener.

Chocolate - carob, cocoa powder, nutrasweet, many dietetic varieties, health store varieties, hot cocoa or shake mix, homemade recipes using these ingredients, small amounts of "the real thing"..

Cookies - health store or reduced-calorie versions, oatmeal, whole grains, fruit sweetened, new fat-free varieties, convert your favorite recipes using healthier ingredients.

Cream sauces - skim or 1% milk, evaporated skim, Butter Buds, whole grain flour, fat-free cream cheese or sour cream or ricotta cheese or cottage cheese or yogurt as a base, tomato sauce base, pureed beans or pureed veggies, instant soups, mustards.

Donuts - lower-fat varieties, eggless health food, bagels, homemade pita pastries, frozen dietary varieties, fat-free muffins and pastries.

Eggs - egg substitute, egg whites, a mixture of these, low cholesterol eggs, powdered vegetarian egg replacer for recipes, applesauce, prune puree or yogurt in recipes.

French fries - fresh homemade baked without oil, frozen bake at home type.

Fried foods - baked varieties, sautéed, breaded or crumb-coated and baked.

Frosting - frozen fruit juice or nutrasweet as sweetener, skim or 1% milk, pumpkin puree base, fat-free cream cheese or ricotta cheese or yogurt cheese, skim milk powder, dried fruit puree .

Gravy - low-salt bouillon or homemade broth as bases, arrow-root, cornstarch or potato water to thicken, herbs and spices in place of salt, whole grain flour, toasted dried onion, skim all fat, refrigerate to harden fat on top for easy removal, gravy separator.

Hamburger - ground turkey breast or extra lean beef, mixture of beef and turkey, veggie or bean (homemade or health food varieties), soy-type, lots of fresh veggies (lettuce, tomatoes, sprouts, etc.), diet buns, whole grain buns, pita pockets, fat-free or low-fat mayo or thousand island dressing, low-salt mustard, low-sodium pickles, grill or broil.

Ice cream - non or lower fat varieties, ice milk, sherbet, sorbet, low or non-fat frozen yogurt, pureed frozen fruit, dietary shakes, cream fluffs (recipe section), lower fat types in frozen food section (watch sugar).

Pancakes - whole grains, add ricotta cheese, pureed fruit, egg substitutes, skim milk, potatoes, oatmeal, egg whites, mashed banana, fruit toppings (recipe section), reduced-calorie syrups, non-stick butter-flavored cooking sprays, butter sprinkles, non-stick cookware.

Pasta - whole wheat, spinach or vegetable varieties, tomato based sauces, low or non-fat cottage or ricotta or cream cheese or sour cream bases, spaghetti squash (mix ½ & ½).

Pastries - homemade (recipe section), non-fat ricotta cheese filling, health food varieties, fruit toppings, frozen dietary types, top toast, bagel or English muffin with cream cheese or ricotta and jam or Fruit Topping or Equal and cinnamon.

Peanuts - defatted, freeze-dried, garbanzo nuts (roast cooked beans), low-fat peanut butter.

Pies - fruit, rhubarb, pumpkin, grapenut or flake cereal crust, graham cracker crust, yogurt cheese layer, diet margarine, crumb toppings, homemade recipes, fruit juice sweetener.

Ribs - use healthy cooking methods, lean cuts of beef, remove fat, homemade marinades and barbecue sauce.

Sour cream - non-fat sour cream or cottage cheese or yogurt, yogurt cream cheese, homemade.

Stuffing - whole grain breads, butter substitutes, diet margarine, eggplant, apple, celery and other vegetables or fruits, rice, shredded carrots, raisins, broth to moisten, butternut squash.

Sugar - frozen fruit juice concentrate (apple, orange, etc.), grape juice, honey, maple syrup, fruits and fruit sugars, raisins, carrots, molasses, nutrasweet, grain sweeteners (barley, rice, etc.), sucanat, Fruitsource, Dr. Bronner's barley malt powder, Sweet One.

Syrup - fruit toppings and syrups (recipe section), low-calorie types.

Tap water - bottled spring or distilled, low-sodium mineral water, home purified.

Whipped topping - skim milk recipes, evaporated skim milk, powdered skim milk, fruit juices or nutrasweet to sweeten, egg whites, low-calorie frozen type, new non-fat aerosol.

Whole milk - 1% low fat, skim milk, mixture diluting the higher fat varieties, evaporated skim, powdered skim, light soy or rice or almond based beverages (Rice Dream or almond milk).

In A Nutshell

1) You can learn to have your cake and eat it too!

2) Check the Food Substitution Chart for ideas to get you started.

3) Review Chapter 34 "Sodium and Salt vs. Herbs and Spices".

4) Cut back on offenders such as salt and fat gradually see section on Ease in Chapter 5.

5) Learn lighter cooking techniques.

6) Use suggested serving sizes for accuracy.

7) The more you look for healthier alternatives, the more there seem to be! Have fun!

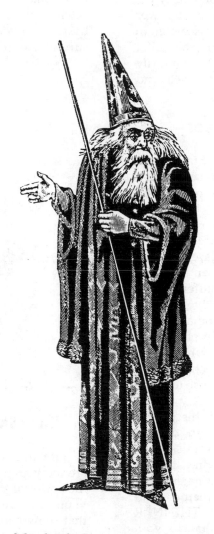

"Finding healthy foods isn't magic, it's just common sense."

Fat and Cholesterol   32

"Who's your fat friend?"
Beau Brummel (referring to the Prince of Wales)

Many people find it easier to stick with a program when they understand the "why" of a system. That's the basis of the entire THINNER WINNERS program, and this chapter will give you a better understanding of the "why" relating to fat and cholesterol. There are some pretty scary facts here, but the motivation and understanding gained has been worth it for me ... and I hope for you, too. The point is not to scare the fat off of you (well, maybe just a little), but to inform you and empower you with the knowledge as to why it is better to choose certain foods and lifestyles over others. I'm not doing this just to be a health nut! I voluntarily and joyously choose positive health for myself, and you can make the same choice.

One Million of Us Each Year

Half of all deaths in the United States each year are caused by coronary artery disease. That's over 1 million deaths annually ... more than all other causes of death combined. Over 1.5 million people suffer heart attacks in America each year and 5.5 million additional Americans are estimated to be suffering from coronary heart disease, detected or undetected. These figures represent an alarming epidemic. And a lot more. The pain, suffering and tragic impact of these facts on the lives of the patients and their families is unfathomable. The loss of a full, productive family life and replacement with a disabled half-functioning health cripple or worse yet, an empty chair at the dinner table ... the loss of a parent or spouse to guide and travel with through life.

The real tragedy is that much of this misery can be avoided by simple changes in dietary lifestyle. This doesn't have to be a miserable, pinched diet pattern. Believe me, I couldn't stand to have one of my favorite pastimes eliminated from my life (eating, of course!). The recipes and alternative foods discussed in the THINNER WINNERS program should prove that to you. Merely an awareness of the changes needed and how simply they can be incorporated will help to bring your diet and lifestyle into line with an acknowledged healthful one ... as opposed to a lifestyle that will put you and your family into the category of statistics mentioned above.

The really scary part about heart disease for

me came when I discovered that even with 90% blockage of an artery, you may still "feel fine" ... and get a passing-with-flying-colors report from your doctor based on a treadmill stress test or a resting EKG. It is not until the disease is very advanced (90-95% blockage) that you begin to feel pressure in your chest upon exertion or have other symptoms. Recent research has indicated that at least some of this blockage may be reversible, if you catch it in time. However, 50% of all first-time heart attack victims die and up to 33% of those that survive die in the first year following their attack.

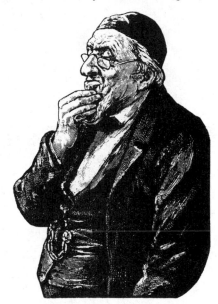

*"Hmm, maybe I'll pass
on the fried cheese logs in butter sauce today."*

Early Studies Link Diet and Health

If you think that you or members of your family are too young to worry about these things, consider that arterial plaque has been found in infants as young as 3 years old! Studies have been conducted that show coronary artery blockage in a fetus. And according to Dr. Forest Adams of the Pediatric Arteriosclerosis Clinic at UCLA, by the time an American child is ten years old, it is now common for the disease to be present.

Also consider the study of young servicemen, our nation's finest, sent over to the Korean and Vietnam Wars. Autopsies of these apparently healthy soldiers indicated that in 77% of the men "gross evidence of coronary disease was demonstrated". The conclusion was that 35% of these young men had severe coronary heart disease. Their average age was 22. Dr. William Enos, who conducted this study also autopsied young Japanese males between the ages of 20 and 30. He found no significant arterial closures. His conclusion was that the American diet and lifestyle caused these differences in heart health.

This early study prompted other researchers to test the conclusions. The much-discussed Seven Countries Test was conducted using almost 13,000 men ages 40-49 in the United States, Japan, Finland, the Netherlands, Italy, Greece and Yugoslavia. The study showed that the higher the percentage of fat in the average diet, the higher the incidence of heart disease and, conversely, the lower the percentage of fat in the diet, the lower the incidence of heart disease. The highest percentage at that time was in the Netherlands with 40% of the diet consumed being fat. The average American diet has been 42% fat, until just recently when it began to drop slightly.

Two further significant early studies, much reported, really started the ball rolling in linking diet with health. Dr. Ancel Keys at the University of Minnesota studied men in the 40-60 age range for a period of 15 years. The men who suffered heart attacks during that time were found to have significantly higher levels of fat and cholesterol in their blood than their counterparts who did not have heart attacks. This was the first study to link cholesterol with heart disease in humans and led to further studies.

The second notable and famous study was the Framingham Study started by the Public Health Service in Framingham, Massachusetts in 1948. This was a very large study involving 5200 individuals who were given physical exams every two years over a 12 year period. Men and women in the 30-49 year age group with a cholesterol level of 260 were shown to have four times the rate of heart attacks as compared to their counterparts with cholesterol

levels of 220. The conclusion? The higher the cholesterol, the higher the risk of heart attack.

Many further studies have confirmed these findings year after year. Dr. Keys has studied over 25 populations that were on low-fat diets and his conclusions were always the same. Lower fat and cholesterol levels equaled a lower incidence of heart disease. To answer the question of the role of heredity in the level of cholesterol, he performed a study with 3 groups of Japanese. Each group was in a different dietary environment. Group One lived in Japan and ate the traditional low fat diet. Group Two lived in Hawaii and had a mixed diet of partly traditional Eastern, partly American. The third group lived in Los Angeles and ate the typical American diet high in fat and cholesterol. The level of cholesterol in the blood and rate of coronary heart disease increased proportionately to the increases of fat in the diet. The conclusion was that heredity played a much smaller role than previously thought. Diet was the determining factor in the disease.

The Standard American Diet (S.A.D.)

What the average American eats results in poor health! Are you surprised that in this prosperous, abundant country we are so lacking in awareness of the truly healthful foods that we are basically a sick and malnourished people, suffering far too many illnesses and diseases? I was. The organizations that study these matters periodically update their recommendations to stay in line with the research and have been steadily moving toward a simpler and more healthful pattern such as the one outlined in the THINNER WINNERS program. The American Heart Association, the American Cancer Society and the U.S. Senate's Select Committee on Nutrition and Human Needs have all made recommendations for national dietary goals that are quite different from the average American diet. Consider the figures below to see what we are eating as a nation and what is the recommended diet.

S.A.D.	Recommended diet
42% fat	15-30% or less total fat
16% saturated fat	10% or less saturated fat
800 mg cholesterol	300 mg or less cholesterol
18% refined sugar	10% or less refined sugars
8,000 mg sodium	1100-3300 mg sodium
10 g fiber	20-35 mg fiber

No wonder that Dr. John Farquhar, Director of the Stanford Heart Disease Prevention Program stated, "The American diet may be hazardous to your health".

America and the World

The normal mean for cholesterol in the United States is 250 mg. This means that a person with a cholesterol level of 250 has 250 mg of cholesterol in a deciliter of blood serum. The higher the number, the higher one is at risk for heart disease. According to a study by the National Institute of Health, a 1% reduction in blood cholesterol results in a 2% reduction in the risk of heart attack. In the past, a cholesterol of 300 or more was considered to be a high risk category while a level of 200 or below was considered to be a low risk. As the health profession has become more aware of the effects of cholesterol upon health through research these figures have changed dramatically and are likely to continue to become lower in the future.

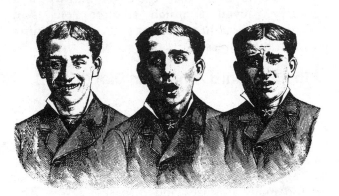

"My cholesterol is what?!"

Americans have among the highest levels of cholesterol in the world with proportionately high percentages of deaths from heart disease. In Japan the normal mean level is 163. In South America, Asia and the Mediterranean the levels are between 150-180. Italy, 175. India, 146, and most of the vegetarian Third World nations come in at only 100-140! Why then do American physicians consider a "normal" range to be 225-275 mg? Are we so physiologically different from the humans in other countries? What about our "melting pot" sociological makeup? Because of our high cholesterol and fat diets, evidently the "norms" have risen as the averages have also. As evidenced by the high levels of coronary disease and deaths, proven by research to be directly related to the levels of cholesterol in the blood, these high figures can no longer be considered normal or healthy. The level which we should use as our goal range is between 150-180 mg. Anywhere above that level is a compromise to your health and an increase in your risk for heart disease. The good news is, you can get there and stay there with the THINNER WINNERS recommendations. Just a bit of awareness

and a desire to consciously control your health will get you there sooner than you might think.

Can Damage Be Reversed?

Many studies have been done on the reversibility of cholesterol levels and triglycerides. And there is very encouraging news! Reducing fat percentage in the diet can reduce cholesterol levels in the blood dramatically in very little time. Consider the study conducted and retested by Dr. J. M. Beveridge. When subjects of different age groups, sex and race were placed on fat and cholesterol-free diets, their cholesterol levels dropped 25% on average in just four days! When he increased their dietary fats and cholesterol, their levels shot back up again in 95% of the cases. So don't think that this health pursuit needs to take years for real results to be accomplished. Some simple changes right now could help save your life. Dr. Dean Ornish, director of the Heart Health Institute at San Francisco State University, has brought this news to the public eye in his book Reversing Heart Disease. His work documents dramatic proof that diet and lifestyle changes can actually reverse damage!

Now we know that arteriosclerosis or hardening of the arteries causes coronary heart disease and that high levels of cholesterol and fat in the blood causes arteriosclerosis and also cancer, high blood pressure, diabetes and stroke among some of the more impactful diseases. And we know that diet can effectively reduce those dangerous levels to ones of safety and health. But just what is cholesterol and fat?

What is Cholesterol?

Cholesterol is a waxy substance, actually called a sterol, not a fat as is commonly thought. It is found in every cell of the body. Our bodies make what little they need and we also can get it from foods of animal origin. There are two types of cholesterol. **"Bad" cholesterol, called low density lipoprotein or LDL (remember L for Lousy),** has a thin protein coating and as it travels through your blood stream it may deposit itself on the walls of your arteries causing plaque, a waxy buildup. **"Good" cholesterol, high density lipoprotein or HDL (H for Healthy),** carries the cholesterol package out of the bloodstream. This may sound simplistic, but basically this is the relationship between HDL and LDL. The higher the HDL the better, since it actually prevents the negative actions of the LDL by escorting it out of your bloodstream more quickly. The higher the high and the lower the low the better off you are! Although

HDL in their bloodstream. LDL can effectively be reduced by diet. However, the best way to increase your HDL level is not only through your diet, but regular aerobic exercise as well. This is discussed in excruciating detail in Chapter 21 "Get That Body Movin'".

The American Heart Association recommends no more than 300 mg of cholesterol daily in our diets. Other health professionals consider anywhere from 100-300 mg to be safe according to your age and other health risk factors. The average American now consumes 800 mg daily and this contributes greatly to the fact that 1 out of 158 Americans over the tender age of 15 are at serious risk for heart disease right now. We're talking about ninth graders!

Types of Dietary Fats

In understanding dietary fats (we do want to, don't we?), we find there are three primary types: (1) monounsaturated, (2) polyunsaturated, and (3) saturated.

1) **Monounsaturated oils** are liquid vegetable oils that have been shown to be effective in lowering blood cholesterol LDL's but not HDL's. Olive oil and canola oil are in this category.

2) **Polyunsaturated fats** are oils from vegetable products and fish. They are usually liquid at room temperature. Although unsaturated oils help lower LDL's, they also lower HDL's. Included in this category are safflower, sunflower, corn, soybean and cottonseed oils. Omega-3, a part of fish oil is also an unsaturated fat and has been shown to reduce the risk of heart attack by almost half when just two fish meals are included in the diet weekly, according to the New England Journal of Medicine. Good sources are salmon, mackerel, lake trout, whitefish, fresh tuna and herring. If you don't care to eat fish there are fish oil capsules available as well as flax seed oil for vegetarians.

3) **Saturated fat** is the dietary fat that raises the level of cholesterol in the blood and can also cause arterial plaque by raising the level of LDL's. Characteristically, this type of fat usually hardens at room temperature. Saturated animal fats are found in meats, whole and low-fat milk and dairy products and egg yolks. Saturated vegetable fats are found in solid and hydrogenated shortenings, coconut and coconut oil, cocoa butter, palm oil and palm kernel oil. Forty-four percent of all fat in the American diet is saturated.

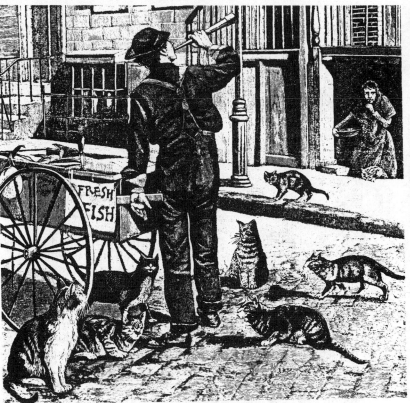

You may not have heard about omega 3 oil, but your cat has.

4) A somewhat sinister and misleading variety of fats are the **hydrogenated fats or "trans fats"**. These are oils and fats changed from liquid form to solid form through food processing methods. Included are most margarine's and shortenings. They may be partially or completely hydrogenated. According to the American Heart Association, you should completely avoid hydrogenated fat as, in the body, it closely resembles saturated fat. Margarines containing partially hydrogenated oils may be acceptable if they contain at least twice as much polyunsaturated as saturated fat. Check the labels.

How Much Fat Should You Eat?

While you need to keep an eye on the types of fat that you consume, the overall amount is also an important factor. Total fat content should be in the 10-20% range, with the lower end best. If you are 5-15 pounds overweight, aim for 20% or less total fat. If you are 15 or more pounds overweight, 10-15% fat is your target. Stay at these levels until you have burned off and used up most of the excess fat that you are now storing on your body. Saturated fat should be no more than 10% of the total calorie intake and less is better. Americans now average 42% fat intake in their diets and the dire health statistics prove it.

42% fat intake in their diets and the dire health statistics prove it.

Calculating the fat content in any given food is simple using the following formula. There are 9 calories in one gram of fat. If the food in question has 100 calories per serving with 5 grams of fat per serving (read the label!) then simply multiply 9 x 5 and you get 45 calories per serving from fat. Divide the fat calories by the total calories and you get the percentage of calories derived from fat. Therefore, the food is 45% fat! Put it back and find something healthier to eat.

Here's how to calculate the fat percentage in foods

1 gram of fat = 9 calories
100 calories total in the food, with 5 grams of fat (read the label)
5 gms of fat x 9 cals per gm of fat = 45 calories from fat
Divide calories from fat by total calories or 45/100 = 45% fat in the food

---

Most labels now provide this information, but it's always good to know how they arrived at the figures. For foods without this information, you can now calculate it easily for yourself.

Get a good food count book and read food labels carefully. (This is a good habit to develop as I have emphasized. You cannot really become aware of what you're eating until you read the labels!) Incidentally, protein and carbohydrates have only 4 calories per gram. That makes fat over twice as concentrated in calories along with all the other disadvantages. Or the way I see it, I can eat two servings of carbohydrate or protein for the same calories as one serving of fat! My whole, wonderful salad has no more calories than 1 TBL of fatty dressing. And most people average 4 TBL of dressing per salad! Not a very wise or informed choice.

Look up foods that you eat most frequently. That may be a shocker. Turn your shock into resolve to find comparable foods that are better for you with less fat and cholesterol. Most people only eat about 100 foods on a regular basis, so pretty soon you will know which ones are better for you and you won't need the guide as much.

Matching Fat Grams to Weight Loss

A simpler way to reduce fat in your diet is to keep track of the grams of fat in the food you eat. You can do this easily with a pocket fat gram counter. The lower your calorie intake, the lower your fat gram intake should be . Use the chart below to determine the amount of fat grams you should eat. For instance, if you're eating 1200 calories daily and want to stay around 20% fat, then choose no more than 27 grams of fat daily. Larger people and pregnant or lactating women can eat at the higher range of calories according to your personal needs and goals and directions from your health care professional.

Desired Fat Percentage in Diet				
Total Daily Calories	10%	15%	20%	25%
1200 cals	13gms	20 gms	27gms	33 gms
1400	16	23	31	39
1600	18	27	36	44
1800	20	30	40	50
2000	22	34	44	56

You may lose weight faster by eating less fat, but be sure to eat enough to satisfy yourself. Also, some fat in your diet is necessary for certain functions in the body, such as absorption of fat-soluble vitamins. Don't be tempted to cut out fat entirely. Keeping track of fat grams is the fastest and easiest way to eliminate excess fat, and to begin losing weight without a lot of calculating and hassle.

Fat is Fat

There is no longer any question about the dangerous health risks we bring on ourselves by a diet high in fat. But there's something more. As Covert Bailey, the popular MIT biochemist shows in his book Fit or Fat?, fat makes fat people fatter. Fat that you eat is fat in your body (and unfortunately on your body). So my suggestion ... avoid fat in your diet like the plague, especially during the fat-reduction phase of your weight control program. When you reduce the health-compromising habits that got you fat in the first place, and replace them know just what to do with that scoop of French Chocolate ice cream. Until then, your body just stores it, and that is definitely not what you want or need. So hang on, retrain your body and look forward to a more balanced relationship with fat in the future. If you follow the principles in this program, you can become one of those people who can indulge occasionally and stay slim. I know, I'm one of them right now. Join me.

In A Nutshell

1) Coronary artery disease is epidemic in the United States, killing 1 million people annually. Many early studies pointed to diet as a cause of heart disease and following studies confirmed the link.

2) "Normal" cholesterol for Americans is not the norm in other countries. The Standard American Diet (S.A.D.) is not healthy. Americans have among the highest cholesterol levels in the world and proportionately high rates of heart disease.

3) Reversing heart damage is now a proven reality.

4) Good cholesterol (HDL) and bad cholesterol (LDL) are discussed.

5) There are three types of dietary fats: saturated, polyunsaturated and monosaturated. Hydrogenated or "trans fats" are oils or fats that have been changed from liquid to solid and act like saturated fat.

6) Fat is fat! Avoid it like the plague. Calculate the amount of fat in your food so you know what you're eating or just count fat grams.

7) Dietary recommendations for fats:
   a) Total Fat Intake: 13-27 gms daily for women, 18-36 gms daily for men, depending on how much you are overweight.
   b) Polyunsaturated or monosaturated fat: 10-20% or less of your total calorie intake,
   c) Saturated Fat: 10% or less of total intake.
   d) Cholesterol: 100-300 mg daily according to age & risk level (Americans consume about 800 mg daily).

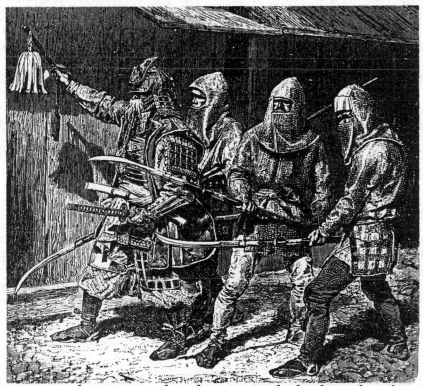

Some people go to great lengths to purge the fat from their diet.

Fiber is Your Friend   33

"My vegetable love should grow, vaster than empires ... "
Andrew Marvell

There is so much current information regarding fiber that it's easy to be confused about this vital component of a healthy food style. However, a good understanding of fiber's role in our diets will serve you well. I consider fiber so important that I have included it as one of "The Fabulous Five" which you will find in Chapter 38 "Secrets of Successful Maintenance". Let's sort out the facts and find out what this fiber controversy is all about.

What is Fiber?

Dietary fiber is the part of plant foods that we cannot digest. There is no fiber in any animal foods. There are two types of fiber: soluble and insoluble. Soluble fiber forms a gel in water and slows down food absorption. It benefits diabetes control and helps lower blood cholesterol, thus reducing the risk of heart disease. Sources include oats, barley, psyllium, beans and whole fruits, especially apples. Insoluble fiber is woody-looking and absorbs water as it moves through the digestive tract. It speeds elimination, relieving constipation and may prevent some types of cancer. Sources include bran cereals, whole grain breads, vegetables and nuts.

How Much Fiber Should You Eat?

The Food and Nutrition Board of the National Academy of Sciences recommends between 20-30 grams of fiber daily. But you should not exceed 35-40 grams since there is some evidence that more than this could interfere with the absorption of certain vitamins and minerals. The average American now consumes about 10 grams a day, so don't worry that you'll get too much. It's not that easy.

In addition to the benefits mentioned above there are several reasons why addition of fiber to your diet promotes positive health. Foods high in fiber are usually low in fat and calories. The fiber makes you feel full and satisfied so you tend to eat less. Foods high in fiber take longer to chew so you eat more slowly. I particularly had a problem with eating too quickly. Suddenly, the food was gone ... and there was no choice but to have another helping to satisfy me! When I increased the foods containing high fiber, I couldn't consume all the calories needed to stay at 272 pounds! I still need to feel full to feel satisfied, but now I fill up on high fiber

foods. There is also a faster transit through the intestines so fewer calories are actually absorbed.

Problems related to low fiber intake include obesity, diabetes, gallstones, coronary artery disease, constipation, hemorrhoids, diverticular disease, appendicitis, cancer of the colon, heart disease and high cholesterol! With all that going against you and such great tasting foods and benefits going for you, why wait another day to add plenty of fiber to your diet?

Add Fiber Slowly and Drink Water!

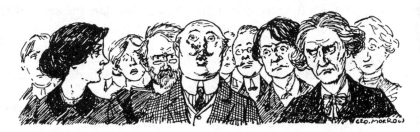

It is very important to add fiber slowly to avoid any uncomfortable side effects that "too much, too soon" could cause. First, determine how much fiber you get on an average day from your 3-day nutritional assessment in Chapter 4. Then increase fiber slowly in your existing diet by adding about 5 grams in a day. Stay at that level for a week or more allowing your body to adjust to the increased amount. When you feel comfortable with that, then add 5 more grams the next week until you are at the desired level. Think EASE.

Be sure to add lots of water to your diet. If you are not already doing so, drink at least 6-8 glasses daily of water, mineral water (low sodium) or herbal tea. This assists the fiber in its work. If you increase the amount of fiber you are getting without increasing the water at the same time, you may actually slow down the movement of food through your intestines and be quite uncomfortable. This is a major reason why people give up trying to add extra fiber. Not enough water and initial discomfort. Keep at it, this is worth it.

Many of the recipes in this book are high in fiber. I have found that fiber is fun ... and what a joy to find something I needed to add to my diet instead of taking away! I consider fiber, as well as water, exercise, fat regulation and a great attitude to be the basis of my new way of life.

Benefits of Fiber

* Usually found in foods that are low in fat and calories
* Makes you feel full and satisfied so you eat less
* Takes longer to chew so you eat more slowly
* Faster transit through your intestines so fewer calories are absorbed
* Regulates elimination
* Lowers blood cholesterol, reducing the risk of heart disease
* Benefits diabetes control
* May prevent some types of cancer
* Is vegetarian

Good Sources of Fiber

* Bran cereals, bran and psyllium (go for 10 grams of fiber for breakfast)
* Whole grain breads, cereals and pasta, popcorn
* Beans and lentils, kidney, lima, black, pinto, etc.
* Berries, pears, prunes, apples, strawberries, bananas
* Grapefruit, oranges
* Carrots, potatoes, corn, peas, yams, pumpkin
* Broccoli, cabbage, spinach, artichokes, asparagus
* Nuts and seeds (watch fat grams)
* Ground spices such as chili powder, cinnamon and paprika

Problems Related to Low Fiber Intake

* Appendicitis
* Cancer of the colon
* Constipation
* Coronary artery disease
* Diabetes
* Diverticular disease
* Gallstones
* Hemorrhoids
* High cholesterol
* Obesity

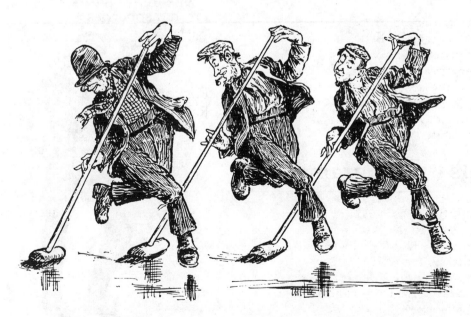

Think of fiber as an internal broom ... sweeping you clean.

Compare this high fiber menu with the low fiber one.
Some simple, informed choices really make a big difference!

Low Fiber   High Fiber

Breakfast
Orange juice, ½ cup	= 0.5 g	Whole orange, 1	= 4.0 g
Corn flakes	= 1.0 g	Raisin Bran	= 2.5 g
Milk	= .0 g	Milk	= .0 g
White toast	= .0 g	Whole wheat toast	= 2.0 g
Jelly	= .0 g	Whole fruit jam	= 0.5 g
Total	1.5 g		9.0 g

Lunch
Cheese sandwich/		Bean Burrito/	
sourdough bread	= 2.0 g	whole wheat tortilla	= 4.5 g
Potato chips	= 1.0 g	Carrot/ jicama sticks	= 2.0 g
Apple juice	= 0.5 g	Whole apple	= 4.0 g
Total	3.5 g		10.5 g

Afternoon Snack
Candy bar	= .0 g	Dried figs	= 2.0 g

Dinner
Regular pasta	= 0.1 g	Whole wheat pasta	= 2.2 g
Reg. spaghetti sauce	= 0.2 g	Chunky spag. sauce	= 2.0 g
Plain lettuce salad	= 0.7 g	Salad w/ green peas, tomatoes	
Garlic toast, white	= .0 g	& mushrooms added	= 3.4 g
Raspberry sherbet	= .0 g	Whole grain garlic toast	= 1.0 g
		Fresh raspberries	= 3.0 g
Total	1.0 g		11.6 g

Evening Snack
Crackers	= .0 g	Popcorn	= 2.0 g
Jelly	= .0 g	Raisins	= 3.0 g
	.0 g		5.0 g

Daily Totals   6.0 grams   38.1 g

"See for Yourself."

In A Nutshell

1)   Fiber is only found in plant foods, not animal foods.

2)   There are two types of fiber: soluble (gel in water) and insoluble (woody-looking).

3)   20-30 grams of fiber daily are recommended.

4)   Do not exceed 35-40 grams per day.

5)   Americans average only 10 grams daily.

6)   Many health problems are associated with low fiber intake.

7)   Many health benefits are associated with high fiber intake.

8)   Fiber is low in fat and calories and helps you feel full longer.

9)   Good sources of fiber are listed.

10) Add fiber slowly so your body can adjust. Five grams extra daily for a week at first.

11)   Drink lots of water to aid the fiber in its work.

12) Stick at this. It is worth it!

Sodium and Salt vs. Herbs and Spices   34

"Distasted with the salt of broken tears"
William Shakespeare

Taking Sodium Off the Podium

I find that a meal must have zip and zing to really satisfy my taste buds ... it must make them want to sing! Spicy Mexican, unusual curries, sweet sauces, pungent dishes and fragrant baked goods make food special and eminently satisfying. Unfortunately, many traditional American dishes seem to depend on salt for that flavor enhancement, but there is a better way. Great chefs and good cooks everywhere know that herbs and spices are subtle flavor-enhancers, not a heavy-handed mask like salt. Salt can add water weight to your body and make you look and feel puffy, too. It can also contribute to high blood pressure, certain heart disorders and even can cause food cravings. Instead, I use lots of herb and spice combinations plus a few condiment-type ingredients such as fresh lemon or vinegar to zip up the foods. Before we get into this fun topic , let me fill you in on the definition of salt and sodium and why it is so important to your health to develop alternative seasonings.

The Difference Between Salt and Sodium

Just what is the difference between salt and sodium? Sodium is a mineral and occurs naturally in some foods. We get most of our sodium from salt, though. Either salt added at the table, in cooking or in packaged foods. Salt is a chemical compound, sodium chloride, made up of 40% sodium and 60% chloride. One teaspoon of salt equals 2000 mg of sodium. Salt as a flavoring additive is second only to sugar in usage in the U.S. today. Food labels show the amount of sodium in milligrams in the food. Milligrams of sodium is what you should watch.

Why You Should Avoid Sodium

I was amazed to find that the average American consumes 10-20 times more sodium than he or she needs! Your body only needs about 200 mg daily to maintain the functions of fluid balance, nerve impulses and muscle contractions. However, we now consume an average of 4,000 to 8,000 mg daily. Since one of the characteristics of sodium is that it holds water, a diet high in sodium causes retention of large amounts of fluid. This can cause

several health problems. Excess sodium is eliminated through the kidneys and over a prolonged period of overwork they can be strained to the point of kidney damage or failure.

Heart disease, stroke, edema and hypertension (high blood pressure) are also potential health problems related to high sodium intake with hypertension being the most serious health consequence. This disease causes 150,000 deaths annually in the U.S. and affects 60 million Americans (one out of every four of us). Excessive amounts of trapped water and sodium in the bloodstream cause a rise in the volume of blood circulated by the heart, which must work harder to create the pressure to move this additional fluid through the bloodstream. However, at the same time, the small blood vessels constrict due to the excess sodium, thereby increasing resistance to blood flow. There is a corresponding increase in pressure in order to push the fluid through the body, and the heart is again overtaxed. High blood pressure is often referred to as "the silent killer" since there are often no symptoms. Over the years the pressure slowly increases until the victim has an "event" such as a stroke or heart attack. By this time it's too late to repair damage done to the heart, kidneys and blood vessels. It is estimated by the National Institutes of Health and the American Heart, Lung and Blood Institute that 50% of all Americans who have hypertension are not even aware of it and are increasingly at risk for stroke and heart disease. These are pretty heavy statistics and I wanted to find out more about this seemingly "harmless" substance that contributes to these health problems.

How Much Sodium Do You Need?

How much sodium is recommended? The Food and Nutrition Board of the National Academy of Sciences and the National Research Council have issued reports stating that a "safe and adequate" level of sodium intake is between 1100 and 3300 mg of sodium daily. The American Heart Association recommends limiting sodium intake to 1 mg for each calorie consumed. So, if you consume 1500 calories daily then you should consume no more than 1500 mg of sodium daily. There is a growing consensus among health professionals that this figure should be adjusted drastically downward to the neighborhood of 220 mg daily. It seems the lower your sodium intake, the better your health. What little sodium we actually need is readily available even in an only-fresh-foods diet which precious few of us follow regularly.

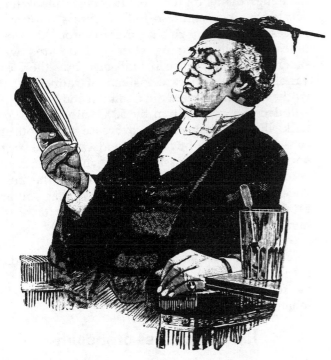

"Hmm, I didn't know that about sodium."

The Potassium Connection

Potassium works together with sodium in your body to regulate blood pressure and the balance of fluids. It also acts to maintain a regular heartbeat, plays a role in nerve functions and muscle contractions, makes sure oxygen gets to your brain so you can think clearly and even helps your body cleanse away wastes! Recent studies have shown that a diet high in potassium but low in sodium can actually lower blood pressure significantly. It also appears that potassium can help cancel out the effects of even a high sodium diet by encouraging normal fluid balance and thus normal blood pressure. People who cut their sodium intake to control hypertension do even better when they also increase their potassium intake at the same time.

The need for blood pressure medication can also be affected. In one study, over 80% of the people following high potassium diets for one year were able to cut their blood pressure medication in half. Nearly 40% of them were able to drop their medication entirely. They weren't on any supplements, but merely included 3 or more servings of high potassium foods in their diets daily. In another study, a single serving of high potassium

food resulted in a 40% reduction in risk for fatal stroke. Powerful impacts from simple changes.

Potassium deficiency can be brought on by many circumstances such as excessive sweating from exercising or on a hot day, or fluid loss from diuretics, cortisone medications, excessive caffeine or alcohol consumption or diarrhea. Low potassium levels can cause muscle weakness or cramps, dizziness, fatigue, constipation, slow or weak pulse and mental confusion. You retain more sodium and lose more calcium, too. It is estimated that 65% of women and nearly 40% of men don't get the potassium they need daily, yet it is readily available in fresh, whole foods like those recommended for THINNER WINNERS. If I get too much sodium, usually from eating out in a restaurant, I make sure I get plenty of fluids and include extra potassium foods the next day.

If you have a salt tooth now, you might want to try a potassium-sodium blend that cuts the sodium, boosts the potassium and still has a salty flavor to help wean you off the sodium. But the best way to get more potassium is from the great variety of foods that contain this vital mineral. There is no Recommended Daily Minimum for potassium, but the estimated minimum daily intake is 1,600-2,000 mg. The best sources are potatoes (840 mg for 1 medium) and cantaloupe (825 mg for ½). Foods that provide from 400-650 mg per serving include tomato or orange juice or the whole fruits, yogurt and skim milk, dried fruit, dark green leafy vegetables, snapper or salmon, lima beans, sweet potatoes, acorn squash, turkey, broccoli and of course, bananas.

Where Does All that Sodium Come From?

Recipes in the THINNER WINNERS program use no added salt in their preparation, and whenever processed (canned, packaged or frozen) foods are called for, they are of the low-sodium or reduced-sodium variety. There are also ways to reduce or dilute the sodium content of foods that are not already reduced. About 10% of our sodium intake, or 200 mg (all that we really need), comes from natural food sources such as fruits and vegetables, meat and fish, dairy products and drinking water. Another 15% is from table salt used in cooking and at the table. But the majority of our sodium intake, 75%, is derived from canned, frozen and packaged foods. There are many reasons why processed foods contain so much sodium, not all of them the most socially conscious ones. Food preservation is the most obvious reason, although with the plethora of reduced sodium products (with curiously inflated prices) on the market, it has been shown that a reduction of sodium for this purpose is possible. Another reason for adding sodium to food is that salt, like sugar, is an inexpensive filler, adding weight (and profits to food processors).

However, the main reason we have dangerously high levels of sodium in our processed foods stems from the fact that foods often suffer greatly in flavor (as well as nutritional content) after being processed. To overcome this, the foods are highly salted and we, as a nation, have been conditioned for a lifetime to this salty taste. Salt can be addictive and once our taste buds are used to a certain level of salt, they begin to crave even more. Babies are not born with this preference for salty taste. It is developed beginning with the salted baby foods which taste better to Mommy when she tests the food for baby. We are doomed from the start it seems to crave that salt.

But wait! The good news is that since salt preference is an acquired taste and mainly a habit, we can also reverse the process and slowly reduce our craving for salt to a manageable level. Your taste buds are retrainable!

What can you do to help reduce the taste for salt in yourself and your family, greatly reducing the risk of serious and irreparable damage to your health? First, you must become aware of the sources of sodium in your diet. Let's look at the obvious sources and the hidden sources of sodium.

Obvious sources of sodium

Cheese and cheese foods.

Processed or smoked meats such as ham, bacon, sausage, luncheon meats and hot dogs.

Restaurant items such as fast food hamburgers, pizza, Mexican and Chinese food and just about everything not freshly prepared.

Salty condiments such as seasonings containing salt, soy sauce and bouillon cubes or powder, mustard.

Salty foods such as chips and pretzels, salted nuts, pickles, olives and pickled foods such as herring and sauerkraut.

Canned and dehydrated soups.

Table salt either added at the table or during cooking.

Use your nutrition guide containing the sodium contents of common foods, both natural and processed. Look up foods you usually buy before your next shopping trip. You may be surprised that different brands of the same product contain significantly lower milligrams of sodium. For instance, a 6-oz can of Hunt's tomato paste contains 620 mg of sodium while the same size can of Del Monte's contains only 90 mg. Manufacturers may provide you with information on their product if you write to them. Sodium content is now required information on the new nutrition labels introduced in March 1994.

If you can't find the sodium content for a food, try to substitute another brand that does provide that information. If salt is listed as one of the first three ingredients on the label it is best to look for a substitute. You can also reduce excess sodium in processed foods by rinsing them thoroughly three times in fresh, running water. I do this with sauerkraut when I use it (and also buy the fresh variety in the deli case instead of canned). This works well with canned tuna, salmon and beans. You will decrease the sodium by 50% with this simple trick. But the best way to decrease your sodium consumption is to buy fresh foods and cook from scratch whenever possible. As your taste buds become retrained, you start to appreciate the fresh, delicious, unique flavors of the foods that you are eating and preparing. Everything won't taste the same anymore!

Now for the real culprits ... foods that we don't even suspect pack a wallop of salt. Here are a few of the foods to look out for with hidden sources of sodium:

Hidden sources of sodium

Baked products (commercially produced) such as crackers, bread, pastries, desserts

Baking soda - 820 mg per teaspoon

Bread - up to 300 mg per slice (average 175)

Cheeseburger (fast food) - 1,510 mg or more

Chicken dinner (frozen) - 1,150 mg or more

Cottage cheese - up to 850 mg per cup (even non-fat!)

Dill pickle - 925 mg each

Drinking water and softened water

Drugs such as aspirin, antacids, laxatives and cough syrups

Eggs - 70 mg each

Macaroni and cheese (packaged) - 1,086 mg per cup

Margarine - 120-200 mg per tablespoon

Meats and fish (canned), packed in oil - 430 mg (3 ounces tuna)

Oatmeal (instant) - 374 mg per cup

Salad dressing (bottled) - 150-300 mg per tablespoon

Soy sauce - 1,380 mg in 1 tablespoon

Tomato products (canned)

Vegetable juice or tomato juice - 882 mg (8 ounces)

Vegetables (canned) - 450-900 mg per cup

If you really want an eye-opener, chart your sodium intake for three days using your nutrition guide (this is part of your Nutritional Analysis in Chapter 4). I was amazed at the amount of sodium I was consuming on a regular basis, even though I felt I was avoiding the obviously salty stuff. When I finally got a handle on it, I began to feel so much lighter ... and looked firmer instead of puffy. I even lost several pounds. I know, I know, just water weight. But it's always nice to lose a few pounds permanently and feel lighter, too. It made me feel good and that can't be bad, right? And of course, the burden on my heart and other organs was lightened.

Easing Up on Sodium and Salt

I know what you're thinking, but food prepared without salt doesn't need to be bland or tasteless at all! Just take it easy and don't try to cut out all salt at once or your taste buds will rebel and send you back to the salt shaker. First, gradually wean yourself away from added salt at the table and in cooking by cutting by ¼ the amount of salt you use. If a recipe calls for 1 teaspoon of salt, use ¾ tsp. Recipes in the THINNER WINNERS program use no salt in preparation. I suggest making them as written first, then adding salt if you feel it is necessary, tasting after each light addition of salt to make sure you get just enough to satisfy your taste. Stay at this level of salt intake until it becomes quite comfortable for you, perhaps 3 months. Then try cutting down another one-fourth If the recipe calls for 1 teaspoon of salt, try using just ½ tsp. at this point. Stay at this new level until you are comfortable. Continue in this way until none or very little salt is needed. I know it doesn't seem like it , but your taste buds will adjust and food will taste even better as your taste buds reawaken.

As you cut back on the obviously salty foods you will automatically be directing your attention toward the flavor of foods. As an interesting experiment, after one year of conscientious salt reduction, try one of your previous salty favorites. You will probably notice that the food will taste decidedly too salty. Some of the foods I previously found tasty now taste like they are soaked in brine and are actually no longer edible!

This method can be used for the elimination of fats and cholesterol from your diet, also. Skim milk and non-fat dairy products are often difficult to adjust to for those who are used to whole milk and dairy products. Cutting down first to low fat products and allowing the taste buds to adjust before moving on to the nonfat ones makes the transition a bit slower, but easier. You are not racing anyone to change your habits, with the exception of a major health problem like I had. If you are in reasonably good health, there is no reason why you can't allow your tastes to acclimate to new habits over a year or so.

You can use this technique of easing in to something new for increasing fiber in your diet, increasing your water , increasing exercise ... all sorts of great, healthy things that you may have had a bit of trouble getting to stick in the past ... if you're like someone else I know! Moi!

Learn to Use Herbs and Spices

Another decidedly delicious way to help cure yourself of sodium overuse is by learning to use herbs and spices. We tend to take these wonderful foods for granted in our modern everything-at-our-fingertips society. However, great civilizations of the ancient world were immensely effected by the spice trade and the history of these effects is quite fascinating. (Columbus was following the spice trade to India when he stumbled onto the Caribbean cruise ship routes.) Today in America we have a huge variety of aromatic and flavorful spices and herbs available that offer much to the taste buds. The fun of experimenting with new flavors and the satisfaction of coming up with a new taste treat that your family loves should not be missed for fear of failure. As you get to know the different tastes better you'll develop an almost instinctive feeling as to which spices and herbs would be good in a certain dish.

However, until you're ready to do it on your own, here are some suggestions to get you started. There are several manufacturers who are putting out excellent salt-free blends of seasonings. I especially like Mrs. Dash and McCormick's line of Parsley Patch seasonings. The latter comes in a wide variety including All-Purpose, Lemon Pepper, Garlicsaltless, Sesame All-Purpose, It's A Dilly, Popcorn Blend and Spicy Cinnamon. In this way you can get a blend of flavors without having to be an expert. McCormick also has a "spices of the World" cookbook that lists all of the spices and general uses for them. Additionally, on spice and herb labels you will often find suggestions for uses. I found these quite useful when I was just starting to experiment. Celestial Seasonings also publishes a chart of spices and herbs that you may find useful.

On the next page you'll find some of my favorite herbs and spices and how I use them.

Herbs and Spices

Basil	Aromatic, mild mint-licorice flavor	Common in Italian and French cooking, seafood, soups, stews, sauces, salads, tomato dishes, most vegetables.
Bay Leaves	Aromatic, woodsy	Essential to soups, stews. Also good for poultry, fish, gravies, marinades.
Chili Powder	Spicy	Actually a blend of chili peppers and spices. Mexican dishes, chili, stews, soups, sauces, dressings, relishes.
Cinnamon	Warm, spicy	Baked goods, desserts, cereal, fruits, spiced beverages, chicken, stews, carrots, winter squashes, sweet potatoes.
Cloves	Hot, spicy, penetrating	Use sparingly in desserts, fruits, sauces, baked beans, carrots, winter squashes.
Curry	Fragrant, exotic, warm	A blend of many spices. Stews, eggs, fruit, poultry, dressings, sauces, shrimp, beans.
Dill	Aromatic	Dressings, dips, seafood, poultry, cottage cheeses, salads, vegetables, soups
Garlic	Pungent, aromatic	I love this healthy herb and find new uses daily! Italian, Mexican and Oriental cooking, sauces, fish, poultry, vegetables, dressings, dips, soups, etc.
Ginger	Aromatic, sweet, spicy, penetrating	Oriental cooking, stir-fries, curries, chutneys, baked goods, fruits, poultry, stews, cereal, beets and yellow vegetables, dressings, cheese sauces, marinades.
Marjoram	Delicate mint-sage	Fish, poultry, soup, stews, cottage cheese, green salads, dressings, vegetables, omelets (egg whites only, of course!).
Mint	Fruity, distinctive, aromatic	Teas and drinks, salads, fruit, desserts, cottage cheese, sauces, fish, soup, cabbage, peas, beans, carrots, potatoes.
Nutmeg	Spicy, sweet	Desserts, fruits, beverages, cereal, breads, stews, soups, sauces, vegetables.
Oregano	Pungent, pleasant	Italian and Mexican cooking. Salads, sauces, tomato dishes, soups, dips, spreads, fish, poultry, eggs, vegetable dishes, mushrooms.
Parsley	Sweet, spicy	Very versatile herb. Spreads, dips, soups, salads, breads, omelets, fish, poultry, vegetables, as a garnish, chew as a breath sweetener, juice.
Pepper	Pungent, strong	Kitchen essential. Experiment with black, red, white and green varieties. Can be used in almost anything.
Sage	Pungent, warm	Fish, stuffings, poultry, soup, chowders, gravies, green salads, tomatoes, carrots, lima beans, peas, onions, Brussels sprouts, eggplant, Italian and Middle Eastern cooking.
Thyme	Pungent, pleasant	Fish, gumbo, soups, sauces, poultry, tomato dishes, cheese, eggs, beans, artichokes, mushrooms, potatoes, onions, carrots.

In addition, there is a variety of wonderful natural flavoring extracts available. Flavors include the ever versatile vanilla, almond, rum, chocolate, orange, lemon, peppermint, banana, coconut and many others. Buy the all-natural varieties without added sugars and artificial ingredients.

Enhancing the Flavor of Food

Here are some suggestions on how to season particular foods:

Beans - Thyme, coriander, garlic, bouquet garni (parsley, thyme, bay, red pepper)
Broccoli - Tarragon, onion, mustard seed, lemon, oregano
Cabbage - Caraway seed, mint, nutmeg, allspice, ginger, savory, dill, tarragon
Carrots - Bay leaf, dill, mint, marjoram, thyme, sage, oregano
Cauliflower - Celery or caraway seed, tarragon, cumin, curry, mace, dill, mustard
Cucumber - Mint, basil, dill
Egg dishes - Pepper, nutmeg, parsley, onion, chervil, vegetable flakes, dill, garlic, curry
Eggplant - Italian seasoning, oregano, marjoram, basil, garlic, sage, cumin, lemon, curry
Fish - Basil, dillweed, ginger, garlic, fennel, chervil, onions, lemon, capers, celery, cumin, curry, onions, turmeric, savory, rosemary
Fruits - Allspice, cinnamon, nutmeg, ginger, coriander, vanilla, cardamom
Grains - Cinnamon, cardamom, cloves, allspice, cumin, dill, garlic, bouquet-garni, celery seed, curry, turmeric
Mushrooms - Garlic, oregano, paprika, thyme, rosemary
Peas - Mint, savory, rosemary, dill, marjoram, oregano, sage
Potatoes - Onion, chives, garlic, pepper, basil, bay, thyme, caraway seed, mint, oregano, paprika, rosemary, coriander, sage, curry
Poultry - Tarragon, rosemary, curry, paprika, lemon, garlic, mustard, sage, thyme
Soups - Bouquet garni, bay leaves, garlic, onion, dill, parsley, marjoram, basil, thyme, herbs d'Provence (a mixture)
Spinach - Nutmeg, basil, marjoram, mace, rosemary, lemon
Summer squash - Basil, rosemary, Italian seasoning
Tomatoes - Basil, fennel, anise or celery seed, Italian seasoning, oregano, bay leaf, dill, garlic, sage
Winter squash - Cinnamon, allspice, nutmeg, cloves, ginger, fennel

The Difference Between Herbs and Spices

Herbs are the leaves, roots, flowers and seeds of plants that generally grow in temperate climates. Spices are the nuts, fruits, seeds and bark of tropical plants. Buy whole leaves whenever possible and grind or crush just before adding to your dish. Herbs and spices are perishable foods and the whole leaf will hold its flavor longer. Store in airtight containers away from heat and light (never near the stove or dishwasher!). Write the date you purchase each herb or spice right on the container and test for potency after 6 months by crushing a bit in your palm and smelling it. Discard any weak or non fragrant ones. They will add little to your cooking anyway. Identify the herbs and spices you do not use frequently and store the portion you're not likely to use in the near future in a plastic bag in the freezer. Don't buy in bulk unless you intend to freeze some or use a lot. However, you can save a lot of money by buying bulk.

Fresh Herbs and More

I prefer to use a lot of fresh herbs. If you'd like to also, you'll need about 3-4 times as much fresh herb as you would in dry form. Place fresh herbs in a glass or jar of water, stem side down in the refrigerator. Cover the leaves with a plastic bag and they 'll stay fresh for about two weeks. Or if you buy fresh herbs in bulk in season you can rinse well, blot dry and package in plastic bags in the freezer, breaking off only what you need at the time. If you have one of those marvelous kitchen garden windows you can even grow your own fresh herbs. They not only look and smell wonderful, but are the freshest. Herbs to grow include basil, rosemary, sage, thyme, chives, parsley, mint, or if you're really ambitious and your climate is amenable, grow a bay laurel tree in your backyard! Dry herbs by hanging them upside down in a cool, dry, dark place. Store in sealed plastic bags.

Organic herbs and spices can be purchased at local health food sources or from Certified Organic

Farmers such as Sun Mountain Research Center, 35751 Oak Springs Drive, Tollhouse, CA 93667 or Frontier Cooperative Herbs, P.O. Box 299, Norway, Iowa 52318.

Many more seasonings and condiments can be healthfully added to your dishes. Try seasoned and flavored vinegars, salt and sugar free or reduced condiments, lemon, lime and orange juices or zest (grated rind without the white part), Tabasco sauce, Angostura Bitters, natural smoke flavoring (I like Wright's), or Worcestershire sauce in moderation (because of the sodium content). Wines and liquors used for flavorings are wonderful in many ways. They tenderize the fish and chicken, add lovely flavors and are very aromatic as well as being an aid to the digestion. Do not buy cooking wines since they are highly salted. A good table grade of wine will do. Eighty-five percent of the calories and all of the alcohol are removed from the dish at 175°F and above. They are wonderful for sautéing vegetables and stir-fries, also. Fat-free broths can be frozen in ice-cube trays and then placed in plastic bags in the freezer. Whenever you want to sauté or stir-fry just pop one cube into the pan and allow it to melt. (By the way, that's a good method for tomato paste, also.)

As you can see, sodium-free cooking can indeed be varied and flavorful. There are plenty of challenges and discoveries awaiting the healthful cook who decides to throw away the salt shaker and experiment. Do your heart and health a flavor!

In A Nutshell

1)   Heart disease, stroke, edema, kidney disease and hypertension are related to high sodium consumption.

2)   1 in 4 Americans has hypertension.

3)   Americans consume 10-20 times the sodium needed and at least twice as much as recommended.

4)   Sodium is a mineral, salt is a chemical compound.

5)   1 mg of sodium for each calorie consumed is a general guideline.

6)   You can"retrain your taste buds" to be satisfied with less salt. Taste first and then gradually cut down. Give yourself time to adjust.

7)   Read labels looking for hidden sources of sodium.

8)   Buy fresh, cook from scratch whenever possible.

9)   Balance high sodium processed with low sodium fresh foods.

10) Learn to cook with spices and herbs, lemon juice and salt-free blends. Experiment!

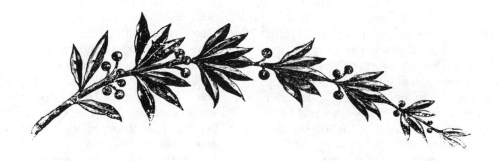

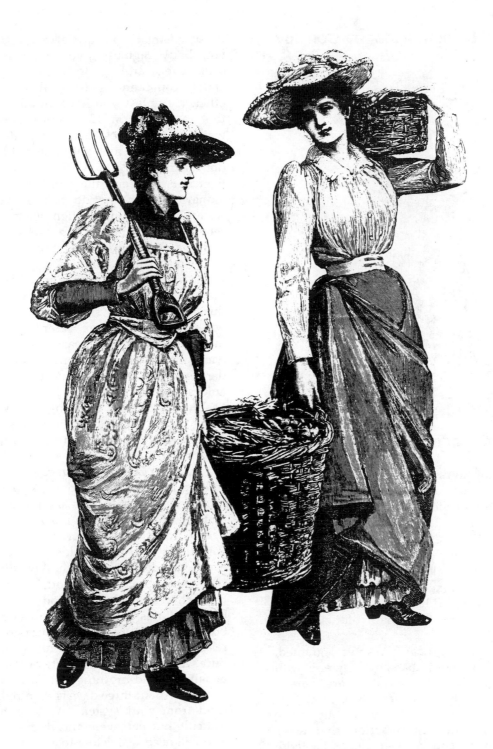

There's nothing quite as good as home-grown herbs and veggies!

Water — The Magic Potion   35

"O plunge your hands in water, plunge them up to the wrist
Stare, stare in the basin, and wonder what you've missed."
                                        W. H. Auden

The Healthiest Drink that Money Can Buy

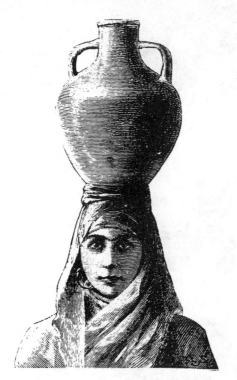

Long before soda pop there was water.

The following information is so unbelievable that it almost qualifies as a real, live "miraculous cure" (just like the magic pill we keep hoping will bring health, wealth and thinness without all that doggone work!). The essential nutrient which has been called the "drink of champions", a "secret ingredient" and the single most important catalyst in losing weight and keeping it off, as well as enhancing endurance and health in many ways is ... are you ready? Water! Yes, plain old everyday water!

Although water is generally taken for granted, your body needs more of it than anything else, with the exception of air (yes, I'm sure there are some of you who don't think it's nearly as essential as shopping malls, bagels or chocolate ... but you're mistaken!). Every chemical reaction that takes place in your body depends on water, including those involving your blood, muscles and organs. Digesting and absorbing food, transporting nutrients through the bloodstream to the cells, carrying wastes out of your body, regulating your body temperature and fluid levels, and lubricating joints all depend on water. You cannot perform these functions at top efficiency unless you have an adequate amount of this incredible stuff. Studies have shown that water also suppresses the appetite naturally and helps your liver metabolize stored fat. Really! I'm not making this up! Without enough water your liver must suspend this function and help out the kidneys which cannot do their job without adequate water. Not drinking enough water can cause water retention which shows up as swollen hands, feet and legs. Bloating, darling. Yuck.

It may sound contradictory, but to lose excess water from your body, you must drink more. A lot more. When you restrict water, your body perceives this as a threat to survival and holds on to the water it has. Water retention. My natural inclination for many years was to drastically cut back intake of any fluids and head for the dangerous "water pills" or diuretics the instant my ankles or face puffed up. Just the opposite of the healthy solution of drinking plenty of fresh, pure water to flush out excess fluid! This is only released when plenty of water is furnished to your system. So drink it!

Another factor that can cause water retention is sodium intake. (See Chapter 34 "Sodium and Salt" for a discussion of sodium and potassium. Since your body can handle only so much sodium at a time, it needs additional water to dilute the excess. Sometimes your body holds onto water stubbornly, even when drinking enough. When this happens you can use a handy method, called "breaking through", to trick your body into letting go of bloating fluids. This method causes the cells of your body to be saturated with enough water so they release the excess. Simply drink one quart (4 cups) of pure water within a 30 minute period, 3 times a day, usually in mid-morning, mid-afternoon and early evening. About three days is required to flush excess fluid from your system. At first this may sound difficult, but persevere and find a convenient time. You will need to be close to a bathroom for about an hour after each quart is consumed, and you'll probably be surprised at how little water is released initially. This method is so much healthier and natural than harsh chemical diuretics. Of course, check with your health practitioner first.

A lot of water is also released during exercise or just by normal perspiration, especially on hot days. Now that I workout every day, I no longer have a water retention problem and believe me, it used to be almost a daily ritual to have to "put my legs up" to relieve the swelling. I almost never drank water and felt that juice, coffee or soda was all the liquid I needed and wanted. No wonder I chronically suffered from bloating, kidney stones, sluggish low energy, constipation, complexion problems and generally a clogged up toxic condition in my overfat body! Water will relieve these and other uncomfortable daily endurances and the resulting miserable feeling that you just aren't healthy.

Constipation is another problem that can be caused by lack of adequate water. Your body gathers water from internal sources such as the colon if it does not get enough from what you're drinking. Pardon the frank talk here, but this causes small, hard stools without the proper lubrication for normal bowel movements. Adequate water consumption will usually return your bowels to normal functioning. Many dieters needlessly suffer this symptom of low fiber and low water intake.

How Much Water is Enough?

Six to eight 8-ounce glasses minimum is generally recommended. However, if you are exercising regularly (you are, aren't you?) or if the weather is hot and/or dry, then you need more. Add an additional 8-ounce glass per day for every 25 pounds that you are overweight. (Let's see. That means I had to drink Lake Michigan daily when at my top weight, right?). If this seems like a lot, or is way above what you have been drinking, then just start wherever you can ... six glasses a day being the absolute minimum. Half a glass every hour. (Come on. You can do that ... didn't you say you would do *anything* to be thin?) A word of caution however: you can go overboard ... don't drink more than about 15 glasses maximum! This could deplete certain nutrients, such as minerals.

It's ironic and surprising that your natural thirst will reappear after you start drinking more. When you're not thirsty this should signal you to drink. Why? Thirst does not keep up with water loss and it will not prevent dehydration. You must monitor your intake of fluids without the aid of natural thirst. Your thirst gets even less sensitive as you get older.

For all the trouble you go to in developing this all-important habit, the benefits are no less than astounding. Fat deposits are metabolized more quickly, facilitating weight loss; water retention is relieved; sagging skin is plumped up, more resilient and healthy looking; waste is efficiently removed causing a feeling of cleanliness and lightness; your complexion appears clear with a healthy glow; energy and stamina is increased as the debilitating effects of dehydration and toxic build-up are counteracted. Worth a try, eh? I consider my water habit as one of the major reasons why I don't look like a bag of skin even after a long-term period of obesity and losing over half my body weight. With water, your skin tones and firms up again. Really!

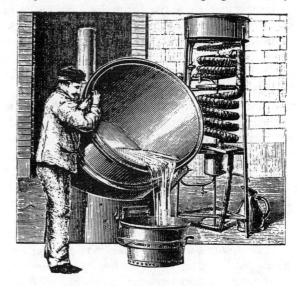

In the beginning 8 glasses sounds like a lot!

How to get all that water down

If you have trouble drinking 6-8 glasses of water daily, here are a few tricks to help you out. However, I'm convinced that as you see how easy it is to add water and the tremendous benefits that follow, you will have no trouble whatsoever. You will, in fact, happily increase your intake of your newly discovered "magic potion". A large, one quart mug is very helpful. Get the kind with a tight-fitting lid and a straw or straw hole in the lid. One of these mugs holds 4 cups (32 ounces) of water and goes very quickly. I drink one in the morning before lunch and again in the afternoon before dinner. They are easy to carry and handy, even in your car. If the taste of water doesn't excite you, try squeezing in a little lemon juice. Some people have tried keeping their whole daily allotment of water in a container on the sink or their desk. That way they can keep track of how much they have consumed during the day. Just ask any healthy person how they drink all their water during the day. They surely will have a trick or two to share. I always keep a 16-ounce squeeze bottle or large mug on hand when working out and sip frequently. Sipping or chugging, your choice. Dehydration during exercise is a common cause of the dragging, can't-go-on feeling half-way through your cha-chas. To counteract this, drink an 8-ounce glass before your workout, an 8-ounce glass for every ½ hour of exercise, and another 8-ounce glass when you finish. Keep sipping during your workout. It sounds like a lot, but you really need it.

Water Quality

Water quality is also very important. This includes the water you use for making coffee, boiling pasta, steaming vegetables and other cooking uses. The Environmental Protection Agency has issued reports stating that at various times the 50,000 existing city and town water supplies in this country not only carry contamination from parasites, viruses, bacteria, algae, yeast and molds but also many are liberally laced with asbestos, pesticides, heavy metals such as lead and cadmium, arsenic, nitrates, sodium and a variety of chemicals that are known carcinogens. In other words, tap water can be, and more often is, dangerous to your health. The treatments used to "purify" our public water sources, such as fluoridation and chlorination possibly pose further health risks. The Public Health Service states that several million Americans are right now drinking water that is hazardous to their health due to chemical and bacterial contamination. Both of these organizations urge Americans to take the responsibility for safe drinking water into their own hands, since the problems are simply too large for any one organization to handle.

What can you do to make sure that your water is safe? To test the purity of your tap water there are two booklets that will be helpful. From the League of Women Voters Education Fund, 1730 M Street, N.W., Washington, D.C. 20036, request a copy of "Safe Drinking Water for All: What You Can Do" for 25 cents. From the Water Supply Division, Environmental Protection Agency, Washington, D.C. 20460, request a single copy (free) of "Manual for Evaluating Public Drinking Water Supplies". This manual can be used to compare the test results of your public drinking water with the standards of the Public Health Service. The administrator in charge of water quality in your city or town or the local water company can be contacted with a request for the results of water sampling tests. If you live in a county area, I have found the county government to be very helpful in providing this information and even to provide free testing services if you have a well.

Another way to insure safe drinking water is to buy bottled water either at the supermarket or

through a company that supplies homes. But be sure you check with the manufacturer as to the water's source, the type of processing and, again, results of water sampling tests. The EPA has conducted surveys showing that some bottling plants put out bottled water that was contaminated with intestinal bacteria due to unsanitary conditions in the plants. Remember also that many plants are located in industrial areas and get their water supply directly from the tap. You can purchase a home "purifier" which may employ various purification methods (steam distillation for example). The EPA and Consumer Digest both have extensive results from testing various devices. Check with them before investing in a purification system.

You can buy distilled water from the supermarket or use a home distiller. Some find that distilled water has a flat taste due to the removal of minerals, but I enjoy the taste. The minerals we need are more efficiently and consistently derived from food we eat and supplements we take than from water.

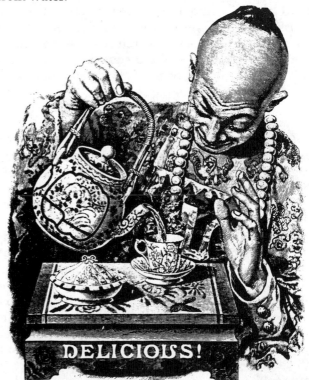

"Ah, herbal tea. Delicious!"

More Ways To Get Your Water

Other fluids you can drink as well as pure water include mineral water and herbal teas, either hot or cold, made with pure water. I drink at least one quart a day of mineral water. Many great flavors are available and I serve them up in a crystal goblet with a strawberry or lemon slice for a special touch. There are even stores now that carry only water from different sources from around the world. Now is a great time to become a connoisseur of fine (and healthful!) water.

Caffeine-containing beverages (coffee, tea, cola and cocoa) and alcohol shouldn't be used as part of your water requirement. However, in the beginning, or if you are really having a tough time getting all your water down, you can count half of any fruit juice or liquid milk as part of the 6-8 eight-ounce glasses that you need. You will be much better off, however, and the weight will be easier to lose, if you drink the full amount of pure water. Think of it as an internal bath.

Take This Habit-Changing Challenge

This habit is so important in permanently changing your health that I challenge you to try this experiment. For the next 21 days, follow the above recommendations exactly. Whatever it takes to overcome any obstacles that arise, determine right now that you will drink 8 glasses minimum of pure water a day. Period. Now, at the end of these 21 days, I believe you will enjoy all the benefits outlined and that you will feel, as I do, that this very important and underrated habit will be easy to continue considering the results. It's worth it! I personally drink quarts of pure water every day, no matter where I am. Good health begins with pure drinking water and plenty of it. So get a cup right now and start drinking your way to better health. (Wasn't there a "Drinking Man's Diet" once? I don't think they were talking about water though.)

In A Nutshell

1) Water is the single most important catalyst in losing weight and keeping it off.

2) Every chemical reaction in your body depends on water, including metabolizing stored fat.

3) Water retention can be caused by not enough water and too much sodium.

4) The healthy way to lose excess body water is to drink more water, until cells are supersaturated and release the excess.

5) Drink a minimum of 6-8 eight-ounce glasses of water daily, with 1 more glass for every 25 pounds you're overweight. Another glass each ½ hour of exercise, or if it's hot or dry.

6) Don't drink over 15 glasses a day. You could deplete certain nutrients in your body.

7) Natural thirst does not keep up with water loss, but it will return when you begin drinking adequate amounts of water.

8) Quality of water is very important to health. Go for the purest and best!

9) Take the 21 day challenge and experience the many benefits of your new "Magic Potion".

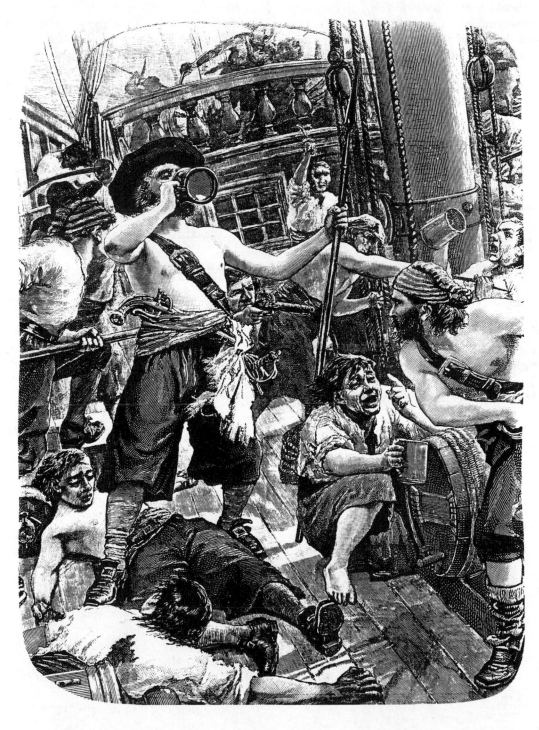

"That's got to be seven ... I'm sure I've had seven glasses by now!"

How to Survive Eating Away from Home   36

"Give me the clear blue sky over my head, and the green turf beneath my feet,
a winding road before me, and a three hours' march to dinner ... and then to thinking!"

William Hazlitt

Plan for Success

Whether you're eating in a restaurant, going to a party or just dining with a friend, this is a time for special care and planning. You are faced with an incredible challenge every time you leave the serenity and control of your own safe and sane home. The atmosphere in the "outside" world is usually jovial, fun and relaxed and the food and drinks are abundant. Nobody seems to care about the fat, calories, sodium and all that mundane stuff ... that is, until Monday morning when the nation as a whole groans as they step on the scale.

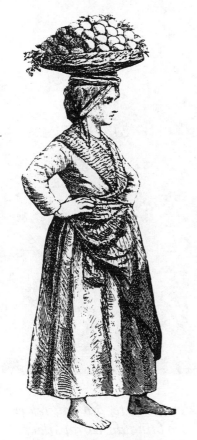

"This? Oh, I always take fresh fruit when I travel."

This atmosphere can cause you to become somewhat lax about what you are eating, to say the least. But there are specific ways you can stay focused on your new healthy outlook.

The key to success in these situations is to PLAN AHEAD. Think out a strategy. The suggestions below will help you to be prepared before stepping out on the town. Stick at it until you've got it right. Don't expect to learn it all the first time out (that's like expecting to shred down the "Expert's Ecstasy Totally Vertical Downhill Daredevil Ski Run" at 100 miles per hour the same day you graduate from the "Snow-Plowing Made Easy" class at the base of the bunny slope). You will make some good choices and you'll probably make some not-too-great choices, too. Don't expect to be instantly perfect and you won't become discouraged. Do the best that you can, and make each choice by conscious decision, not just habit. Stay aware.

Restaurants

We all love to eat out in restaurants (for one thing, no dishes!). It can be quite a challenge ... since many restaurants don't offer common items found in home kitchens, like steamed veggies, non-fat milk or yogurt. Keep asking though. If they know what we want, they will begin offering it. They also seem to have cooking methods developed in the favorite kitchens of famously fat Diamond Jim Brady (he was known to eat six bowls of soup and four complete chickens before he got down to the main course). It may take you several tries to get it right, but it will feel great when you do. By sticking to your goals, you'll gain confidence that you can make it work whenever and wherever you are away from home.

The best way to deal with eating out at a restaurant is to plan your meals carefully the day you will be going. Eat a good breakfast (as usual, right?), and a light but satisfying lunch. Don't go to the restaurant famished. Eat a light salad before you go, or an hors d'oeuvre, appetizer, yogurt, serving of bulky vegetables such as raw cauliflower, spaghetti squash or the like. If you go out hungry, you are likely to eat even more than you intended. And that basket of greasy chips or hot garlic bread and butter is going to do you in before the menu has even arrived.

If possible, know approximately what items on

the menu you will be having. This will help you greatly in planning.   While you are actively involved in losing weight, as opposed to maintaining, it would be wise to avoid the all-you-can-eat buffet style restaurants since they can tax the resolutions of a saint! Fast food establishments are improving, but they're still a challenge. Note the "Fast Food Strategies" later in this chapter. Just about any other type of restaurant will be able to offer you some healthy choices ... if you seek them out.

Restaurant Survival Kit

Always take a "Restaurant Survival Kit" with you. Carry one in your car or purse, so if you decide to go out to eat on the spur of the moment, you'll always be prepared.

In this kit, have several individual packets of reduced-calorie salad dressings so you won't be limited to lemon juice or vinegar. However, those can be quite tasty, also. Include a few individual packets of butter-flavored sprinkles. Before they were available in packets, I just took the bottle (about the size of a spice bottle). A bag or two of herbal tea can be nice and hot water can be ordered everywhere. A bottle of salt-free seasoning. An envelope of reduced-calorie hot cocoa mix is not only a milk serving for the day but also a great, satisfying dessert to enjoy while my cohorts have their Hogs-R-Us Heavenly Horror dessert.

If you're going to the restaurant directly from home, take along a small plastic container of your favorite low-fat salad dressing, cottage cheese, low fat cheese, sour cream or reduced-calorie cream cheese for your baked potato or salad (condiments really make a difference). I recently started taking along a plastic bag full of crisp carrot and celery sticks or peeled baby carrots to Mexican restaurants. I got tired of feeling out of control with the chips. Wonder of wonders, I wasn't the only one at the table who reached for the carrots to dip in the salsa. Now I have to take twice as many to have enough for the whole gang to munch! Instead of feeling obligated to eat all those chips, that greasy basket of high-fat calories left the table almost untouched ... which used to be about as rare as leftover breadsticks in an Italian restaurant. Get creative. It's your meal and your health.

The Right Attitude

Before heading out the door, dress up in your best outfit. Remember look good, feel good? (See Chapter 17 "Rewards".) My outfit always includes a belt that is non-expandable. This acts as a little reminder should you begin to overindulge! Kind of

like a food chastity belt. Also, if your source of support happens to be going along, be sure to clue them in as to what you hope to accomplish at the meal. No one else needs to know about your "diet" if you don't want them to ... and I recommend that you don't share the fact that you are on a weight control program. This is generally not a popular dining topic, as it tends to draw attention to what everyone is eating, and makes some people very uncomfortable, to say the least (they're often overweight). So just keep it between "you and yourself".

Finally, as part of your preparations, think about why you are going out. Is it just simply to stuff as much food into your mouth as possible? Certainly not! You want to enjoy good, satisfying food served in an appetizing way. But also, you're there to enjoy the company and the atmosphere of the establishment. These are the real reasons besides satisfying your need for a meal. Keep this in mind, and become involved in the conversation and appreciate your surroundings. Enjoy the total experience, not merely the food!

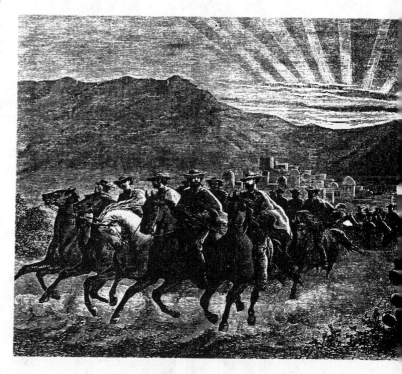

"Hey Hombre, did you remember to bring the carrot sticks?"

The Healthiest Restaurant Foods to Order

Listed below are foods that are your best choices for lower fat, cholesterol and sodium and higher nutrition and fiber in different types of restaurants. Ask about the method of cooking, specific ingredients and order any sauces served on the side ... so you control the amount .

You may feel that all this is a lot of bother so I will offer you a noteworthy example of the benefits that you can check out at your local video store. In the movie "When Harry Met Sally", Billy Crystal accuses Meg Ryan of being a "high maintenance" person after she gives a waitress some very specific instructions in a restaurant. And she is indeed a "high maintenance" person who's not so easy to please. But open your eyes and look ... Meg Ryan looks pretty good, doesn't she? Sure, it's "just a movie", but do you think the "real" Meg Ryan orders high fat, maximum meals or frequents all-you-can-eat joints? I doubt it!

Mexican

Salsa, salads, black bean soup or gazpacho, steamed corn tortillas, frijoles (beans) served whole, refried beans (sparingly ... watch for lard), burritos or soft tacos with vegetable filling, white meat chicken or seafood, grilled fish, Spanish rice, chicken or seafood fajitas made with "just a little oil please", white meat chicken or seafood enchiladas. Ask for light cheese, hold the sour cream, guacamole, fried anything including chips and excessive cheese. Beer and chips are a lethal combo for overdoing, so opt for iced tea (with a tiny paper umbrella) and a party hat. You'll thank me the next day.

Chinese

Steamed anything is good including vegetables, dumplings, rice and white meat poultry or seafood. Veggie mooshu (rice pancakes you roll up at the table) are my favorite. Veggie chow mein or chop suey with tofu, chicken or seafood. Ask for no oil, MSG or soy sauce to be used in the cooking. Veggie dishes of all kinds made this way are great. I season with a touch of concentrated hoisin sauce or hot mustard and they usually add a little broth in the cooking. Don't forget your fortune cookie and tea! Avoid fried anything, greasy meats, egg dishes, nuts and seeds, cream sauces, duck and other dark meat poultry. Rice noodles are okay, but not egg or fried noodles. Wonton soup for a treat.

Italian or Pizza

Black bean soup (hold the sour cream), minestrone, Italian bread or breadsticks, one glass of wine, pasta with tomato-based sauces, veggie pizza with light cheese or hold the cheese (trust me, this grows on you), grilled or steamed seafood or white meat poultry, salads with garbanzo, kidney beans or seafood, pickled veggie appetizers (beware of

sodium), sorbet, creme caramel for a treat, espresso or cappuccino with skim or low-fat milk. Avoid anything fried, smothered with cheese, with a cream-based sauce, butter, rich desserts, stuffed anything including calzone, lasagna or ravioli unless they have a light version, cold-cut toppings on pizza, excessive pesto (some to season is nice, though).

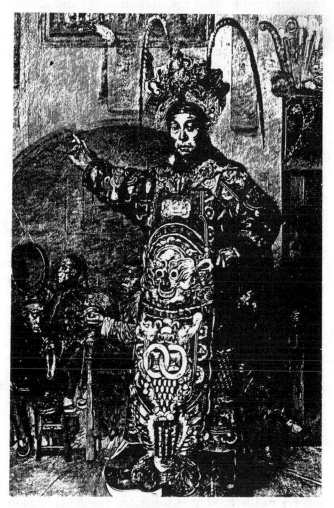

"No MSG!"

Steak House

Non-creamed veggie, lentil, bean or seafood soups such as Manhattan clam chowder, onion soup (hold the cheese) if you don't have a sodium problem, salad bars or fresh dinner salad, seafood salad, French or Italian bread or plain dinner rolls, round steak or filet mignon, plain baked potato (top with cottage cheese, vinegar, steak sauce or ketchup, and chives), rice, grilled or baked (without sauce) fish or poultry breast (remove skin), glass of wine, sorbet or sherbet. Avoid creamed soups, heavy dressings and sauces, prime rib, sirloin,

T-bone steaks, French fries or cottage fries, anything fried, sour cream, butter, garlic toast (unless you can get them to leave off the butter), hard liquor, stuffed dishes and anything sautéed in butter, heavy desserts and after-dinner drinks.

Indian

Veggie soups such as mulligatawny or lentil, steamed rice, white meat chicken, seafood or veggies, chapatis (puffy whole wheat flatbread), dal (thick bean sauce), raita (cukes in yogurt), tandoori dishes (ask for minimum oil and sauce), curry dishes not in cream sauces, chutney, fresh fruit or fruit desserts, tea. Avoid anything fried or in a cream sauce, dark meat poultry, nuts, coconut and butter.

I'll Have Health, Please

When you're finally at the table, look over the menu. In most of the places I frequent, I know just about what I'll be ordering each time and I even have a few places where the waitress knows I will be having "the usual". But let's assume you are going there for the first time as a health conscious person. Pick out dishes that are prepared as simply as possible, such as steamed, broiled or baked without added sauces, gravies or butter. Be the first to order when the waiter comes so you will not be tempted by what others order.

Narrow your choices to two or three and discreetly and pleasantly ask the waiter or waitress how they are prepared, to further help you decide. Ask that the dish be brought without added sauces, that the vegetables be steamed or cooked without butter, and that the condiments be served on the side. Be very specific about any changes that need to be made. Be pleasant, but firm. Sometimes I'll mention that I'm following a "special diet" and this can help the process go more smoothly (nobody wants a person to get sick in their restaurant). Most wait persons really do want to serve you the food you want and need ... after all, their tip largely depends on pleasing you. Be nice to them ... they're your link to the chef.

Start with non-creamed soup or a salad ordered with extra veggies on top, such as sliced tomatoes. Soup can be high in salt so watch it if you're salt sensitive. Cheese-based soups are the saltiest. If your meal comes with vegetables, ask for a double serving. Sometimes you will not be charged for this since you're omitting the sauce or sour cream, etc.

Order a glass of wine, wine cooler or spritzer, light beer, or drink if you wish. Just note the additional calories carefully. If your group orders a second round, make yours a club soda, soda, mineral water or juice. Know your limit. Mine is one. If I have more than one drink my judgment gets a little fuzzy, and all this health stuff (and everything else for that matter) just starts to seem a little silly.

Place your planned serving of bread or chips on your bread plate. Then move it to the other side of the table, so you can't get at it so easily, or have the waiter take it away. In its place, order herb tea (or hot water if they don't have it and use the herb tea bags you brought), decaffeinated coffee or a fancy glass of mineral water.

When your order comes, be sure to check it carefully and if it's not prepared the way you ordered it, then firmly, but in a pleasant way, tell the waiter that you cannot eat it, and that you would appreciate it if he or she would return it to the kitchen and make the corrections. You're paying good money for your meal and you should get what you ordered ... a meal you can eat and feel good about. You will soon see why it is important to be very specific when ordering. If the serving looks too large, decide before you begin how much you want. Move that part of the meal to one side of the plate and reserve the rest to take home.

If your companions urge you to try a certain dish or taste their yummy cheesecake, politely say "no thanks" and be sure to act like you've got the best meal in the place. If you wish, you may have a small serving of the rich food. "Just a taste" really satisfies me. I get lots of variety and don't have to eat the whole thing (this is similar to "high gourmet" style of eating where you're served 63 courses and each one is the size of one bite).

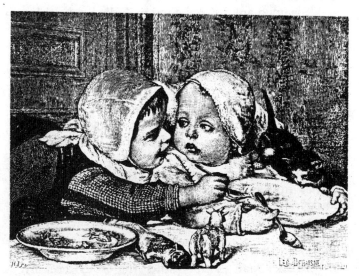

"Mind if I have a bite?"

If you sit there, drearily picking at a plain plate of lettuce, then you will not only be miserable, but may possibly put a damper on the whole event. So unless you are martyr, relish your food, talk, laugh and enjoy! Attitude, darling. Often times, I have others at my table eyeing my plate with more than a little envy because the food looks so appetizing and I'm obviously enjoying every bite! Sometimes I have to share!

Try to eat as slowly as possible, alternating your bites with mineral water or nibbling on the extra vegetables. It takes about 20 minutes for food to reach your stomach and signal your brain that you're getting full. Take a trip to the restroom to freshen up at mid meal. This way, others at the table who may have more to eat than you will not have half their meal left when you're done. If that happens, order a pot of hot tea and enjoy the conversation. Ask the waiter to wrap up your extras and enjoy a yummy lunch tomorrow.

Fast Food Strategies

If you're going to a fast food restaurant instead of a more elegant one, use the same techniques described above. Many places now have absolutely fabulous salad bars with a veritable potpourri of fresh, colorful veggies, several sources of good protein such as beans and cottage cheese or cheese, although the latter two are usually of the full-fat variety so limit them to smallish servings. You almost always have to bring along your own dressing so carry little individual packets. Cottage cheese mixed with a dressing packet makes a creamy topping for salads or baked potatoes. Keep a copy of your food pocket guide in your car so you can check foods out carefully. This won't always be necessary, since you'll probably order similar items each time and will get to know which things are best. Use this guide to help plan your meal.

Sometimes you must use your own best judgment as to the ingredients. Consult a cookbook to get a general idea of the contents, if necessary. Keep the serving size in mind when choosing. Try breaking a dish into its individual parts and figuring out what's in each part. For example, to determine how much a slice of pizza will "cost" you, break it down into crust, sauce and toppings. The 14" thin crust (go ahead, measure it!) will be about $1\frac{1}{2}$ breads per slice ($\frac{1}{8}$ of the pie). The sauce will be tomato sauce or paste and the topping will be about 1 ounce of cheese per slice. Add any other toppings such as pepperoni or sausage (about one ounce per slice) or veggies. Now add it all together. The tendency will be to estimate low, but it will be much better for your weight control program if you estimate high. Studies have shown that most dieters underestimate their calorie and fat intake by nearly 50%! If there is a question in your mind as to whether a food has $1\frac{1}{2}$ breads or 2 breads then go with the 2 breads.

You can have grilled hamburgers or garden burgers, burritos and even pizza at your favorite fast food places. Avoid fried foods and be aware that fast food is usually high in sodium (their definition of flavor), so balance your intake for the rest of the day or the week to avoid water retention (see Chapter 34 "Sodium"). Since fast foods also tend to be high in fat, limit fat whenever possible by eating where they grill instead of fry, and having them "hold the mayo". Go light on the cheese.

I think you'll be surprised at the healthier foods being offered at many fast food restaurants: lower fat burgers, vegetarian garden burgers, reduced calorie and fat shakes and cones, fat-free muffins, cereals, fresh juice, salads and salad bars, stir-fries, steamed rice, light cheese, bagels, low-fat milk, baked potatoes, low-fat chili (and even lower fat fries? ... well, maybe in the future on those fries). The demand for improved health and convenience has brought these to the marketplace at last. Now you can feel right at home ordering healthy foods.

A Job Well Done

Leave the restaurant with a warm feeling of satisfaction, knowing that your planning kept you in control. It beats walking out of a restaurant like some people do ... with a heavy burden of too much food, too much drink, guilt from "losing control again", and the painful prospect of facing the scale in the cold light of morning. Not you! You can enjoy the satisfying fact that you have successfully learned how to survive in a restaurant. Congratulations! Your new habits will become second nature in time, just as they are for thin folk ... because you will be a "thin folk", too. Reward yourself for your effort! How about a world cruise, a two carat diamond or even a new house plant with the money you saved on drinks and dessert? We have a lot of house plants ... living reminders of success! Choose a reward that suits you.

Parties and Other Gatherings

Holidays, family celebrations or get-togethers with friends are other occasions that may challenge your new eating patterns. Especially the first few times that you're confronted with them, when you don't know yet how fun and easy they can be to manage. If you're the host or hostess, of course you will have a better chance at selecting foods to cook and serve that will fit your weight control plan. Take this opportunity to cook up special dishes that you ordinarily wouldn't make ... since too many goodies lying around the house would be overly tempting. This especially goes for desserts in my case. If I left a chocolate marble cheesecake in the refrigerator I might have some trouble controlling myself. But since I know my guests will eat it all, or I can send it home with them, I'm safe while still being able to enjoy my just desserts. If you are not the one in charge of the food, then, first of all, reread the section above on eating out in restaurants. The information there can also be put to use at special occasions and parties.

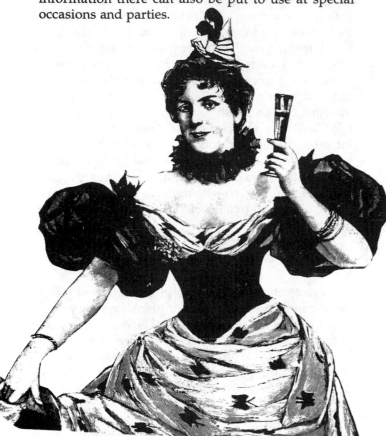

With the right hat nobody will suspect you of drinking mineral water at the party.

A good plan and a good attitude are most important for success. Know ahead of time what you can eat and estimate what is likely to be offered. Determine this by the time of day of the gathering and who is hosting the event. If it's Friday night at Mom's house, then you know for sure or can readily find out what the fare will be. Contact the host or hostess to ask what will be served. Take your own casserole or dessert to a pot-luck or get-together. That way you're assured of having something delicious and healthy.

Office parties may be entirely different. Make allowances in your daily and weekly menu plan so that you'll have plenty of choices. Again, you may wish to eat a salad or other such light but filling food before you go. You don't want to arrive ready to eat the world. "A few drinks" has been the downfall of many a good intention. One drink, then switch to mineral water, diet soda, club soda or juice. Stretch your favorite drink by mixing it with water or soda. Nibble on fresh veggies. Keep track of how many hors d'oeuvres you're eating or chips, nuts and other higher-fat foods. Talk to everyone. Mingle and no one will notice what you're eating. Be a social butterfly.

Buffets can be difficult so plan, plan, plan. A good strategy is to take a look at the buffet before starting through the line and decide on your best choices. Go through once and hit the salad section hard. Bring along your emergency kit of salad dressings, etc. Try to avoid the "trough and brew" mentality that seems so rampant in our culture ... like sharks at a feeding frenzy. Big hotels in gambling towns like Las Vegas prey on this by offering huge "all you can eat" buffets for super low prices. After you've eaten so much that your eyeballs look like pinwheels and you can hardly budge, you waddle out into the never-never land of the casino, where you end up paying the true cost of your discount hog-out. If this sounds like you, maybe you should eat elsewhere.

See Your Success

Picture yourself making the right choices. Then it will be easier for you to sail through confidently, since that's what you will be expecting (see Chapter 6 "Great Expectations"). Put this concept to work for you. Spend some time before the affair visualizing yourself there and making healthy, pro-thin choices. Visualize yourself leaving the event with the entire occasion having been a complete success! See yourself with a smile on your face and a feeling of calm, perfect control, as well as having had a terrific time with the people, food and party experience. Healthy and happy! (See Chapter 7 "Visualizations".)

With a bit of practice and perseverance you will learn how to eat your favorite foods both at restaurants and parties. When you first begin, it will take effort on your part to get the hang of it, but pretty soon you'll be able to judge which items on a menu will be the best for you. When the food arrives you will be able to "eyeball" the portion that is an average serving. Eventually this will become a habit and you'll be able to eat anywhere ... confident that you can maintain your slimness forever. It can be done and you can learn to do it with flair and style. Don't forget to reward yourself for success. You deserve it! Share your accomplishment with your support person to get reinforcement and recognition. Happy celebrations!

In A Nutshell

1) The key to success is to PLAN AHEAD. Think out a strategy.

2)   Give yourself time to develop techniques and change habits.

3) Take a "Restaurant Survival Kit" and your pocket nutrition book.

4) Dress up and wear a belt!

5) Know how to order and what to order ... be specific.

6) Don't mention your "diet". It's a party pooper.

7) Enjoy the atmosphere, food and people at the restaurant.

8) Practice at home to become familiar with serving sizes and approximate ingredients.

9) Parties follow many of the same rules ... watch alcohol!

10) See yourself ahead of time succeeding ... with healthy choices and a great attitude!

11) Reward yourself and share your accomplishments!

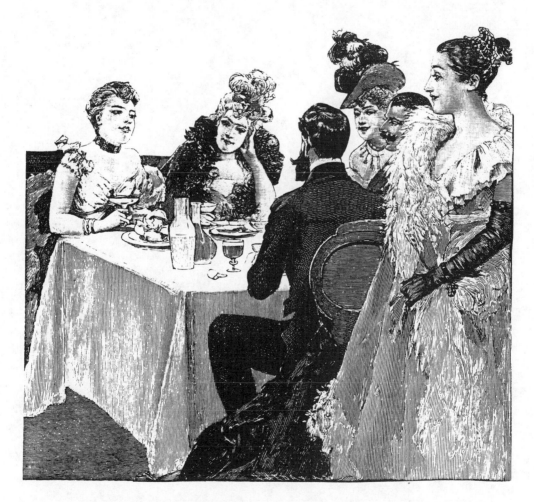

Enjoy the company when you eat out, as well as the food.

Part VI

Additional tools
and
Resources

Accelerated Weight Loss Plan   37

"There is more to life than increasing its speed."
Mahatma Gandhi

What about the times when you want or need to take off weight and trim up fast? Everybody wants to know how to speed up the process once in a while. This is not a regularly recommended practice as you almost certainly will regain weight taken off quickly ... since you did not develop any habits to keep it off or retrain your body to handle excess fat and calories. But there are certain situations where you can take off 10-15 pounds without doing too much damage ... if you follow some very specific guidelines. You may want a speedy start to your program or have an upcoming event such as a wedding or reunion in your near future. You can choose to follow this accelerated plan for a limited time only ... a maximum of two to four weeks. You can also use these guidelines if you're stuck on one of those famous plateaus where the pudge won't budge and you are in danger of abandoning your effort. It would be better just to hang on and realize that this adjustment is only temporary as long as you are staying with the program. However, a few days or a week on this accelerated plan might give your body a little extra push to get on with it and give you a psychological boost as well. Use this approach sparingly.

Before you begin this accelerated plan, ask yourself the following questions about how you are progressing in your program. They can help you pinpoint any weak areas or trouble spots. Perhaps some minor adjustment is all that you need.

Questions for Evaluating Your Current Program

1)   Are you keeping track of everything that you eat and writing it down every day? It's easy to lose track if you don't. At the very least, keep a Daily Success Planner one day a week just to check up on yourself. The better you get at keeping track mentally, the longer you can go without a "tune-up". If you find yourself slipping, do this first. Your Personal Journal can also help you identify possible problems or patterns that may be making the weight stick. Reread Chapter 12 "Your Personal Journal" and Chapter 18 "Daily Success Planner".

2)   Have you weighed and measured all your foods lately to check portion sizes even if you think you can judge them correctly? Weigh and measure everything once a week or if you're unsure of a portion. It's amazing how portions can get way out of line fairly quickly. Always measure highly concentrated foods such as oils or mayonnaise or other fats.

3)   Are you keeping the boredom out of your meals by choosing a variety of foods each day and trying new recipes at least once a week? Variety is the spice of life, and your diet! Keep your interest high. At the very least try a new condiment or spice. Reread Chapter 29 "Sample Meals".

4)   Are you limiting sodium and salty foods? Water weight often causes the scale to show pounds that are just temporary but nonetheless discouraging. Use your sodium counter for a checkup. Reread Chapter 34 "Sodium and Salt vs Herbs and Spices".

5)   Are you drinking all of your water or herbal tea everyday? This helps flush out excess fluids in your system. Remember "to lose water, you must drink water". Reread Chapter 35 "Water: The Magic Potion".

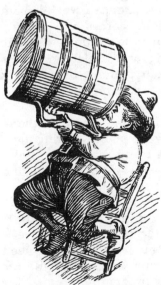

6)   Are you using affirmations, your Dream Book, Treasure Maps and visualizations as instructed to keep up your attitude and keep a thin future foremost in your mind? If you see yourself thin and act thin, you will eventually be thin! Review the section on Attitudes and Personal Development.

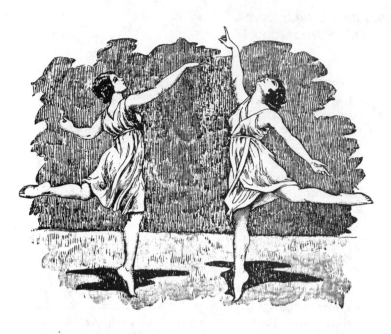

Frieda and her friend frolic on their Free Day

7)   Are you meditating daily and practicing your stress reduction techniques? Reread Chapter 11 "Breathing and Meditation" and Chapter 14 "Taming Your Stress".

8)   Are you weighing yourself on the same scale at the same time ... once a week maximum? Wearing similar weight clothes and having eaten similar foods? Don't be a daily weigher. It can be discouraging and deflating. Study your weight chart for your patterns of weight loss. Use other guides to judge your progress.

9)   Women, is your period on the way? Your body may add several pounds during the week preceding it. Be patient and you'll probably have an extra good loss next week. Meanwhile, limit caffeine and salt. Exercise and drink your water.

10)   Are you doing more activity than usual and exercising at least three times a week (with firming and toning moves also)? You need to exercise to maximize your weight loss. Reread the Exercise section of the program.

11)   Are you sharing your thoughts and progress with your support person on a regular basis? Talk it through. A fresh perspective and empathetic ear often works wonders. Reread Chapter 16 "Creating a Powerful Support System".

12)   Have you given yourself enough time? Don't fall into the trap of weighing yourself several times a week, or even a day, hoping the scale will show a drop each time just because you're being "good". Remember, this is a lifelong lifestyle, not an overnight fling. Be patient! Concentrate on increasing your health and educating yourself about your particular health issues. Stick with it, it's worth it!

13)   Have you had a "FREE DAY" in the last month? Sometimes pushing too hard can set up resistance. Lighten up, relax a day, enjoy your progress so far.

If you answered "No" to any of the above questions, that may be the area where you need to step up your concentration. Any one of them could be holding you back from a steady weight loss and a positive attitude about losing and progressing. If you're faithfully following the program and have not been losing weight or inches at all for the last 2 or 3 weeks, then look over the following suggestions and choose some that feel comfortable.

Acceleration Techniques

1)   Food
Do not stop eating! This is the biggest mistake you can make! Remember that if you limit your intake to much below 1200 calories daily your body will automatically slow down to conserve itself, and you will not lose much weight ... just metabolism points, muscle and water. You want this to be permanent weight loss, not temporary. Keep your intake around 1000-1200 calories minimum for women, 1400-1600 for men. Smaller people can eat the lower amounts.

Limit fats, but don't eliminate them. Count your fat grams. Lower fat to 10 grams daily if you want, but no lower! Increase veggies, especially raw ones, and soups, which are very filling. People who have soup daily eat less, are more satisfied, and lose more than those who don't. Try it! A soup and salad meal is the perfect combination for maximum satisfaction and weight loss. Increase fiber and bulk any way you can to make yourself feel fuller and satisfied with less actual calories and fat. Many of the THINNER WINNERS recipes and tips are designed with this in mind, since I love to feel like I'm getting a lot of food. Cut out 1 bread a day if you're eating 4-6 servings. Increase your water to 8 glasses minimum daily and your vegetables to 6 servings minimum daily.

Stay home and cook for a while, and avoid restaurant food (with ingredients that you can't control). Cook plain and simple meals avoiding high salt, sugar or processed foods such as packaged and frozen items, packaged meats, pickled foods and olives.

Now is a good time to break the caffeine habit since caffeine has been shown to be an appetite stimulant. Switch to water, herbal tea or water-process decaffeinated coffee. Eat three well-planned meals a day and snacks at your most vulnerable times. Don't eat for at least three hours before you go to bed (remember those Sumo wrestlers). Have a satisfyingly large breakfast and lunch and a fairly light dinner. If you get hungry in the evening have a container of non-fat yogurt, a Cream Fluff (see Chapter 30 "Basic Recipes") or whole-grain crackers and a cup of hot herbal tea or low-sodium bouillon.

There are times when I enjoy having nothing but freshly made juices for one whole day. I call this my "juice day" or "cleansing day" since I feel so light and refreshed, both mentally and physically, for several days after. By eliminating all fat and sodium from your system in this manner for a day, you give your digestive system a break also ... kind of a breather for your whole body. Never do this for more than one day per week or you will run into toxic build-up problems and really jolt your metabolism in the wrong direction. To do this, consume 1000-1500 calories a day of freshly-made-only fruit or vegetable juices. Canned, frozen or bottled juices will not do here at all. Juice loses a significant amount of nutrients within twenty minutes of being processed! Use a high-quality juice extractor to get the most vitamins, minerals, fiber and other nutrients from fruit as possible. Diluting a little with fresh water and sipping slowly is even better as this allows your body to assimilate the juice more slowly. Sip a glass whenever you feel hungry throughout the day. Add a frozen banana half to the juicer if you're really hungry. My juice extractor (a Champion machine) also processes frozen fruit into fantastic fresh fruit "ice cream". I simply freeze the whole fruit the night before (bananas, strawberries, blueberries, pineapple ... whatever your favorites are). Then I process combinations of different fruits about 3 or 4 times during the juice day. It doesn't even feel like "dieting" at all. I think of it as something wonderful I do for my body. Be sure to drink 6-8 glasses of water during the day and do some light stretching and mild aerobics. To help fill in the time which you will not be spending cooking, eating and cleaning up make this an especially busy day ... not one where you are just hanging around the house asking for trouble. Have several projects going and the time will fly by. This is one of the best methods for calming and de-stressing that I know of. It really gives you a break from all the harried concern over food, food, food all the time. Instead of a whole day, consider trying this for only one meal during the day, such as breakfast. You absolutely must check with your health pro before using a juice day as an acceleration technique.

2)   Exercise

Increase your exercise by one session over what you are doing now, or to at least 4-5 times regularly each week. You should already be doing 3-4 sessions minimum weekly. If not, now is the time to get going! Spread the sessions out so you never go more than two days in a row without some aerobic workout. This fuels your metabolism on a more regular basis instead of letting the fire completely burn out. Increase the length of time spent in each session by 10-15 minutes. A longer, lighter aerobic session is much more effective in burning fat than shorter, more intense sessions (see Chapter 21 "Get That Body Movin'"). Increase activity during the day and don't just plop down in front of the TV at night for several hours. Keep active and moving around. Now may be the time to start walking for 30 to 60 minutes every night after dinner.

Aerobic exercise will burn calories, tone muscles and increase cardiovascular fitness, but does little to build muscle tissue ... the actual metabolic machinery of your body. Only specifically working the muscles will do that. So start lifting some light weights 3 times a week following a beginners program carefully. Guidelines can be found in video tapes or books and magazine articles. Or see a professional at a gym. Stretching and breathing help to relax and de-stress your mind and body. Give yourself a ten minute full body stretch-out every day, preferably as part of your cool-down after your walk or workout. Try breaking your workout into 2 sessions daily (30 minutes mid-morning and 30 minutes after dinner).

3)   Attitude and Behavior

Keep it up! Now is the time to reward yourself for all the good work you've done so far! Buy a new piece of exercise wear, such as matching headband and socks, a new sweat shirt or a new leotard. Have your hair done. See yourself as a healthy, active person with a temporary weight problem. Keep that image of yourself always in your mind's eye. Read your affirmation cards often and concentrate on believing them fully. Allow yourself to spend at least $\frac{1}{2}$ hour a day alone ... just thinking and contemplating positive, peaceful thoughts. Gaze up at the sky and daydream for awhile. It is very refreshing and uplifting. Meditating for 20 minutes twice daily will decrease stress and induce harmony in your thoughts and reactions, even regarding food! Take a "Breathe Deeply" break several times a day. Talk to your support person or group about your feelings ... that's what they're there for. Stay around positive, supportive people and happy situations. Don't seek out partners for your personal "poor me, pity party". Good friends won't let you get away with it (not for very long anyway). Write down your feelings during this time or work in your Personal Journal. Create a Treasure Map and a Dream Book. And give yourself a break! All this thought and work you are doing is great and you deserve to acknowledge your efforts. It's pat on the back time.

Remember, if this is a plateau, it's only a temporary glitch. You are going for the permanent solution (see Chapter 13 "Troubleshooting Guide"). Give yourself the time you need to develop the habits that will take you over the finish line and into the THINNER WINNERS circle. You must meet, face up to and conquer each of the rocks set in the pathway leading to your goal. There is no "quick" permanent solution ... only true awareness and understanding will lead you to Thinland forever. So use this accelerated plan sparingly, then get on with the real work that will take the weight off for good. Be patient with yourself and the results that are on the way, instead of being "a patient" for your doctor!

In A Nutshell

1)   Use these acceleration techniques sparingly for 2-4 weeks maximum.

2)   First evaluate your current program by answering the questions.

3)   Do not skip meals or stop eating. Do not decrease total calories below 1000-1200 for women and 1400-1600 for men. Monitor fats closely staying at 15% maximum (don't go below 10 grams a day!). Increase veggies, fiber and water.

4)   Add one session of aerobic exercise weekly and/or increase length of sessions by 10-15 minutes each. Be more active in general.

5)   Attitude - Stay positive by employing the methods listed.

6)   Give yourself time to develop new methods of dealing with food, food issues, emotions and situations. Remember:

"Sow an action, reap a habit.
Sow a habit, reap a character.
Sow a character, reap a destiny!"
Zig Ziglar

"Healthy days add up to healthy lives!"
Roseanne

Secrets of Successful Maintenance   38

"For more than five years I maintained myself ... "
Henry David Thoreau

It's really not so difficult or secretive to maintain your hard-earned new body. Let's take a closer look at the people who are doing it successfully, and see exactly what it is they do differently from those who habitually "put it all back on and more".

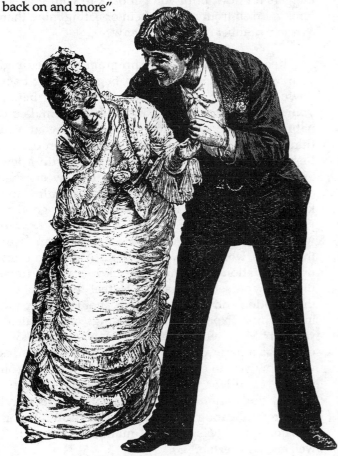

"Is that a rib I feel?"

Take It Off the Right Way

First of all, you have taken your weight off at the recommended rate of 1 to 1½ pounds per week, right? Right! So to lose 15 pounds it has taken you about 10 weeks. The habits that you have developed over these weeks are becoming pretty well ingrained by now. Habits such as drinking 8-10 glasses of water a day, keeping a Daily Success Planner, choosing lower fat foods at restaurants (yes, even at Greasy Joe's No-Star Cafe) and keeping a healthy kitchen stocked with all the right munchies.

By looking through your nutrition guide on a regular basis you have learned a lot about what foods have in them and you're more aware when shopping. By reading labels, planning meals ahead and shopping with a list, less "surprises" land in your cart. Cooking healthier and skinnier is almost second nature by now. You always remove skin and fat before cooking, and let the fat drip off your food with a rack or broiler pan. You mainly steam, bake and microwave. You rarely use much oil or fat to cook with or use on top of foods.

You've even had time to convert a few favorite recipes into healthier versions. Aunt Tessie's Two-Ton Fruitcake is now a manageable and scrumptious Two-Fruit Cobbler and you love it! Exercise is a daily ritual that you look forward to as special energizing and relaxing time for yourself. You realize that your walk will clear away the cobwebs from your thoughts and give you lots of energy for the day or evening ahead. You feel great and look terrific! Your self-esteem and attitude are both pretty good these days and you have a calm knowing that you have learned much that will help you stay in this new and wonderful place.

Now, I understand that when you hit that magic goal weight on the scale, there is a tendency to say, "Okay, I'm off the diet now and can go back to eating whatever I want!" Hold on! That's not the way it works. If you haven't gotten this yet, get it now! You have been changing your habits and lifestyle, and absolutely have *not* been on a traditional "diet". Yes, you will be able to eat more now that you are no longer trying to lose weight, but **if you eat, think and act like you did before, you will eventually weigh what you did before**. Pretty logical, eh? It's also absolutely true. It seems simple, but some people just don't seem to get this basic fact. To change your body permanently, you must change your habits, including eating, permanently. Don't bother reading on until you have repeated that last highlighted sentence at least 10 times out loud and are absolutely certain you understand it and believe it!

This doesn't mean that you can never have Triple Choco-Bliss Pie ever again. You can, and anything else you want also. But now you will plan for it ahead of time and enjoy it as part of a well-balanced diet that satisfies your body, mind and your need for yummies.

By learning and using the THINNER WINNERS principles in this book you have built a strong, solid foundation. If you're reading ahead just to see what maintenance holds for you, this should convince you that those habits you are working on so diligently are absolutely essential!

What is "Normal"?

It's important that you don't get too fanatical about keeping your weight within too strict a range. Understand that most "normal" people have weight fluctuations of 2-8 pounds at different times of the year (gaining in the Fall, slimming down in the Summer) or after certain special events such as vacations or holidays. Don't be too hard on yourself if you gain this much. Otherwise you may go into I-feel-so-bad-I-blew-it-I'm-going-to-eat-the-world mode. Just acknowledge the weight without judgment and say, "Okay, it's time to take a look at my food intake", step up your exercise, if necessary, and see what other areas you need to pinpoint. I call this process **"Tightening Down My Weasels"** because there are about 7 or 8 weasly little tendencies that go out of balance for me personally if I don't pay attention to them. They're kind of like unruly kids who need a little straightening out from time to time, and then they're fine for a while. Eventually they'll grow up!

Your weasels will be yours alone, but for the sake of example I'll list some of my common weasels and how I approach tightening them down when they get out of line :

The Weasels   How to Tighten them up :

Bagels - don't buy more than one if you eat them until they 're gone or they call to you. Same with bags of cookies. Buy just one and eat it.
Crackers - the same for certain kinds of crackers and chips... you know the ones.
Extra "bites" or nibbles - one of my joys and ways to increase variety is to taste whatever Howard is having. But limit to one taste per meal.
Fat grams - Limit to 10% of total calories when weight is up.
Frozen yogurt cones - two per week as a treat. Don't bring home a half gallon.
Movie popcorn - a sneaky killer. Bring your own (air-popped) or take a cup and measure. There are 3.5 grams of saturated fat in every cup of this stuff!
Peanut butter - sometimes it's okay, other times better not to buy it at all.
Restaurants - When you are advanced you can deal with these more easily, but they're still a challenge. Use all you have learned to survive or just eat at home for awhile.
Sugar (mints, maple syrup, etc.) - they're small and tend to sneak in so just don't buy them for now.
Wine - one glass on the weekend or just avoid for now especially if alcohol effects your judgment and lowers your resistance to overeating or over imbibing.

These are mine. Get to know your weasels, too! Basically, when you're in the process of tightening down your personal weasels, either avoid the buggers for now, until you get back to your goal, or limit yourself from buying them or eating more than a certain number of servings per week.

Keep your attitude and program balanced and your weight will stabilize and begin coming back down again. But whatever you do, do not berate yourself for gaining. It's okay. It's normal and natural to experience fluctuations. It's what you think about that extra weight that's important. Remember, you are a thin person now with a few extra pounds, not a fat person who blew another diet. This attitude is crucial. Remain calm and know this is natural, make a plan and be good to yourself. I always give myself a big, juicy reward whenever I find I have become aware of an issue that needs work, like weight gain. And absolutely no deprivation or blame. It backfires every time. Blaming yourself causes you to feel terrible about the situation and what you think about will expand in your life. Expand terrible feelings and what do you get? More terrible feelings. However, thinking of this as a natural cycle that everyone experiences will allow you to expand that thought instead. You will be confident that you're just experiencing a natural fluctuation and it is okay. Less stress and less stressful eating will happen as a result. This is a major secret of successful maintainers. Learn it well and be one, too.

Another cycle that has revealed itself over the last six years of successful maintenance for me has been different food intake on different days. Many times I am so busy or just into the routine on weekdays that I eat standard (but yummy!) fare. Cereal and fruit, a salad or sandwich, baked potato and veggies, yogurt and fruit. And this is just fine. I'm comfortable with it and it's easy. On the weekends however, we often go out to restaurants and that's when I have my richer or more plentiful foods. Find your balance with your particular schedule. After a while it will just be second nature for you.

I notice that each year it gets easier to

maintain my weight as I continue to manage these habits. Experience pays off with weight control and self-awareness as with anything. I'm The Boss now! I worked my way up from the mailroom and I don't ever have to go back. I know the ropes.

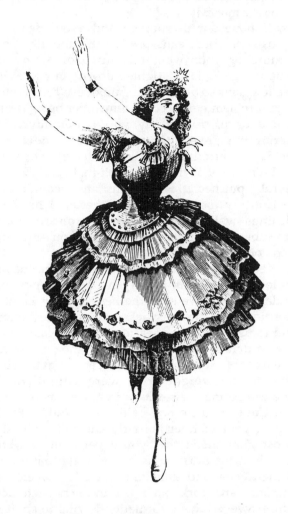

"I'm at goal, and I feel pretty, oh so pretty ..."

I'm at Goal — Now What?

When you first begin to eat more, be prepared for a slight gain on the scales ... about 2-3 pounds due to water and more food volume. This can be disheartening and even scare the bejessers out of you if you're not prepared. Again, this is natural. You may choose to lose a couple of pounds extra if it's very important for you to maintain at a certain weight. Let's say you are aiming for 135 pounds as a goal weight. After beginning to add more food volume you will probably gain 2-3 pounds and end up stabilizing after a week or two at 137 or 138. If you would rather stabilize at 135, then stay on the losing plan for a few more weeks until you weigh 132 or 133. That way you will stabilize at about 135.

When you begin eating more than the reducing plan, add calories and fat like this:

Keeping careful records with your Daily Success Planner, raise your calories 100 per day and fat level by 5%. For example: weight loss plan =1200 calories, 10% fat. **Week 1** of weight maintenance =1300 calories, 15% fat. If at the end of the first week you are 2-3 pounds heavier, that's natural and normal. This weight will not convert to fat as long as you continue to exercise and drink water.

The **second week** on maintenance, add 100 more calories a day (1400 total), but keep your fat at the same level (15%). When you weigh after the second week of maintenance you should have stabilized at 2-3 pounds above your lowest weight ... not gaining or losing. If you gained 1 pound or more the second week, remain at 1400 calories and 15% fat during the **third week**.

If you stabilized and didn't gain, or lost weight, try adding 100 more calories a day during **week 4** (now you'll be at 1500) and going to 20% fat if you want. 20% fat is the maximum, and you may have to cut back to 15% to maintain at your goal. I maintain at about 10-15% fat with comfort, but I know all the tricks by heart. You would too if you wrote this book.

As you can see, stabilizing your maintenance level is a process of fine-tuning certain factors such as fat and calories. Continue adding calories at this rate (100 per day) until you gain 1 pound or more for the week. Then go back to the previous week's calories and fat percentage. That is your personal calorie and fat percentage requirement to stay at your desired weight right now. It may seem like a feast after the reducing plan! And a well-earned feast, too, so enjoy! Of course, there are other factors that determine if you maintain your weight, primarily your activity level, but this will give you a good base from which to work.

What types of food can you eat now? I re-e-ally hope you don't even have to ask this question. But just in case you do, let me refresh your memory. All the foods that you have been learning about in this program are recommended for your maximum health, not just weight loss. These foods contain the high quality, vital nutrients needed for all of us to be the healthiest we can be. They are foods with low fat (especially saturated or hydrogenated fat), high fiber, low sugar and other refined carbohydrates, low sodium, and high in complex carbohydrates. They are as fresh as possible, well-prepared to preserve vitamins and minerals and eaten with moderation, variety and balance in mind. These are exactly the foods you will continue eating to maintain your weight and your health.

But what about cookies or pizza? Can you have those again? Of course! As you were losing weight, you could have chosen to have those things and I hope you did once in a while. Because then you learned how to fit them into your food plan and still lose weight by balancing them with other more healthful foods. That is exactly what you will be doing now. However, you can probably indulge a little more if you choose since you aren't trying to lose any more weight, and you're in full swing with your daily exercise. Add a goodie in, here and there, and see what it does to your weight and attitude. If you can handle it, great! Watch your too-hot-to-handle foods carefully (see Chapter 15 "Managing the Food-Food Connection"). Sometimes I can handle peanut butter and sometimes I can't. Don't deprive yourself but don't go overboard either. I find eating quality, well-prepared foods helps my satisfaction level stay high so that I don't keep eating just to satisfy "something" I can't even put my finger on. This is how permanently slim people do it. Indulge when you really want to and enjoy every bite. This is the process of learning your limits, which all maintainers have to deal with.

Stay in Touch with Your Weight

It is vital that you keep track and not lose touch with your weight. Research has shown that people who weigh themselves weekly tend to adjust their habits accordingly to compensate for any gains. Any longer than that and you may gain too much to easily take off. It can discourage you. Some people just keep putting off getting on the scale until "next week" or Monday or some other future alternate universe. However, "the new slender you" knows that keeping track of your weight is a key to maintaining your permanent slimness. So, pick a day of the week (mine is Saturday morning). You will always get on the scale that day (in front of a witness if necessary) and record your weight in writing. Always, no matter what has gone on the week before.

It is very important to keep a record. That way you will see gaps in your charts if you miss a week and also patterns will emerge over time. If you do miss a week, just write down your best "guesstimate" and make a brief note such as "vacation", "sister's visit" or "too chicken". This will help you maintain a balance later and give you the long-term picture. Keeping your weight where you want it is a long-term project, dare I say life-long? You'll be able to compare where you were last year at this time and be able to spot trends.

Another excellent technique for keeping track of your size is a perfect fitting pair of blue jeans. Not slacks or a skirt, which tend to be more forgiving, but a size 8 (or your perfect size) pair of regular jeans (not baggies, relaxed fit or stretch fabric ... nice try!). I slip mine on every Saturday morning to do a few errands around town. I know right away if I've gained an inch. Snug pants do a great job of keeping you on the money!

Be honest with yourself and avoid denial at all costs. If your jeans are a little too tight one morning or your weight is up 3 or 4 pounds, acknowledge it. Then "tighten down your weasels" for a few days so your small gain doesn't turn into a bigger problem next week. I remember being nearly at goal once, during my yo-yo diet days, and wearing this great little pair of bikini underwear. One day I noticed just a little flab hanging over the top. I remember saying "Oh, isn't that cute", when I playfully pinched it. Six months later I couldn't get them on my toe. Now I know better. I heed my warnings well. Tight clothes are one of them. Remember, you can't change it unless you see it first! Keep your eyes open ... stay aware!

Keeping your Daily Success Planner has helped you lose your weight. If you have been keeping one regularly, you have seen the benefits first hand of recording your meals, snacks and activities among other things. Planning is easier and you really know how much you've had, with no guessing. Researchers recently discovered that dieters resistant to weight loss were found to be underestimating their calorie intake by as much as 50%! Could you be one of them? (Who, me?) By keeping your Planner honestly and faithfully, it is almost guaranteed that you'll get slim and stay there. But, for most of us, we lose the habit after getting to goal and stabilizing for a few weeks. It's just plain hard work and a pain in the bagel to keep it up. However, this information is vital to spotting trends (such as peanut butter binges, emotional situations, sweets indulgences, skipping breakfast, etc.). So continue to write in your Daily Success Planner at least 1 day a week. Perhaps the same day that you weigh would be convenient. This will keep the structure in your mind more clearly for the rest of the week.

The whole point is to "nip it in the bud" if an upward weight trend or eating cycle begins. It will also keep your attitude focused on being in control of your weight. If you let it go too long ... well, we all know what happens when you get on the scale and have gained 10 pounds or more. You eat to numb that horrible feeling of guilt and disappointment and, "Oh, no! I swore I'd never weigh this much again!". With weekly monitoring you can go a long way towards averting that big "surprise", which can lead to depression, bingeing or the classic, "What's the use, I'll just eat it anyway" attitude.

The Fabulous Five

There are really only five things that you must do to attain and maintain your new slim body. I call these the Fabulous Five and here they are ... in order of importance.

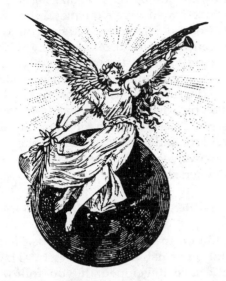

1)   Attitude is top banana!

With a strong, centered attitude, well-powered by all the principles taught in this program, you can weather anything that life can dish out and still land on your feet, slim and trim. It's the source and the power of all that drives you to maintain your health. The depth of your work on your attitude will directly impact your ability to remain balanced. If you haven't gotten this yet, go back to the Attitude and Personal Development section of the program to more fully understand your mind/body connection. What you perceive and know about yourself will reflect very clearly the new, improved person you are becoming. If you've got any doubts remaining, reread Chapter 5 "Motivation and the Success Mindset".

2)   Activity

If you can do nothing else that this program recommends, at least increase your activity. It is the most important thing you can do to get in touch with your body, and it will lead to a better attitude, more efficient system and other strengths that can help you. Find an aerobic activity (or preferably several) and do one every day for at least 30 minutes. Even if you can't do the whole 30 minutes, do 5 minutes at the time you said you would. This may not seem like much, but researchers have found that the daily habit of thinking about exercise, and then following through (no matter how briefly) helps to get that routine set in your daily schedule. Keep trying.

The best activities (the safest and easiest) are walking fast, biking (either indoors or outside), aerobic tapes or classes (low-impact or bench-step are safest), other exercise machines such as skiers or rowers or combination machines, jogging (for the more advanced, less overweight or under 30 crowd with no lower back or joint problems), or anything that you love and keeps you sweating continuously for 30 minutes. I have a friend who twirls a hula-hoop and works up a great sweat. Don't feel obligated to do the same thing every day. You will inevitably get bored and only work one set of muscles. Choose several activities you enjoy and are fun and you'll be more likely to stick with it for life.

Begin adding a light weight routine 3 times a week to tone and increase your muscle tissue. Focus weight training on your upper body since most aerobic activities will already be working your lower body. A daily abdominal routine is necessary to flatten and strengthen your stomach and help protect your lower back. Many people complain of lower back pain, but a strong abdomen will go a long way towards eliminating this.

Take it slow in the beginning, but get active now! It's the best thing you can do for yourself and your health. I couldn't walk even one block when I started, so that's no excuse. And I know women with kids, careers and households to run who find and make time every day to exercise. You can too if you don't look for excuses and problems, but instead seek solutions to the challenges this habit change will inevitably bring. Talk with your health professional, then get started.

3)   Low Fat / High Fiber Intake

The third important factor for losing fat and weight is your fat and fiber intake. Fat first. You learned how to calculate the conversion of fat grams into calories in the chapter "Cholesterol and Fat". Again, about 10-20% fat (with just $\frac{1}{3}$ of that coming from saturated or hydrogenated fats) is all you should be eating while you are actively losing fat. This is easiest to accomplish if you simply don't put any added fat into or onto your food. Use the many guidelines and tips in this book to substitute other foods and techniques. After you have reached your goal weight or fat/muscle ratio , then increase your fat intake to 15-20%, if you choose, for lifetime maintenance. Be strict on this and you will notice a big difference. Replace your fat calories with complex carbohydrates such as potatoes and other starchy vegetables, whole grains and cereals, beans and other legumes. You'll actually get to eat a lot more since fat is over twice as concentrated in calories as carbohydrates.

Fiber intake is also an essential factor for healthy weight maintenance. Consuming more veggies, whole grain foods, whole fruits and beans will ensure you get more fiber, both the soluble and insoluble varieties. And it will help you even more if you eat fewer low fiber foods (fat, sugar, dairy and meat). High fiber foods will move through your system faster and act as an internal "broom", sweeping out the residues to keep you clean and light. It keeps you filled up, gives you lots to chew and helps protect against the build-up of toxins. Be sure to drink plenty of water (and less caffeine ... a diuretic). If you are not used to extra fiber found in natural foods, add it slowly until you are at comfortable levels. Remember, ease into the plan and you will be much more likely to stay with it until you automatically live the THINNER WINNERS lifestyle.

4)   Water

Number four of the Fabulous Five is that magic elixir, water. So simple, but very, very powerful in its ability to help your system run smoother in every way. It helps metabolize foods more efficiently, hydrates all your internal organs and tissues and keeps you filled up while suppressing your appetite naturally. Drop in a slice of lemon if the taste of your tap water is odd at first, or make decaffeinated herbal tea (hot or iced). Mineral water (with no sodium) is excellent also, but more expensive. Eight to ten glasses of water a day will do wonders for all phases of losing weight and maintaining health. Consider this absolutely necessary for the THINNER WINNERS program. I have long ago conquered the inconveniences of this habit, and reaped giant benefits in health and slimness. You can, too! Start right now.

5)   Stress Management

The last Fabulous Five component, but certainly not the least, is your ability to effectively manage your stress. You need to develop effective coping skills to get a handle on your own stress so that it does not interfere with your health and weight.

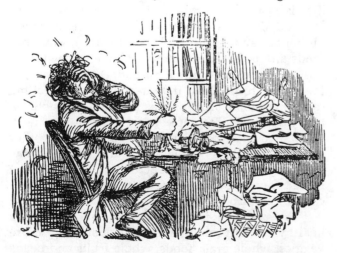

There are no advantages to being out of control.

Some form of meditation and proper breathing is essential for a healthy lifestyle. So is peace of mind and a sense of being in control of your life. There is a calm energy center within your mind that is independent of all the trials and tribulations of daily life. You can tap into this renewing energy reservoir by meditating on a regular basis. You will discover that it will give you the ability to view your life from a quiet perspective. You will feel more in control and more in touch with your essential core self. In the course of your daily activities you can maintain this sense of calm control by learning to breath properly. Breathe deeply and you bring more oxygen and fresh air into your system. Please refer to Chapter 14 "Taming Your Stress" for additional suggestions and exercises to become aware of stress and develop your own stress-reduction methods.

More Habits to Stay Slim

In addition to the above Fabulous Five, there are several other habits that successful THINNER WINNERS have developed. If you follow along with their proven success strategies, you can join their healthy group, too.

Develop an active lifestyle.

Don't sit around on the couch or lounge in a chair for hours. Twenty or thirty minutes is about the limit for inactivity. Then, get up, move around, get a glass of water ... anything to keep your body in motion. If you are brave and determined, hide the remote control! If it's a nice day park your car at the far end of the parking lot, walk or bike to the store, or walk during your lunch hour. Malls are fun for this (avoid cinnamon roll shops and cookie stores, however!). Look for and find ways to stay active. It may be hard at first, especially with extra pounds to lug around, but watch a slender person for a while. They are active, and this habit helps keep them burning calories and revving up their metabolisms.

Learn to eat and cook the lighter way.

Try the techniques suggested for eliminating fats and frying from your cooking. Develop healthier recipes for your favorite dishes by using your Food Substitution Chart. Learn to recognize restaurant "fat traps" such as sauces, gravies, dressings and fried foods. Order what you want specifically. Request your dressing "on the side", and your entree broiled or steamed, not fried. Skip the sauces and melted butter. Just knowing about the biggest offenders can help you avoid them. Experiment a bit and you'll find many very tasty, delicious alternatives.

It saddens me to think that lots of fat people stay fat even though they are trying to choose better foods just by simply not knowing that 1% milk is really 40% fat and that "healthy" peanut butter is 75% fat! Be aware, read labels and don't fall into common traps that can keep you fat for life instead of thin forever.

Reward yourself regularly

Few people would work at a job if they didn't get paid periodically. The same principle holds true for dieters. You need regular reinforcement to acknowledge your efforts. Whether it's money, vacations, new clothes or a long, hot, undisturbed bath, find out what really motivates you to give the extra effort ... and use it as a reward. In between your big payoffs, find some small prizes that make you feel special and remind you that you're doing a great job. The key to long-term weight control is to successfully modify your behavior so that your habits are serving your purposes. Behavior modification reinforcement techniques may be a mouthful to say, but they really do the job.

Share your success with others

Overcoming difficult problems often leads to great learning, growth and wisdom. When you have learned to control your weight at the levels you want you will have seen a lot of light along the way. You will have a stronger sense of "The Big Picture". You'll realize that the way to truly get the most out of life is by sharing with others. When you run across someone who is struggling with weight and health issues you can share the benefits of your wisdom and in doing so you will help make the world a healthier place. Your work to regain your health is validated when you relieve the pain of others with your knowledge.

Follow an individual plan ... adjusting to your lifestyle

The best insurance for truly being a THINNER WINNER is a complete, personalized, all-inclusive, flexible plan that covers the important personal issues and can be used as a guide for the rest of your life. It is holistic in nature, just like you. There is a synergy to all the techniques, which expands to encompass all possibilities. This is the real secret. Aha! You are more than just the food you eat, the activity you engage in, the thoughts you generate or the feelings you have. You are all these things and more. You are a whole person with many complex issues and needs. You are unique ... and your needs and issues will change as you travel through life. The plan you follow needs to be flexible enough to adjust to these changes. The ideal weight control program is not one that you go on and then off. It is a flexible, fluid process which allows for changes. To truly be effective, your plan will help you develop the habits you need that will enhance your health to its maximum level possible during a lifetime of change.

Be intelligent, realistic and patient.

You are doing this for a lifetime. Studies have proven, with virtually all people who have lost their excess weight and kept it off long-term, that gradual and realistic plans work best. Radical quick-loss approaches are dangerous and offer only short-term results for all that risk. Any extreme changes in what you eat, or large weight losses in a short period, are doomed to failure. But you've heard this before and I'm convinced you know it by now. So decide here and now you will do it the right way this time, and get it done once and for all. Then you can move on to enjoying your food, your body, your health and your wonderful new THINNER WINNERS lifestyle.

The most important factors in losing fat permanently are gaining gradual control, learning to cultivate a livable set of positive habits and having a pro-health attitude (often referred to as wellness). With this approach you'll win the goal you want and safely and sanely be able to stay thin for the rest of your life.

Good luck to you and let me know how you're doing. I always love to hear from people who are using these techniques and learning to reshape their lives and their bodies ... to become THINNER WINNERS.

In A Nutshell

1) Taking off weight the right way initially is the essential groundwork needed for successful maintenance.

2) To change your body permanently, you must change your habits, including eating, permanently.

3) A 2-3 pound gain when switching from losing to maintenance is to be expected.
   Heed the warning of weight gain, tighten down *your* "weasels" and maintain without pain.
   It's natural and normal to experience weight fluctuations of 2-8 pounds.

4) A plan is outlined to gradually add back calories and fat until a balance is reached.
   To maintain, add in foods of the same healthy nature that you have been eating to lose weight.

6) Nip any gain in the bud by:
   a) Weighing weekly and keeping a record to reveal long-term patterns and trends and to stay aware.
   b) Own a perfect-fitting pair of jeans and test the fit weekly.
   c) Keep your Daily Success Planner one day a week (minimum).

7) Use the Fabulous Five as your essential structure for maintenance:
   1) Attitude is top banana!
   2) Activity and Exercise level
   3) Low Fat/High Fiber foods
   4) Water
   5) Stress Management

8) Other stay slim habits are reviewed.
   * Develop an active lifestyle
   * Learn to cook light and order right in restaurants
   * Use rewards and recognition to give yourself a pat on the back
   * Share with others the knowledge and understanding you have gained
   * Customize this complete plan to your own needs and be flexible when necessary
   * Be intelligent, realistic and patient. You're working for a lifetime worth of glowing health!

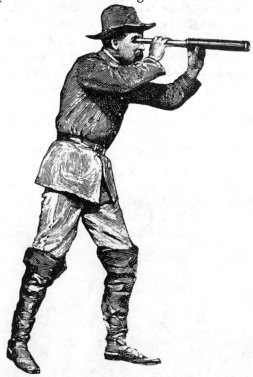

"Sa-a-ay, she HAS lost weight!"

Top Ten Greatest Hits For Weight Control 39

"Nothing great was ever achieved without enthusiasm."
Ralph Waldo Emerson

Here is a concise summary of the top ten areas you need to concentrate on to reach your goal of a permanent, thin life in the steadiest possible way. These are capsule versions ... detailed information on these topics is provided in other chapters.

Make it a habit to practice all ten and you will not only be very busy, you will be rolling along toward your dream at a nice, quick pace! If you're just starting out, don't try to do everything at once, just add a little each day from one or more of the power-packed sections below. Pick your weakest area and concentrate on strengthening that first.

Write all the titles of the ten "greatest hits" on a 3 x 5 card. Carry it with you or put it someplace where you will see it often. Mentally go over the ten steps and always be thinking of improvements or personalized additions you can make. That's how to get the very most from this list of Top Ten Greatest Hits For Weight Control and turn your hard work into glorious success at the scale and in the dressing room!

This first one is a biggie so hold on, be strong. Get this clear and you're on your way with a solid foundation!

1. Set the Stage for Success with a Positive Attitude

First, focus precisely on what you're doing. Decide that you really want to lose your extra weight and keep it off for good. Do it for yourself .... no other source of motivation can even come close to your own burning desire to succeed. If you can't firmly feel this commitment in yourself, then you must explore this issue and discover why you really won't commit to losing the weight. Try to isolate specific reasons and then work with those until you are free to truly make the decision to lose the weight for yourself.

Once you have decided that you want to lose the weight, then you must decide that you can. You must be absolutely convinced in your mind and heart that it is possible for you. Others have done it, why not you? Remember, if you think you can do it, then you can! If you think you can't, then you can't. Your beliefs predict your future.

Attitude is everything ... it determines your success. Guard it carefully and never let yourself sink into self-pity or negativity. It will just slow you down. If you catch yourself thinking or saying something negative or self-defeating about your program (and we all do from time to time!), then gently remind yourself that this is a counter-productive habit you're breaking and replacing with a more productive one. Get rid of the "diet mentality". You are putting together a program and a set of positive habits that will shape your life from this point forward. This is no mere diet to go on and off. Choose to change your attitude and you are choosing to change your life.

Create an inner image of yourself as thin ... and visualize yourself thin often. Spend time each day imprinting the image into your mind ... perhaps first thing in the morning before you get up, or last thing at night before you fall asleep. Relax, breathe and see yourself being thin and happy, feel yourself there. Watch your thin self go about daily tasks ... realize this is the real you and your fat is only a temporary condition. "Be" as a thin person to become one.

Above all, resolve to never give up, ever ... and ultimately you will remove all the obstacles and achieve your goal. It's inevitable.

2. Develop a Support System

Gather support around you. Find a person or a group who will take the time to understand your program fully and watch your progress with you. If one person isn't enough, then go for several or a group approach. Get together on a regular basis (say once a week) with this person or group solely for the purpose of discussing your program and how it's going. Talk, listen and ask questions. Share your thoughts, triumphs and concerns. Be sure you can contact them at all times, by phone at least. This is a vital tool to get you through any rough times.

With your supporters, set specific short-term and long-term goals in each of the four areas of the program. Put them in writing and have deadlines for their completion. Review them together every month at least. That way you can refine your step-by-step plan to reach your goals. Surround yourself with positive people, books, TV shows and activities. Shun the things that bring you down from your position of confident belief in your permanent success.

3. Get Moving

In virtually every instance where a formerly overweight, out-of-shape and unhappy person transforms into a thin, healthy, happy one, exercise is involved. How have people who previously would have eaten dirt before they would go to an exercise class changed into activity-loving folk? Here is a major secret that can be the key to your success. The fact is, exercise feels good, right and natural when your body is well-nourished.

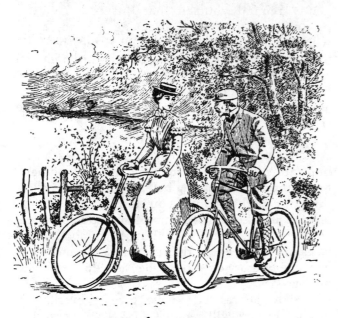

*"You know, my Dear,
you're the first person I've ever known
who could ride a bicycle side-saddle."*

A body over-stuffed with unhealthful foods that make it feel awful, goes numb and is unaware of the normal need for activity. It's a terrible and vicious cycle that keeps fat people from feeling the real needs of their bodies, and it is the reason that so many people can't even stand the thought of beginning an exercise program. Unfortunately, it takes a while before the effects of a balanced diet and regular exercise coordinate in the body and mind, and those essentials become necessities to well-being.

Your body will begin to heal itself on this program and to release your anesthetized senses from their long sleep. While you're waiting for this to happen, begin to know your body by stretching gently every day. Long, slow and careful stretching will go a long way to put you in touch with your physical self. It feels good and will help relax and release tension from your muscles.

Next, find an activity that you enjoy. It doesn't have to be a standard form of exercise. Just something that you enjoy and gets you moving. Walking has been the choice of many for its safe, pleasant qualities and the ease with which you can begin (see Chapter 21 "Get That Body Movin'" for a detailed description of exercise). As you get into the habit of being more active on a regular basis, your need for activity will increase and you will naturally seek more activity. Don't push it or force yourself or you may soon give up. Just listen to your body especially after your walk or other activity. Notice that you feel good and relaxed.

You will discover paradoxically, that exercise increases energy and the need to be active. That is the key and the secret to becoming active and thin. Eventually, if you exercise regularly, your positive habit will not allow you to not exercise without feeling like something is missing. You will begin to miss your workouts if you skip them. Honest.

4. Self-Discovery

In these amazing yet confusing times in which we live it's almost impossible to turn around without being told how we should look, feel and act in almost every situation. We're inundated with "ideals". The "best" jobs, places to live, interactional styles and looks are constantly blasted into our faces by movies, television and the print media. Be this, do this, look like this! This is what we are told directly ... and, of course, the hidden message is that if we don't ... well, then we're bad, wrong or inadequate. The people who convey these messages are all trying to sell products or ideas. If they're successful, we buy. If not ... they just keep on trying. Heaven knows that they keep trying.

But what about you? Most likely you're just trying to live the best life you can ... in the best way that you can. In the midst of all this hubbub it's really important to get to know yourself ... your real self. Who are you, and why do you do the things you do? What's your big dream in life? Write it down ... that's the perfect place to start. Why is it important to you? Do you know the steps that will take you in the direction of your dream? There are a lot of questions for you to try and find answers to in this life. And it really is important for you to try to find your own answers. It's your life, after all.

But this doesn't mean that you have to do it all on your own. There are many sources of help that don't have hidden agendas (people, books, audios and videos). Don't be afraid to explore yourself ... your body, your mind, your soul. It's the greatest adventure available to anyone. Begin. Right now. You deserve this.

One of the smartest things you can do is take control of the pace of your life. Just because the advertisers are throwing a thousand images into a

15 second commercial doesn't mean you have to watch it. Instead you can turn off the tube and take a good deep breath. Fill your lungs with the stuff of life and feel the oxygen rushing through your body. Take a few more deep breaths and relax those tense muscles. You owe yourself a little peace. In fact, the best thing you'll probably ever do for yourself is to learn how to meditate and breathe. Recharge your mental batteries. Identify your stressors and find some new coping skills that allow you to smile more as you go through life.

5. Read, Study, Learn

The more you know about a subject, the more you can control the way it affects your life. This is particularly true for weight control, attitudes, behavior, nutrition and exercise. The more you know about the ways that your thoughts, food habits and activity affect your health and your mood in direct ways, the more you will see the importance of mastering these subjects.

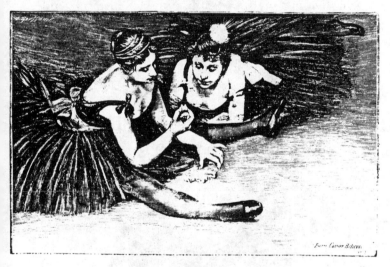

*"My fortune cookie says,
'dancers have thinner futures.'"*

With the THINNER WINNERS program you are getting a sneak preview of the prizes that wait behind "door # 1" (where the good prizes are hiding). This program is based on published research and it has been tested on real people. It works! It takes the guesswork out of your future. But the same information and books that we have studied are available to you. We share the condensed highlights with you ... but you owe it to yourself to really understand what makes you tick.

You already know that picking "door #2" (the Standard American Diet and an inactive lifestyle) results in too much weight and poor physical and mental health. Expand your awareness ... not your waistline.

6. Nutrition Commitment

Don't eat anything you don't like! Learn to cook your favorite foods, at the very least, and have them often. Decide to learn enough about cooking to know what low-fat, healthy food looks and tastes like and make it taste great!

Experiment in your kitchen, even if it's only with a microwave and refrigerator! Buy magazines and books on healthy cooking and peek into them once in awhile. If you are more dedicated, you could even try a recipe or two. Learn to season without the salt-shaker by finding a few herbs and spices that you like and using them to season your food. Cut the fat and pump up the fiber! Boredom with food can be alleviated by eating a variety of foods. Try at least one new food or recipe a week.

7. Keep a Daily Success Planner and Personal Journal

In the beginning, write down everything that you eat, the water you drink and your exercise. Especially if you slip away from the program, keep writing down what you're doing. It is important to monitor your weight control program because of the invaluable lessons you can learn from the information. There is a strong connection between your eating and activity patterns and the way that you respond to them. Write down the emotions you were feeling or the situation that triggered the slip. At your weekly meeting with your support person or group, get some feedback about your diary. What did you do right? What problems did you encounter? Exactly where were you when the problem started? Use your Daily Success Planner as a mini-Personal Journal if you would like to keep your entries brief . This also keeps everything all in one place. The important thing is to record what's happening with you. This can be a great help when looking for ways to improve and quicken your pace. They are great learning tools.

8. Drink Water

Review Chapter 35, "Water — The Magic Potion" to see why water is so wonderful! Then get a glass and start reaping the benefits right away. Drink at least six 8-oz glasses of pure water every day, plus an extra glass for every 25 pounds you are overweight, and an extra glass or two when you exercise. Your water glass should be your constant companion. If you can't get down the water in the beginning, try hot or iced herbal tea, flavored mineral waters and club soda (low-sodium varieties). Coffee, regular tea, juices and soda do not count. Believe it or not, soon you will look forward to your water and find it cleansing and refreshing. It's one of the very best things you can do for your weight control and your health in general.

9. Reward Yourself Often

Always have a reward picked out for your next accomplishment. This not only assures you'll have something to work towards, but you'll be having lots of fun thinking about getting there, too! This program should be fun ... never dull or boring! Make a list of the goodies that you want, big and small and then wrap them up and give them to yourself as you earn them.

Never punish yourself for slipping up. That's the worst thing you can do. It sets up a negative emotional state related to the idea of losing weight. Instead, forgive yourself, "confess" to your support person, learn what you can and then reward yourself for getting back on track. Love yourself for all the effort you are putting out.

Every day should bring you lots of little reminders that you are doing a great job: gold stars, heart stickers, cash or anything that will make you feel good and happy about your progress. You will be increasing your sense of self-worth and having some fun while taking loving care of yourself.

10. Remember "The Tortoise and The Hare"

Everyone knows the old fable about the hare who raced ahead of the plodding tortoise ... and then got overconfident, slacked off and lost the race. So what's the message in this for you? Well, let's see ... do you want to lose weight fast or do you want to win the weight control derby?

OK, let's pull out our racing form and see what the odds are. Hmm, Diet Pills looks like a real winner ... fast out of the chute, quick around the first turn ... but not many wins, lots of injuries and usually winds up at the back of the pack. Real long odds

against winning. So who's next here? Liquid Protein ... word on the street says this one moves out like lightning. But this baby seems to have some health problems ... low energy, intestinal blockage and possibly death. Poor overall record. Maybe not today. Number three looks like Latest Fad Diet. A lot of skinny ad men have money riding on this pony ... Hmm, seems to do best on a diet of pure promotion. Always seems to win at home track in Beverly Hills. Lousy record most other places. Very inconsistent. And finally we have Well-Balanced Plan ... a real plodder. Look at these times, they're so slow. But holy mackerel, this diet has the best long-term win record in the bunch. It must be this training schedule ... consistent eating and exercise program, juiced up with rewards and a good attitude. Well, it seems to get regular, predictable results, too! I think I'll put my money on a Well-Balanced Plan. How about you?

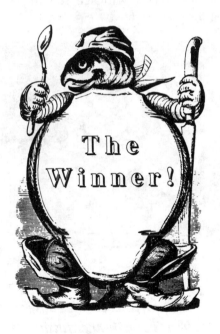

Top Ten Greatest Hits Success List

The following series lists many of the thoughts, actions and attitudes that you'll need to put into practice to become and stay a lifetime THINNER WINNER. Note the items that you've accomplished so far. Look up the information on the items you haven't yet achieved and keep working at it! Never give up!

1)   Setting the Stage for Success - Decisions, Attitude and Image

I have decided I want to lose the weight.
I have decided I can lose the weight.
I have decided I will lose the weight.
Attitude is everything! I guard my attitude carefully from negative or self-defeating thoughts.
What I think about expands, grows and takes root in my life ... so I only think about what I want to happen.
I am developing a set of positive habits to replace those that keep me fat.
I have created an inner image of myself as "THIN" and I hold that image strongly.
I never give up! Ever!
I don't just dream it ... I am my dreams, I do what it takes and I make them happen.

2)   Get Some Support

I have a supporter who shares my progress with me.
I surround myself with "positives" ... books, tapes, videos and people.
I talk about my progress and feelings regularly with my support person or group.
I set specific goals ... both short and long term, with deadlines for accomplishment.
I follow a specific plan and review it at least once a month.

3)   Get Moving

I realize exercise feels good to a healthy body.
I know my body was designed for activity and movement.
I realize that proper nutrition encourages exercise.
My body will begin to heal itself with proper nutrition.
I stretch every day to feel in touch with my body.
I have found something ACTIVE that I enjoy doing.
I enjoy walking because it is safe, pleasant, easy and effective.
I never push or force myself ... I enjoy my exercise! But I do work hard and sweat.
I listen to my body.
I feel good, relaxed and energized when I exercise.
My exercise is self-reinforcing ... the more I do, the more I want to do.
I realize that exercise is one of the SECRETS of getting thin.

4)   Self-Discovery

I realize that finding out who I am is important to being totally healthy.
My first step is having personal goals ... I write them down.
I allow myself to get help from people, books, cassettes and videos.
I know it's my life and I live it to the best of my abilities.
I have learned to breathe properly and meditate.
I have identified my main stressors and found ways to cope that are meaningful to me.

5)   Read, Study and Learn

I realize that attitudes, food and activity directly affect my health and mood.
By mastering my thoughts and actions I am mastering my life.
I take the guesswork out of my future ... I put myself at the wheel.
I am expanding my awareness not my waistline.
I read and study all I can about attitude, behavior, exercise and nutrition because I know that the more
    I learn and understand the more successful I will be.

6)   Nutrition Commitment

I never eat anything I don't like!
I have learned to cook my favorite foods in healthy ways.
I have learned to replace sodium and salt with herbs and spices.
I eat a wide variety of foods ... trying something new at least once a week.
I have cut the FAT!
I have pumped up the FIBER!

7)   Keep a Daily Success Planner and Personal Journal

I write down everything that I eat and know what I'm putting in my body.
I keep track of the water I drink.
I keep an exercise log.
I know which parts of my program are working because I write down what I'm doing!
I monitor my progress closely.
I make suggestions for ways I can improve my program. I work my plan.

8)   Drink Water

I realize that water is a "Magic Elixir" and a necessity for health and thinness.
I drink at least six 8 ounce cups every day ... plus one 8 ounce cup for every 25 pounds I am overweight.
       More if it's hot or I'm exercising a lot.
I drink extra water when I exercise.
I realize that water is cleansing, refreshing and healthful.

9)   Rewards

I preplan my next reward because it helps motivate me ... and I deserve it!
I keep my weight control program fun (maybe even a little silly).
I never punish myself for slipping up. I just get back on track, and give myself a reward for sticking with it.
I work at increasing my self worth. I know I deserve rewards for work well done.

10)   The Tortoise and the Hare

I realize that other diet methods sound fast ... but I now know they're a fast way to poor health and
       staying on the weight loss roller coaster.
I realize that a program of good nutrition and exercise coupled with positive attitude and consistent
       productive behaviors is a winner every time!
I practice the principles of a THINNER WINNER daily because I am one!

In A Nutshell

1) What you think about takes root, grows and expands in your mind. Set the stage for your success with a positive attitude. Don't just dream it ... be it, do it and make it happen! You can do it.

2) Develop a strong Support System. Set goals and follow a plan.

3) Get your body moving with activities and exercise.

4) Get to know yourself, set your own pace and start following your dreams. Learn to breathe properly, meditate and reduce your stress.

5) Read, study and learn about health, nutrition and how your body and mind work.

6) Make a nutrition commitment to learn to cook low fat, high fiber, low sodium foods.

7) Keep a Daily Success Planner and Personal Journal to refer to and learn from later.

8) Drink plenty of water.

9) Reinforce your accomplishments with rewards often. Never punish yourself.

10) Remember "The Tortoise and the Hare" ... slow and steady wins the race.

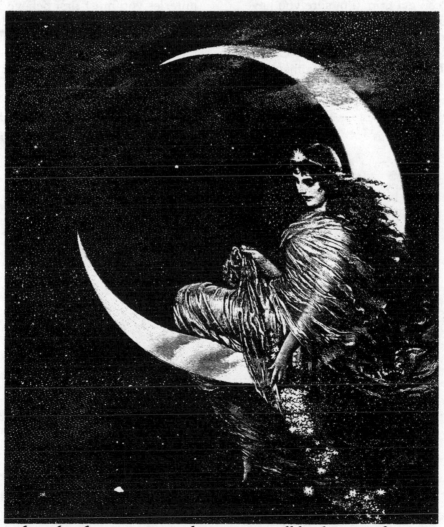

Shoot for the moon! Even if you miss you'll land among the stars.

A Final Word

It gets easier. Really it does, I promise. Be patient with this process and just know you are going the right way...the only way to really permanent change. All this work you are doing will pay off big time. Your new habits will begin to feel right after a while and the old ones which caused you to be fat won't. Health and fitness become more comfortable than junk food and TV, and they feel a whole lot better, too. As you shed your fat and release the thin, light person inside, your body, mind and heart lighten and you begin to feel that things are as they should be again.

This "miracle" will take time on your part... time to accept and love yourself. You're a trooper for finishing this whole book. There's a lot in here! It takes real guts to face and conquer this fat issue instead of burying your head in the sand of denial or trying another diet wonder plan. I congratulate you for your courage and I have nothing but respect and love for you.

It should no longer be a mystery to you why you got fat or how you can get thin. (I'm sure you have some good ideas about that sneaky secret by now!) You know the plan to follow for lifelong healthy weight control and happy self-confidence. Choose to face your obstacles now and eliminate them one by one ... or choose to wait until later and face them.

But there is no other way if you are to be thin for life. There certainly is no instant way. You know that! Give all of yourself to this program and become a THINNER WINNER! Other people, including myself, have followed this very method and succeeded. So can you!

I won't wish you luck because now you know you make your own luck. I will wish you lots of happiness along the way, though. Enjoy your blooming into a unique successfully thin person. If you try to pattern yourself after some ideal of perfection, you'll probably be disappointed if you ever get there. Molded, self-styled perfection isn't your goal. Realization of your innate perfection is another thing altogether, though. All that you are is already perfect. Realize your potential and become all you are capable of. Use your talents and they will grow. The more fully you develop them the more you can give and contribute to the growing of all life.

I have no doubt in my mind that you can do this because I have seen the miracle happen to myself and others. It can happen to you, too! Like most miracles you must first believe it will happen. Be a believer. What have you got to lose? Choose to take control right now and make it happen. You deserve the very best.

Reach deep inside yourself and you will reach your potential.

Health, Happiness and Love,

Roseanne Strull

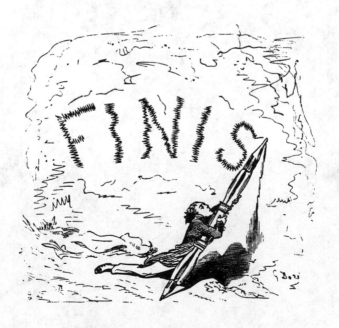

Bibliography

Attitude

Acres of Diamonds - Conwell, 1960, Spire
Ageless Body, Timeless Mind - Deepak Chopra, 1993, Harmony
Creative Visualization - Shakti Gawain,1982, Whatever
Double Win - Waitley, 1982, Berkeley
Each Day - A New Beginning, Hazeldon Meditation Series, Harper
Eat More, Weigh Less - Dean Ornish, 1993, Harper-Collins
Emotional Weight - Sundermeyer, 1993, Perigee
Good-bye Jumbo, Hello Cruel World - Louie Anderson, 1993
Handbook To Higher Consciousness - Keyes, 1987 Ed., Love Line
How to Stop Worrying and Start Living - Dale Carnegie, 1948 Ed., Simon & Schuster
Lighten Up - C.W. Metcalf, 1992, Addison Wesley
Living In The Light - Shakti Gawain, 1986, Whatever
Love - Leo Buscaglia, 1972, Fawcett Crest
Magic of Getting What You Want, David Schwartz, 1983, Berkeley
Move Ahead With Possibility Thinking -Robert Schuller, 1967, Spire
The Path of Transformation - Gawain, 1993, Nataraj
Peace, Love and Healing - Siegel, 1989, Harper
Personhood - Leo Buscaglia,1982 Ed., Fawcett
Power of Balanced Living - Bob & Zonnya Harrington, 1983, Harrington
Power of Positive Thinking -Norman Vincent Peale, 1956, Fawcett Crest
Promise of a New Day: Daily Meditations -Hazeldon Meditation Series, Harper
Psycho-Cybernetics - Maxwell Matlz, 1960, Wilshire
Psychology of Winning - Denis Waitley, 1984 Ed., Berkeley
Psycho-Pictography - Vernon Howard, 1965, Parker Publishing
Real Magic - Wayne Dyer, 1992, Harper
See You At The Top - Zig Ziglar, 1977 Ed., Pelican
Success Through a Positive Mental Attitude -Napoleon Hill & W. C. Stone, 1977 Ed., Pocket
Think And Grow Rich - Napoleon Hill, 1960 Ed., Crest
Wake Me Up When I'm A Size 5 - Cathy Guisewite, 1990 Ed., Andrews & McMeel
Women's Encyclopedia of Health and Emotional Healing - Foley, 1993, Rodale
You Can If You Think You Can - Norman Vincent Peale, 1974, Spire
You Can Work Your Own Miracles - Napoleon Hill, 1971, Fawcett Crest
You'll See It When You Believe It - Wayne Dyer, 1989, Avon
Your Erroneous Zones - Wayne Dyer, 1976, Avon

Behavior Changes

Act Thin, Stay Thin - Stuart, Jove
Breaking Free From Compulsive Eating - Roth, 1984, Bobbs-Merrill
Diets Don't Work - Schwartz, Breakthru
Dressing Rich - Feldon, General
How To Lower Your Fat Thermostat - Remington, 1983, Vitality House
I'll Never Fat Again - Livingston, 1980, Ballantine
It's Not What You Eat, It's What Eating You - Janet Greeson
It's You! Looking Terrific Whatever Your Type - Cho, 1986, Ballantine
Joy of Sex - Alex Comfort, 1972, Fireside
Ninety Days To Self Health - Norman Shealy, 1980 Ed., Bantam
Perfect Health - Chopra, 1991, Harmony
Permanent Weight Control - Mahoney, WW Norton
Raquel Welch Total Fitness & Beauty Program - Welch, 1984, Holt-Rinehart
Stress Management - Charlesworth, Ballantine
Take Effective Control of Your Life - Glasser, Harper & Row

The Thin Book - Westin, CompCare
The Thin Book By A Formerly Fat Psychiatrist - Rubin, 1966, Trident
Thin Within - Wardell, Pocket
When Food Is Love - Geneen Roth, 1992, Plume
Wishcraft - Sher, Ballantine

Activity and Exercise

A Walk Across America - Jenkins, Fawcett Crest
Art of Breathing - Zi, 1986, Bantam
Callanetics - Pinckney , Morrow
Complete Guide To Exercise Videos - Collage Video, (800) 433-6769
Complete Illustrated Book of Yoga - Vishnudevananda, Julian
Energy: Everything You've Always Wanted To Know - Hayden, Kangaroo
Face Lifting By Exercise - Runge, Allegro
Fat Burning Workout - Vedral, 1991, Warner
Fitness Through Cycling - Bicycle Magazine, Rodale
Fitness Walking - Sweetgall, 1985, Perigee
Flex Appeal - Rachel McLish, 1984, Warner
Jane Fonda's Fitness Walkout - Jane Fonda, 1987, Warner Bros.
Mountain Bike Book -Van Der Plas, 1989, Bicycle
Mountain Biking the High Sierra - Bonser, 1988, Fine Edge
New Fit Or Fat - Covert Bailey, 1991 Ed., Houghton-Mifflin
Now Or Never - Joyce Vedral, Warner
Oregon Coast Hikes - Williams, Mountaineers
Personal Trainer Manual - American Council on Exerise, 1992, ACE
Richard Simmons Better Body Book - Richard Simmons, 1983, Warner
Richard Simmons Never-Say-Diet Book - Simmons, 1980, Warner
SuperFlex: Ms. Olympia's Guide to Body Building - Corrie Everson, 1987, Contemporary
Total Massage - Hofer, Grosset & Dunlap
Wandering: A Walkers Guide To Trails in Europe - Rudner, Dial
Weider System of Body Building - Joe Weider, 1983, Contemporary
Yoga USA - Hittleman, Bantam

Nutrition and Food

Aerobic Nutrition - Mannerberg, Berkley
American Heart Association Cookbook - Am. Heart Assoc.,Ballantine
Baking Without Fat - George Mateljian, 1994, Health Valley Foods
Beyond Pritikan - Gittleman, 1988,
Book of Garnishes - Budgen, 1986, HP Books
Brand Name Guide To Sugar - Shannon, Nelson-Hall
Busy People's Cookbook - Nemiro, Random House
Calorie Guide - Kraus, Signet
Canning & Preserving Without Sugar - Macrae, 1988, Globe Pequot
Carbohydrate Guide to Brand Names & Basic Foods - Kraus, Signet
Company's Coming (Light Recipes) - Pare, 1993, Company's Coming Press
Complete Book of Canning - Pisinski, Ortho Books
Complete Book of Food Counts - Netzer, 1995, Dell
Complete Book of Health Plants - Bianchini, Crescent
Complete Fat Book (15,000 Listings) - Bellerson, 1991, Avery
Complete Scarsdale Medical Diet - Tarnower, Bantam
Controlling Cholesterol - Cooper, Bantam
Cookbook For People Who Love Animals - Gentle World, 1989 Ed., Gentle World
Cooking Without Fat - George Mateljian, 1992, Health Valley Foods
Deliciously Low - Roth/Pritikan, 1983, Plume
Diet and Nutrition - Ballentine, Himalayan International Institute
Diet For A New America - John Robbins, 1987, Stillpoint

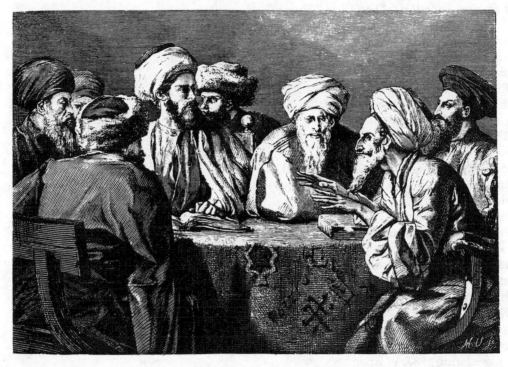

"And then I was amazed to discover that non-fat sour cream is re-e-ally good!"

Diet For A Small Planet - Francis Lappe, Ballantine
Don't Eat Your Heart Out Cookbook - Piscatella, 1987 Ed., Workman
Drinking Water - Donsbach, 1987, Int'l Inst. of Natural Health Sciences
Eating Better For Less - Wolf, Rodale
Eat More, Weigh Less - Dean Ornish, 1993, Harper
Eat To Succeed - Haas - 1986, Onyx
Eat To Win: The Sports Nutrition Bible - Haas, 1985 Ed., Signet
Encyclopedia of Fruits,Vegetables,Nuts & Seeds - Kadans, Parker
Everything You Always Wanted To Know About Nutrition - Reuben, 1978, Avon
Fabulous Fiber Cookery - Groen & Rubey, 1988, Nitty Gritty
Facts About Fats - Finnegan, 1992, Elysian Arts
Fancy, Sweet and Sugar Free - Barkie, 1985, St. Martins
Fit For Life - Diamond, 1985, Warner
Fit For Life II -Diamond, 1987, Warner
Fit or Fat -Covert Bailey, Houghton-Mifflin
Fit Or Fat: Target Recipes - Covert Bailey, 1985, Cookbook
Foods From Foreign Nations - Favorite Recipes Press
Food For Health - Stanford Heart Program, Stanford
Food, Your Miracle Medicine - Carper, 1993, Harper-Collins
F-Plan Diet - Eyton, Bantam
Friendly Foods: Gourmet Vegetarian - Brother Ron Pickarski, 1991,Ten Speed
Fructose Diet Book - Palm, Pocket
Frugal Gourmet - Jeff Smith,1984, Morrow
Frugal Gourmet Cooks With Wine - Jeff Smith,1986, Avon
Grains and Greens - Wright, 1990, Wright
Guaranteed Goof-Proof Healthy Microwave Cookbook - Kreschollek, 1989, Bantam
Guide To Herbs and Spices - Simon & Schuster, 1990, Fireside

Guide to Natural Food Restaurants - Vegetarian Times, 1991, Book Publishing Company
Healing Foods - Hausman, 1989, Dell
Heart Smart - Becker, Pocket
The Herbalist - Meyer, 1950, Meyer
How To Be Your Own Nutritionist - Berger, 1987, Avon
Human Nutrition and Dietetics - Davidson, Churchill
Juice Fasting - Airola, Health Plus
The Juicing Book - Blaver, 1989, Avery
Kathy Smith's Power Foods Program - Kathy Smith, 1990, Media Video
Last Chance Diet - Linn, 1976, Bantam
Let's Cook It Right - Adelle Davis, 1947, Harcourt Brace
Let's Eat Right To Keep Fit - Davis, 1970, Signet
Let's Get Well - Davis, 1965, Harcourt Brace
Living Heart Diet - DeBakey, 1984, Fireside
Low Calorie Sweet Treats - Weight Watchers Magazine, 1987
McDougall Health Supporting Cookbook - John McDougall, 1985, New Century
McDougall Plan - John McDougall, 1983, New Century
May All Be Fed - John Robbins, 1992, Morrow
Moosewood Cookbook - Katzen, 1971, Ten Speed
Muscular Gourmet - Mandy Tanny, 1988, Harper & Row
Natural Foods Cookbook - Hunter, Simon & Schuster
Natural Foods Sweet Tooth Cookbook - Farmilant, Pyramid
Naturally Delicious Desserts - Baker, 1985, Cookbook
Natural Weight Control - Walker, Norwalk
New Laurel's Kitchen - Laurel Robertson, 1986, Ten Speed
New MacDougall Cookbook - MacDougall, 1993, Dutton
New York Times Natural Foods Cookbook - Hewitt, Avon
No More Cravings - Hunt, 1987, Warner
Nutripoints - Vartabedian, 1990, Harper & Row
Perfect Health - Chopra, 1991, Harmony
Pritikan Permanent Weight Control Manual - Pritikan, 1981, Bantam
Pritikan Program for Diet & Exercise - Pritikan, 1983 Ed., Bantam
Pritikan Promise - Pritikan, 1985 Ed., Pocket
Rodale Cookbook - Albright, Rodale Books
Save Your Life Diet - Reuben, Random House
Save Your Life Diet - High Fiber Cookbook, Reuben, Ballantine
Simply Vegetarian - Ananda Publications, 1989 Ed.
Slimming Sampler - Weight Watchers Mag., 1984
Sodium Guide To Brand Names & Basic Foods - Kraus, Signet
Spices of the World Cookbook - McCormick Spices, Penguin
Sundays At Moosewood Restaurant - Moosewood Collective, 1990, Fireside
Sweet and Sugar Free - Barkie, 1982, St, Martins
T-Factor Diet - Katahn, 1989, WW Norton
Tofu - Quick & Easy - Hagler, 1988, Book Publishing Company
Use of Herbs In Weight Reduction - Heffern, 1975, Pyramid
Vegan Kitchen - Dinshah, 1987, American Vegan Society
Vegan Nutrition: Pure and Simple - Klapper, 1987, Gentle World
Vitamin Bible - Mindell, Rawson Wade
Vitamin Book - Wentzler, Gramercy
Vitamin E: Your Key to a Healthy Heart - Bailey, Arc
Weight Watchers - Slim Ways With Pasta - Weight Watchers, 1992, Nal
Weight Watchers 365-Day Menu Cookbook - Weight Watchers, 1983 Ed., Plume
Weight Watchers Fast and Fabulous Cookbook - Weight Watchers, 1983, Plume
Weight Watchers Favorite Recipes - Weight Watchers, 1986, New American
Weight Watchers Meals In Minutes Cookbook - Weight Watchers, 1989, New American
Wellness Low Fat Cookbook - Berkeley Wellness Letter, 1993, Rebus
Whole Heart Book - Nora, Holt Rinehart

Wild Foods Cookbook and Field Guide - Tatum
Wok Cookery - Dyer, HP Books

Miscellaneous

Amazing Food Facts - Chalmers
Animal Liberation and Ethical Treatment - Singer/PETA, Avon
Colon Health - Key To A Vibrant Life - Walker, Norwalk
Colon Health Handbook - Gray, Emerald
Doctors Book of Home Remedies - Prevention Magazine, 1990,
Encyclopedia of Natural Health - Warmbrand, Groton
Fasting As A Way of Life - Cott, Bantam
Fasting Can Save Your LIfe - Shelton, Natural Hygiene Press
Functional Human Anatomy - Crouch, Lea & Febiger
Gray's Anatomy - Gray, Crown
The Green Consumer - Elkington, 1990, Penguin
Magic Medicines of the Indians - Weslager, 1973, Signet
Prevention's Lose Weight Guidebook - Bricklin, 1993, Rodale
Our Bodies, Our Selves - Boston Women's Health Collective, Touchstone
Shopping For a Better World - Economic Priorities, 1989
Survival Into the 21st Century - Kulvinskas, 21st Century

Magazines and Newsletters

American Health Magazine
American Institute for Cancer Research Newsletter
Berkeley Wellness Letter
Bon Appetit Magazine
Covert Bailey Newsletter
Environmental Nutrition Newsletter
Good Medicine (Physicians Committee for Responsible Medicine)
Health & Healing
Health Magazine
Healthy Weight Journal
Johns Hopkins Medical Letter
Living Fit Magazine
Low Calorie Fast & Easy
Nutrition Action Health Letter (Center for Science in the Public Interest)
Obesity and Health Newsletter
Organic Gardening Magazine
Prevention Magazine
Reader's Digest - Excellent stories to boost your attitude
Self Magazine
Shape Magazine
Slim & Fit Diet & Exercise Magazine
Super Good Fast Food, Weight Watchers Magazine
Tufts University Diet and Nutrition Letter
Vegetarian Journal
Vegetarian Times
Walking Magazine
Weight Watchers Magazine *

Audio Cassette Programs

The Awakened Life - Wayne Dyer, Nightingale-Conant (Call 1-800-323-5552 for free catalog)
Balanced Living - Bob and Zonnya Harrington, Harrington
Be-Happy Attitudes - Robert Schuller, Warner Audio
Be More Positive - Success World
The Course In Winning - Moderator Denis Waitley with guest speakers, Nightingale-Conant
Getting Rich In America - Brian Tracy, Nightingale-Conant
Goals - Zig Ziglar, Nightingale-Conant
Insight Audio Magazine - Earl Nightingale & Brian Tracy and guest speakers, Nightingale-Conant
Intuition Workout - Nancy Rosanoff, Aslan
Lead The Field - Earl Nightingale, Nightingale-Conant
Letting Go of Stress - Emmett Miller
Living Rich 365 Days a Year - Bob and Zonnya Harrington, Harrington
Maintaining Motivation - Bob and Zonnya Harrington, Harrington
Personal Power - Anthony Robbins, Nightingale-Conant
Power of the Mind to Heal - Joan Borysenko, Nightingale-Conant
Power of Visualization - Lee Pulos, Nightingale-Conant
Psychology of Achievement - Brian Tracy, Nightingale-Conant
Psychology of Success - Brian Tracy, Nightingale-Conant
Relieve Stress and Anxiety - Success World
Science of Personal Achievement - Napoleon Hill, Nightingale-Conant
Secrets of the Universe - Wayne Dyer, Nightingale-Conant
Spiritual Awakening - Ram Dass
21 Success Secrets - Brian Tracy, Nightingale-Conant
Think and Grow Rich - Napoleon Hill, Nightingale-Conant
Transformation - Wayne Dyer, Nightingale-Conant
You Can If You Think You Can - Norman Vincent Peale, Simon & Schuster
Wishcraft - Barbara Sher

Just in case you were wondering, we actually researched a lot more reference material than what's listed here. But somehow 250 references seemed like plenty. If you have any questions or comments about any of the information in this book please drop us a line.

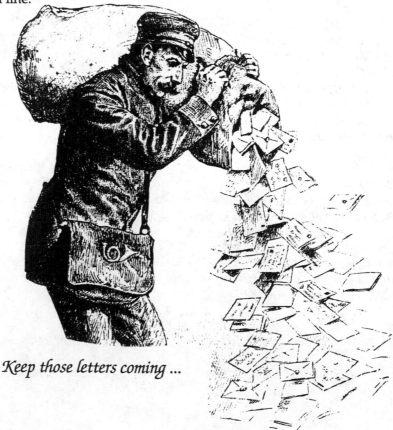

Keep those letters coming ...

APPENDIX

FREE Weight Control Groups

I'm sure you've figured out by now that THINNER WINNERS has a different philosophy from the rest of the people in the weight control world. We're going about our business differently from the rest, too. We are commited to spreading the word about positive health and honest long-term weight control. Because we want you to succeed, and because we want to eliminate as many obstacles from your progress as possible, we have instituted a number of *FREE* weight control support programs. That's right, FREE!

If you are interested in participating in a no-cost THINNER WINNERS study and support group please write to:

THINNER WINNERS Weight Control
22745 Carpenterville Road, Suite 7
Brookings, Oregon 97415
(503) 247-7255

FREE PepTalk Hotline

In Chapter 3 you were given the opportunity to call our FREE PepTalk support hotline. If you haven't called yet, now is the time to get started. There is a new inspirational, informative recording by Roseanne every two weeks. The message is for you!

(503) 471-3922

THINNER WINNERS Newsletter

If you would like a FREE sample copy of the THINNER WINNERS newsletter please write to the address listed above.

Additional THINNER WINNERS Products

The following items are available for your ongoing weight control progress:

THINNER WINNERS — The Complete All-in-One Guide to Lifetime Weight Control
Send your check or money order for $19.95 plus $3.50 shipping ($23.45 total per copy) to the address listed above. If you would like an autographed edition please let us know. Autographed copies are available only if you write directly to our offices.

The THINNER WINNERS Workbook
All the assessment exercises in this book are available in fill-in format with this handy workbook. All the questionnaires, charts, graphs and forms you need to make serious progress are included in this volume. Send $9.95 plus $2.00 shipping ($11.95 total per copy) the address above.

Daily Success Planners
On the next page you'll find a blank Daily Success Planner which you're welcome to copy for your personal use. If you want a bound two-month supply (60 Planners) send $5.00 plus $2.00 shipping to the address above.

To order additional copies of this book by <u>credit card</u> call our 24-hour, 7-day order number: 1 - (800) 852-4890.

See the coupon on the last page for additional order information.

THINNER WINNERS

DAILY SUCCESS PLANNER

Day/Date_____

Affirmation/ Thought:_____

Goals:_____

	Fat	Cals	Fiber	Sodium

BREAKFAST   Time of Day _____

WATER	[ ]	
FRUIT/VEG	[ ]	_____
GRAIN	[ ]	_____
DAIRY	[ ]	_____
PROTEIN	[ ]	_____
FAT GRAMS	_____	
WATER	[ ]	_____
SNACK		_____

LUNCH   Time of Day _____

WATER	[ ]	
VEG/FRUIT	[ ]	_____
GRAIN	[ ]	_____
DAIRY	[ ]	_____
PROTEIN	[ ]	_____
FAT GRAMS	_____	
WATER	[ ]	_____
SNACK		_____

DINNER   Time of Day_____

WATER	[ ]	
VEG/FRUIT	[ ]	_____
GRAIN	[ ]	_____
DAIRY	[ ]	_____
PROTEIN	[ ]	_____
FAT GRAMS	_____	
WATER	[ ]	_____
SNACK		_____

Totals   ____g ____cals ____g ____m g

Grains	[ ][ ][ ][ ] [ ]
Veg	[ ][ ][ ][ ]
Fruit	[ ][ ]
Protein	[ ][ ][ ][ ]
Water	[ ][ ][ ][ ] [ ][ ][ ][ ]
Vitamin/Mineral	[ ]

REVIEWED BY _____

NOTES/COMMENTS:

_____
_____
_____
_____

EXERCISE

GOAL MINUTES_____
ACTUAL MINUTES_____
TYPE_____
PULSE_____

WEEKLY WEIGHT

SUCCESS POINTS

[ ] AFFIRMATION 3 TIMES	(+3)	__
[ ] Met all goals & reviewed	(+3)	__
[ ] COMPLETED PLANNER	(+2)	__
[ ] FAT WITHIN LIMIT	(+2)	__
[ ] CALS WITHIN LIMIT	(+2)	__
[ ] WATER /6 MINIMUM	(+2)	__
[ ] FIBER/25g MINIMUM	(+2)	__
[ ] NO SKIPPED MEALS	(+1)	__
[ ] MEDITATION	(+5)	

SUCCESS SCORE=

(+25 possible)

Index

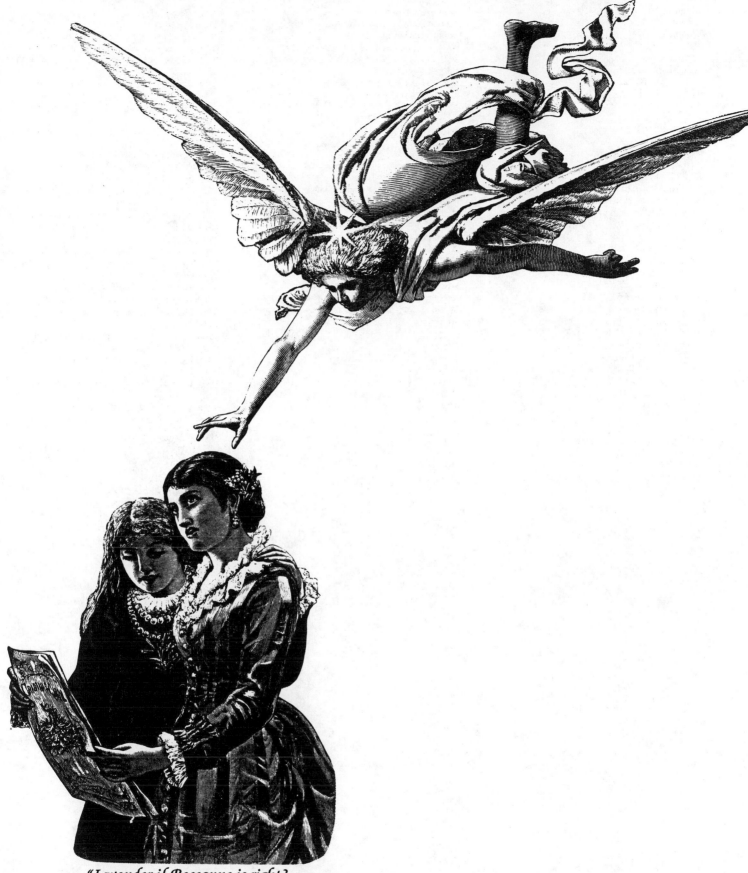

"I wonder if Roseanne is right?
If I start thinking like a THINNER WINNER
will the Universe start moving in my direction?"

THINNER WINNERS
No Risk Order Form

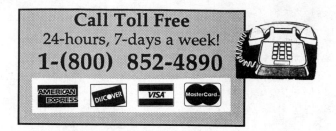

Call Toll Free
24-hours, 7-days a week!
1-(800) 852-4890

AMERICAN EXPRESS   DISCOVER   VISA   MasterCard

Lifetime Guarantee!
If you are unhappy with any of our materials, for any reason, you can return them for a full refund at any time.

You can order **THINNER WINNERS — The Complete All-in-One Guide to Lifetime Weight Control** (336 pages) with our convenient toll free order line. The cost is just $19.95 plus $3.50 shipping for each copy ($23.45 total).

Share Your Success with a Friend!

If you would like to receive an autographed copy of **THINNER WINNERS**, please send your check or money order for $23.45 per copy to the address at the bottom of this page. If you would like to send an autographed copy to a friend please print their name clearly in the space provided below.

[ ]   Please RUSH me _____ autographed copies of THINNER WINNERS. I have enclosed $23.45 per book.

[ ]   I understand that all THINNER WINNERS materials come with a lifetime 100% money-back guarantee of satisfaction. If I am unhappy with any of the materials, for any reason, I can simply return the items and receive a full refund with no questions asked.

Support Materials

The following materials are available by sending your payment to the mailing address below.

[ ]   Please send me _____ copies of **The THINNER WINNERS Workbook.** I have enclosed $9.95 plus $2.00 shipping ($11.95 total per copy)

[ ]   Please send me _____ bound copies of the THINNER WINNERS **Daily Success Planners** (60 pages). I have enclosed $5.00 plus $2.00 shipping ($7.00 total per copy).

[ ]   I would like you to send me information on your FREE support group program.

[ ]   I would like you to send me a FREE sample copy of the THINNER WINNERS newsletter.

Ordered by:	Ship to:
Name	Name
Address	Address
City, State, Zip	City, State, Zip
Telephone	Telephone

Total amount enclosed $ _____   [ ] check or [ ] money order _____

Please send your check or money order (payable to THINNER WINNERS) to:
THINNER WINNERS   22745 Carpenterville Road, Suite 7   Brookings, Oregon 97415